MOTOR BEHAVIOR

CONNECTING MIND AND BODY
FOR OPTIMAL PERFORMANCE

Jeffrey C. Ives

Professor and Graduate Program Chair
Department of Exercise and Sport Sciences
Ithaca College
Ithaca, New York

Wolters Kluwer | Lippincott Williams & Wilkins
Health

Philadelphia · Baltimore · New York · London
Buenos Aires · Hong Kong · Sydney · Tokyo

Acquisitions Editor: Emily Lupash
Product Manager: Matt Hauber
Production Project Manager: Marian Bellus
Design Coordinator: Holly Reid McLaughlin
Illustration Coordinator: Jennifer Clements
Artist: Kim Battista
Manufacturing Coordinator: Margie Orzech
Prepress Vendor: SPi Global

9 8 7 6 5 4 3 2 1

Printed in China

Library of Congress Cataloging-in-Publication Data
Ives, Jeffrey C.
  Motor behavior : connecting mind and body for optimal performance / Jeffrey C. Ives. — 1st ed.
     p. ; cm.
  Includes bibliographical references and index.
  ISBN 978-1-4511-7589-9
  I. Title.
  [DNLM: 1. Athletic Performance—physiology. 2. Psychomotor Performance. 3. Athletic Performance—psychology. 4. Movement.   WE 104]
  612.7'6—dc23
                                                                                    2012038287

LWW.com

To the One whose remarkable design is revealed on every page;
For You formed my inward parts; You wove me in my mother's womb.
I will give thanks to You, for I am fearfully and wonderfully made;
Wonderful are Your works; And my soul knows it very well.
My bones were not hidden from You when I was made in secret,
And skillfully wrought in the depths of the earth. (Ps. 139:13–15)

PREFACE

Motor behavior courses are often thought of as stand-alone courses that little integrate with other exercise science curricula, particularly applied and professional tracks. This book is the outgrowth of over 16 years of teaching motor behavior in a setting that entirely contradicts that notion—a setting in which motor behavior is weaved among biomechanics, sport/exercise psychology, exercise physiology, exercise testing and prescription, and other exercise science courses. The result is a book intended to serve both as a classroom text for courses in motor behavior, motor learning, and motor control, and as a well-worn reference on the shelf of the exercise science practitioner, the physical educator, and other professionals working in the fields of coaching, exercise science, and motor skill training.

The motor behavior field of study suffers a bit of an identity crisis, being called a number of different names depending on the specific focus. *Motor learning* and *psychomotor control* are terms used to describe the more cognitive ("mind") components of motor behavior. These terms are often used in cognitive psychology and physical education. *Motor control*, *neuromuscular control, neuromechanics*, and *movement neuroscience* are terms referring to the more physiological ("body") aspects of motor behavior. These latter terms have found favor in kinesiology and exercise science. The term motor behavior is used here simply because it is more descriptive in identifying the integral physiological and psychological aspects of movement that are inseparable.

AUDIENCE AND PURPOSE

This book is intended for upper level undergraduate students in exercise science or kinesiology, physical education, athletic training, and related allied health professions. It is assumed that these students come with a foundation in anatomy and physiology, and kinesiology or biomechanics. Background courses in psychology (particularly cognitive psychology) and exercise physiology are useful, but such knowledge is not assumed in this book.

The overarching purposes of this book are twofold. The first is to deliberately present motor behavior as a unified mind and body concept, in which one cannot fully understand one without the other. The second is to demonstrate in very practical ways how basic and applied knowledge of motor behavior underlies and enhances clinical, practical, and research skills in those venues served by exercise scientists, physical educators, and related allied health professionals.

APPROACH AND ORGANIZATION

The majority of students in the target audience have access to only a single one-semester course in motor behavior. For this reason, motor behavior texts are decidedly broad in scope to give students a full overview of the topic. This leaves a text shallow in depth, which we feel makes it difficult for students to apply concepts in the field. This book takes a different approach by going into greater depth on fewer selected topics that we have found eminently useful for practitioners. These emphasized topics have been selected based on current research findings, feedback from our alumni in the field and in graduate school, and our own research into the knowledge, skills, and abilities required of exercise scientists physical educators, and allied health care practitioners. As an added benefit, we have seen that students become more excited and more engaged when they can unfold the full spectrum of a specific topic.

The book is organized into three units that cover the body, the mind, and mind–body integration, respectively. Though the emphasis of this book is on unifying mind and body concepts, it is pedagogically useful to present each concept separately, and then bring them together. Specifically, Unit 1 covers the neurological and physiological aspects contributing to movement—which we call motor control—including neurophysiology and muscular physiology. Intertwined within these chapters are biomechanical concepts and the interaction of mechanical and physiological principles. Emphasis is placed on the organization of systems leading to movement production, from the behavior of motor units to reflex movements to the organization of voluntary movements. Another area of focus is the changes in motor control systems with practice and training. The exciting advancements in neurological imaging have revealed just how influential practice and training are on the nervous system. These sections are intended to demonstrate that training and practice sessions train the brain as much as the body, and that how one trains or practices influences brain adaptations and consequently, physiological adaptations. This unit culminates in an in-depth discussion of movement models. Though students are often challenged by these movement models, such as dynamic systems theory, they form a framework for application in the field and in the research environment.

Unit 2 covers motor learning topics, starting off in Chapter 6 with identifying, categorizing, and measuring motor skills and abilities. Depending on the instructor's approach and the background of the students, it is possible to begin the book with this chapter. Within this chapter is a thorough look at individual differences and talent identification. We believe that all instructors, coaches, and leaders involved in sports and exercise engage in talent identification, whether it is instinctual or planned. For this reason, it is important to discuss the uses and misuses of talent identification. Next covered is a description of the motor learning process, including stages of learning and the fundamental concepts contributing to the learning environment. Following motor learning is a specific chapter on information processing, with most of the emphasis placed on memory and attention. The current research and feedback from our alumni practitioners in the field tell us that attention is the most basic and arguably the most important concept for instructors to teach to their students. We culminate the unit with coverage of training and practice and instructional techniques. The endpoint of this unit brings together instructional and practice theories to form a unified model of practice and instruction that readers can take directly into the field. This model is useful in both practice settings and training settings, that is, for developing psychological and physiological capabilities.

Whereas the emphasis in Unit 2 was motor skill proficiency, Unit 3 examines more closely specific motor abilities that underlie successful motor skill performance. In particular, this unit begins with an in-depth examination of postural control mechanisms, followed by postural control training for wellness, injury prevention, and performance. Unit 3 ends with an applied look at functional strength and power training that ties together the psychological and physiological aspects of performance.

FEATURES

Each chapter begins with a set of concrete learning objectives based on purpose and importance of the material. Study questions relating directly to the objectives are presented at the end of the chapter. We believe if students go into each chapter with directed intention to learn the objectives they will assimilate the material more readily and with more meaning.

Other features in each chapter are SideNotes, Concepts in Action, and Thinking It Through boxes. SideNotes are additional pieces of information of general interest and important or timely research findings. Concepts in Action show or illustrate how the topics being discussed are used in real life applications. Thinking It Through boxes pose problems based on the text material for the reader to work through. These problems may ask the reader to engage in various activities such as mini experiments or assignments, and often send the reader off to read the current literature to help in their problem solving.

INSTRUCTOR AND STUDENT RESOURCES

Additional materials and aids for both students and faculty are available on the companion website at http://thePoint.lww.com/Ives. See the inside front cover of the book for details.

The test bank and review questions were prepared by

Tim Hilliard, PhD, CSCS
Associate Professor
Exercise & Sport Science Department
Fitchburg State University
Fitchburg, Massachusetts

ACKNOWLEDGMENTS

This text is an outgrowth of years of interactions with numerous researchers, colleagues, and students. I would specifically like to thank my coworkers at Ithaca College who uphold the standard of excellence for exercise science education and live out the idea of an integrated curriculum. I would also like to thank my Wolters Kluwer Health colleagues who know how to take hold of a vision, and the many reviewers who put considerable thought into their reviews. Most of all, though, I would like to thank my wife and children who have supported my efforts with enthusiasm. Year after year they serve as guinea pigs in all my plots and experiments, and never waiver in their encouragement and love.

REVIEWERS

John Barden, Ph.D.
University of Regina
Regina, Saskatchewan, Canada

Ali Boolani, Ph.D.
Assistant Professor
Oklahoma City University
Oklahoma City, Oklahoma

Jennifer Bridges, Ph.D.
Professor
Saginaw Valley State University
University Center, Michigan

Pamela Bryden, Ph.D.
Professor
Wilfrid Laurier University
Waterloo, Ontario, Canada

Michael Cinelli, Ph.D.
Assistant Professor
Wilfrid Laurier University
Waterloo, Ontario, Canada

Michael Collins, Ph.D.
Professor
Lewis-Clark State College
Lewiston, Idaho

Alberto Cordova, Ph.D.
Assistant Professor
University of Texas at San Antonio
San Antonio, Texas

Steve Elliot, Ph.D.
Associate Director
University of North Carolina Wilmington
Wilmington, North Carolina

Jeff Goodwin, Ph.D.
Associate Professor
University of North Texas
Denton, Texas

Andrea Mason, Ph.D.
Associate Professor
University of Wisconsin-Madison
Madison, Wisconsin

Ben Meyer, Ph.D.
Assistant Professor
Shippensburg University
Shippensburg, Pennsylvania

Jeff Nessler, Ph.D.
Assistant Professor
California State University, San Marcos
San Marcos, California

Rebecca Pena, M.S.
Lecturer
California State University, Northridge
Northridge, California

Kerri Staples, Ph.D.
Assistant Professor
University of Regina
Regina, Saskatchewan, Canada

David Stodden, Ph.D.
Associate Professor
Texas Tech University
Lubbock, Texas

Gregory Wilson, Ph.D., F.A.C.S.M.
Professor
University of Evansville
Evansville, Indiana

CONTENTS

I   Motor Control

Introduction to Motor Behavior and the Mind–Body Connection

PURPOSE, IMPORTANCE, AND OBJECTIVES OF THIS CHAPTER

The purpose of this chapter is to describe the field and study of motor behavior as it relates to kinesiology, exercise science, and sports. In particular, we impress upon the interaction between physiological processes and psychological processes in the learning and performance of motor skills. Without a clear and firm understanding of the way that physiology and psychology interact—in fact they are codependent upon one another—it is impossible to understand the production of purposeful, effective, and efficient motor skills.

After reading this chapter, you should be able to:

1. Define and explain the scope of motor behavior and motor skills.
2. Define and differentiate motor control and motor learning.
3. Explain the concept of psychophysics and the mind-body connection.
4. Understand the importance of skilled motor performance in everyday life.
5. Define and explain the differences between skill and ability.
6. Understand how motor skills become psychomotor skills and why this distinction is important.

Humans move in a vast array of ways, from the slightest twitch using just a tiny portion of a muscle to an explosive action using nearly every muscle in the body. Movements are used to do work, communicate messages, and display emotion. Muscles are also used to internally regulate physiological processes such as moving food through the digestive tract and pumping blood. All of these muscle actions and movements fall under the heading of what we call **motor behavior**. The focus of this book is on **goal-directed movements**, otherwise known as **motor skills**. By definition these are intentional and voluntary acts with an outcome purpose in mind, meaning that the mind plays a fundamental role in how movements are produced and initiated. This separates goal-directed movements from nonvolitional movements in the body, like peristalsis in the gastrointestinal tract, beating of the heart, or pure reflexive action in the skeletal muscles. The terms movement and motor skill are often used interchangeably, but here we define them more precisely. The generic term "movement" may refer to any voluntary, involuntary, active, or passive movement made by the body, and thus, it is necessary to qualify the term, such as "postural movements" or "rotational movements." In the motor behavior terminology used throughout this text, movement generally refers to the subcomponent actions that together make up a motor skill. For instance, a throwing motor skill involves movements of the legs and arms and trunk postural movements. Each of these component movements is purposeful, directed, and even skilled.

In its simplest form, motor behavior refers to the nature and cause of human movement. The term implies both physiological (motor) and psychological (behavior) aspects to movement. Such movements and motor skills include moving the body through space (locomotion), posture and balance, and manipulation (e.g., hand gestures, ball kicking). Movements may be slow, deliberate, and intense with concentration. Movements may be so automatic that they seem to require little or no thought. Goal-directed movements, whether big or small, combine behavioral and physiological elements, and thus, study of these movements must by necessity address both elements.

THE PHYSIOLOGICAL AND PSYCHOLOGICAL COMPONENTS OF MOTOR BEHAVIOR

In studying motor behavior, it is helpful to examine the two basic components of human movement—physiology and psychology—separately and then as a whole. Separating motor behavior in such a way should not be interpreted as motor behavior being two stand-alone components but rather as a way to simplify the study of a vastly complex topic. The physiological component, **motor control**, is concerned primarily with the systems that execute movements and monitor movements, particularly the motor and sensory neurophysiological systems and musculoskeletal systems. The term **neuromuscular control** is used synonymously with motor control. Because these physiological systems act in mechanical and physical manners (e.g., velocity, force) and interact with the physical world, terms like muscle mechanics, neuromechanics, and biomechanics are also used in the study of motor control. In fact, the study of biomechanics and that of motor control are often seen as inseparable. In Unit I we examine how the neurophysiological and neuromuscular systems enable the four movement processes of planning, initiating, executing, and monitoring and how biomechanical and physical properties impose limits or constraints to movement.

The behavioral component, **motor learning**, emphasizes the mind's role in acquiring (i.e., learning), planning, initiating, and modifying movement and how cognitive processing and behavioral states regulate movement quality. In reality, the control and learning components work in combination with one another, as the neurophysiological systems provide the living structures for behavioral functions. Figure 1.1 shows how the study of motor control emphasizes what is happening in the "body" whereas motor learning emphasizes what is happening in the "mind" and that together they form a major part of the **mind–body connection**.

Psychophysics and the Mind–Body Connection At Work

Sensory **feedback** processing typifies mind–body systems at work. Sensory feedback is provided by sensory receptors and the peripheral nervous system. These receptors *detect stimuli* from the external environment like temperature and from the internal bodily environment like muscle stretch. The central nervous system gathers this information and *interprets meaning*, a process called **perception**. Sensation is a motor control process and perception is a motor learning process, and thus, they are not the same. However, the terms sensation and perception are often (and erroneously) used interchangeably only because we often cannot determine what the actual sensation is, only how we perceive it. For example, the sensory system responds to temperature changes, but it is our perceptual system that tells us it is too hot or too cold. The sensitivity and relationship between detection and interpretation are

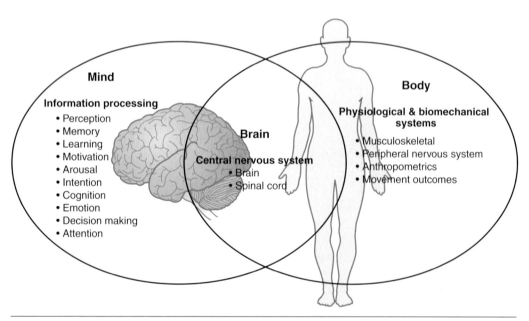

Figure 1.1 • This schematic illustrates the major components of motor behavior and the mind–body connection and how they are studied using the subdisciplines of motor learning and motor control. In this context, the "brain" is considered to be the entire central nervous system (brain and spinal cord) and its associated neurophysiological systems. The "mind" is the function of the brain, which at its core is processing of information. This processing ranges from emotional control to memory storage. The "body" in this scheme is the entire physiological, anatomical, and biomechanical systems in the body other than the central nervous system. The diagram lists only a few of the relevant systems involved in the control of movement. Motor learning emphasizes the brain–mind interaction, whereas motor control emphasizes the brain–body interaction. The study of motor behavior, then, is ultimately concerned with how the mind interacts with the body.

called **psychophysics**. Interpretation is vital because how we interpret the sensory information is more important to our goal-directed actions than is the sensory information itself. A myriad of psychological factors determine what sensory information is used, why it is used, and how it is used. Emotion, reasoning, intention, motivation, and memories of past experiences are notable psychological factors that influence the interpretation of sensory information. These factors determine if information is stored and give rise to meaning and importance. Interpretation of stimuli may be incorrect because of disordered behavioral states and because of inaccurate sensory detection.

Psychophysics is used in many different areas. Among the most common uses is the understanding of pain and discomfort. In exercise science, Borg's rating of perceived exertion (RPE) scale and visual analog pain scales are applications of psychophysics (Fig. 1.2). Graded exercise tests are often stopped when someone points to the highest workload on the RPE scale—even if heart rate and other physiological measures indicate that the person can go longer. In ergonomics, work limits are mostly set according to what is perceived as a work limit, rather than what physiological data may indicate.

Another concept in the mind–body relationship is **perception–action coupling**. Perception–action coupling is when perception of movement-related factors, whether they are environmental obstacles, internal physiological characteristics, or movement goals, is matched with movement actions. For example, a motor action of initiating the first step onto a set of stairs is based on visual detection and then perception of the step height, distance of the step away from the individual, and the timing of the approach to the stairs. These factors lead directly to the subsequent motor action of when and how to

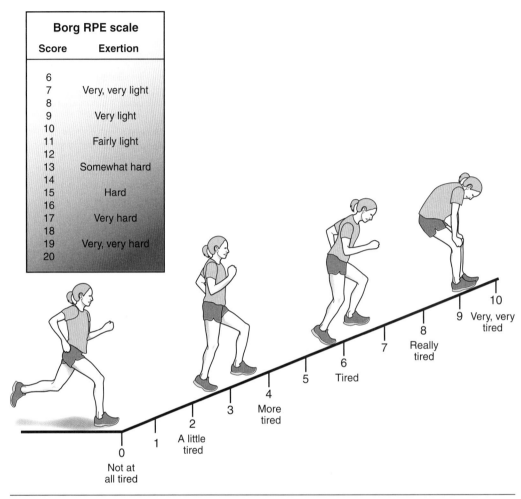

Figure 1.2 • On the top is Borg's RPE scale ranging from 6 to 20. (Adapted from Borg, G. (1970). Perceived exertion as an indicator of somatic stress. *Scandinavian Journal of Rehabilitation Medicine*, *2*, 92–98.) The numbers originally were designed to correspond to heart rate (e.g., 6 = 60 bpm; 20 = 200 bpm), but the relationship between heart rate and perceived effort can vary greatly depending on factors such as motivation and discomfort. Thus, the perception of effort may be greater than the actual physiological effort itself. On the right is a visual analog scale of perceived exertion made for children. Children are able to interpret the posture and facial expressions of the cartoon character and relate that to their own feelings, and thus provide a numerical score. (Adapted from Utter, A., Robertson, R., Nieman, D., & Kang, J. (2002). Children's OMNI Scale of Perceived Exertion: Walking/running evaluation. *Medicine and Science in Sports and Exercise*, *34*(1), 139–144.)

make the first step onto the stairs. Other factors such as fatigue, injury, or a weighted backpack may influence the motor decision that is coupled with the perception of the environmental features.

A clear understanding of the mind–body connection enables mental skills to be exploited to maximize physiological adaptations; in practice this means the development of practice and training programs that are individualized, more functional, and better able to transfer from the training or rehabilitation environment to real life settings. This may sound like overexaggeration, but throughout this text are presented many examples taken directly from the research literature that document this mind–body connection at work.

THE IMPORTANCE OF QUALITY MOTOR SKILLS

The teaching and learning of motor skills are often thought to be important in only three settings: rehabilitation, children in physical education, and athletics. Yet proficient motor skills are essential in all aspects of life across all domains and ages. Motor skills are so important for human functioning that the brain devotes most of its resources to motor acts. The motor system provides the primary way in which humans interact with the world. Consider, for example, that speaking, writing, and "body language" are the main ways humans communicate, and all rely on neuromuscular processes to carry out behavioral intentions. Many of our most beautiful and transcendent accomplishments are carried out through skilled movements, including music, art, sport, and survival. Rage is beat out on drums or with fists, love communicated through tender touches, and joy expressed with jumps.

But is it necessary that relatively healthy persons, apart from athletes, learn to improve movement control aside from that gained during normal day-to-day life experiences? According to Higgins (1991), it is important to enhance movement capabilities because it extends problem-solving capabilities and, by extension, one's ability to interact with the world. Movement quality plays an important role in personal independence, as individuals learn to walk, ride a bike, and drive. The consequences of poor motor behavior in activities like driving can be severe. The decline in movement skills with aging provides a clear example of how poor movements can negatively impact the quality of one's life. In recent years, a growing amount of research has demonstrated that poor movement quality contributes to a decline in "functional health" and overall quality of life, even in relatively healthy adults (Ives & Keller, 2008; Rejeski & Brawley, 2006).

■ Thinking It Through 1.1 Psychology and Injury

Among the most frustrating occurrences for patients following rehabilitation of musculoskeletal injuries is the feeling of not being back to normal and the inability to perform at preinjury levels. Even after extensive rehabilitation from knee injuries or low back pain in which most patients have returned to normal activity, some patients may experience discomfort, anxiety about performance, and poor performance skills. These patients, termed noncopers (compared to adaptive copers), may lack functional coordination skills (Chmielewski et al., 2005) or lack psychological strategies enabling them to cope with their new functional state (Riipinen et al., 2005). Other researchers have found strong relationships among athletic injury rates and negative psychological traits (Johnson & Ivarsson, 2011). Can you think of reasons why or how psychological characteristics may influence movement skill coordination and injuries? For help with your answer, read the Johnson and Ivarsson (2011) article that is listed in the references at the end of the chapter.

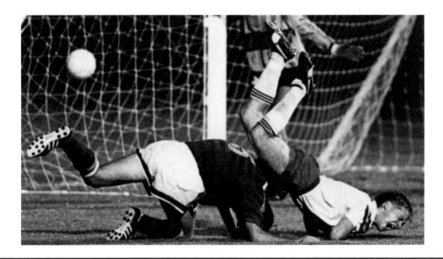

Specifically in the realm of exercise and sport science, it is well known that the primary distinction separating the elite-level athletes from subelite athletes in many sports is motor behavior. In particular, tactical and technical skills, and decision-making skills coupled with coordination, characterize the elite performer in many sports. The most difficult part of many athletic rehabilitation programs is not gaining back physiological capabilities (e.g., muscle strength), but rather gaining back movement control. Neuromuscular and perceptually based training, apart from standard physiologically based training, has been shown to reduce injuries in athletes, improve athletic performance, improve work productivity and lessen work-related injuries, improve physical function in elders, and improve life quality in many populations (Abernethy & Bleakle, 2007; Hewett et al., 2006; Myer et al., 2011; Rejeski & Brawley, 2006). There are other health and wellness implications as well, as those individuals with better movement quality may have fewer risks for things like cardiovascular disease, in part because they are more likely to engage in physical activity (Houston et al., 2002).

DEFINING MOTOR SKILLS

The most practical way to understand motor behavior is by examining and analyzing movement, in particular goal-directed movement. Goal-directed movements, or motor skills, may involve large and small muscle forces, slow and deliberate thought, or rapid reactions. Sometimes they are done without any apparent thought whatsoever. Motor skills can be performed poorly or with great skill. Here we define several terms used to describe motor skill characteristics.

Skill, Motor Skills, Talents, and Abilities

It is important to evaluate the quality of motor skill performance along with the type of movement. The quality of performance is defined as the level of **skill**. Being skilled is separate from having **ability**, which is defined as a general *capacity* of an individual that is related to the performance of tasks. For example, running speed is an important ability contributing to successful performance in long jump and many other sports but in and of itself does not mean that one will have skilled performance. One may have much ability, but little skill. On the other hand, having high levels of skill requires ability. Ability should not be thought of as a genetic component and skill a learned component. Abilities fall into many categories, of which some are genetic, some are learned, and many are a combination of both. These categories of abilities include physical proficiency (e.g., strength, power, flexibility, lung vital capacity), cognitive (e.g., information processing speed, memory, emotional control), and perceptual–motor (e.g., finger dexterity, precision and aiming control, multi-limb coordination, kinesthesia and balance control). The term **talent** is often used to describe specific genetic abilities contributing to performance of a particular motor skill or task, though in Chapter 9 we define it a bit more broadly.

Motor Skills and Psychomotor Skills

Perceptual motor skill and **psychomotor skill** are terms used to describe motor skills with specific features that require a large amount of cognitive effort or sensory feedback to execute. By definition, these terms refer to movements that have any of the following features: a reaction time component (especially choice reaction time); high levels of dexterity, precision, or accuracy; high levels of timing or rate control; or steadiness or speed of the hands or fingers. The term perceptual motor skill is specifically used to describe movements that arise from choices made from interpreting environmental cues (example below). Psychomotor and perceptual motor skills generally exclude movements like running, walking, and whole body balance, but in real life almost any motor skill can be perceptual or psychomotor depending on the circumstances.

SIDE**NOTE**	**WHAT IS COORDINATION?**

Coordination is a term often used in place of skill, but these terms do not mean the same thing. Coordination refers to patterning of the body and limb segments relative to one another and relative to the environment. A coordinated movement takes into account the context in which it is being performed and constraints imposed by the environment. It is often the case that a highly coordinated movement is a smooth, graceful, and skilled movement, but sometimes this is not always true. Elite marathoner Bill Rodgers, for example, overpronated his foot and compensated with an odd and excessive right arm swing that could be described as uncoordinated, yet this did not hold him back from being the most skilled marathoner of his time.

In real life, most motor acts are perceptual in nature. Sports, driving a car, and walking down a busy street all require considerable cognitive control. Vertical jumping provides a good example. In the lab, vertical jumping is not considered a perceptual motor skill. There is little cognitive effort, no reaction to a stimulus, and minimal precision and minimal manual dexterity is needed. On the other hand, vertical jumping in a soccer game as part of a heading movement is psychomotor. The player must anticipate ball trajectory, time the jump, jostle and "feel" for position, aim the jump to position the head, and consider where to head the ball (keeping in mind teammates, defenders, and game situation). The jump is now a complex movement requiring more than explosive muscle strength to be carried out successfully. In fact, it is the perceptual part of many motor acts that determines the efficiency, coordination, appropriateness, and overall effectiveness of the motor act.

SUMMARY

Motor behavior involves study of the physiological systems producing movement and the psychological systems involved in planning, learning, and regulating movement. This connection between mind and body implies that behavioral actions in the mind are transferred to the body, and actions in the body are transferred to the mind. Motor behavior, as much as any academic discipline, examines this relationship and provides insight into practical uses of the mind–body connection. These practical uses center on training or challenging both systems simultaneously to create more effective gains and better performance. How this is done is emphasized throughout this text.

STUDY QUESTIONS

1. Define and describe the differences and similarities between motor control and motor learning.
2. Describe the concept of the mind–body connection. Use the term psychophysics to help explain your answer.
3. Define skill, ability, talent, and coordination, and describe the differences among these terms.
4. Define motor skill and psychomotor skill. Explain the characteristics of a psychomotor skill.
5. Select a motor action and explain it in the context of being a motor skill and in the context of being a psychomotor skill.

References

Abernethy, L., & Bleakle, C. (2007). Strategies to prevent injury in adolescent sport: A systematic review. *British Journal of Sports Medicine*, *41*(10), 627–638.

Borg, G. (1970). Perceived exertion as an indicator of somatic stress. *Scandinavian Journal of Rehabilitation Medicine*, *2*, 92–98.

Chmielewski, T. L., Hurd, W. J., & Snyder-Mackler, L. L. (2005). Elucidation of a potentially destabilizing control strategy in ACL deficient non-copers. *Journal of Electromyography & Kinesiology*, *15*(1), 83–92.

Hewett, T., Ford, K., & Myer, G. (2006). Anterior cruciate ligament injuries in female athletes: Part 2, a meta-analysis of neuromuscular interventions aimed at injury prevention. *The American Journal of Sports Medicine*, *34*(3), 490–498.

Higgins, S. S. (1991). Motor skill acquisition. *Physical Therapy*, *71*(2), 123–139.

Houston, T., Meoni, L., Ford, D., Brancati, F., Cooper, L., Levine, D., & Klag, M. (2002). Sports ability in young men and the incidence of cardiovascular disease. *The American Journal of Medicine*, *112*(9), 689–695.

Ives, J.C., & Keller, B.A. (2008). Functional training for health. In J.K. Silver & C. Morin (Eds.), *Understanding fitness. How exercise fuels health and fights disease* (pp. 71–90). Westport, CT: Praeger Publishers.

Johnson, U., & Ivarsson, A. (2011). Psychological predictors of sport injuries among junior soccer players. *Scandinavian Journal of Medicine & Science in Sports*, *21*(1), 129–136.

Myer, G., Faigenbaum, A., Ford, K., Best, T., Bergeron, M., & Hewett, T. (2011). When to initiate integrative neuromuscular training to reduce sports-related injuries and enhance health in youth? *Current Sports Medicine Reports*, *10*(3), 155–166.

Rejeski, W., & Brawley, L. (2006). Functional health: Innovations in research on physical activity with older adults. *Medicine and Science in Sports and Exercise*, *38*(1), 93–99.

Riipinen, M., Niemistö, L., Lindgren, K., & Hurri, H. (2005). Psychosocial differences as predictors for recovery from chronic low back pain following manipulation, stabilizing exercises and physician consultation or physician consultation alone. *Journal of Rehabilitation Medicine*, *37*(3), 152–158.

Utter, A., Robertson, R., Nieman, D., & Kang, J. (2002). Children's OMNI Scale of Perceived Exertion: Walking/running evaluation. *Medicine and Science in Sports and Exercise*, *34*(1), 139–144.

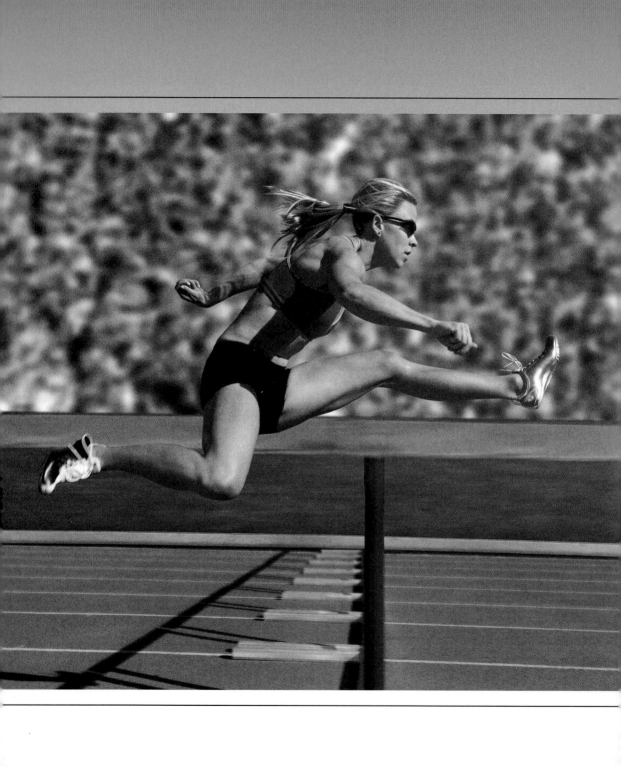

I

Motor Control

The study of motor control concerns the way the nervous and musculoskeletal systems create and carry out movements. In this unit, we focus on how these systems work toward the four main processes involved in movement: planning, initiating, executing, and monitoring. Specifically, in Chapter 2, we look at planning and initiating as central nervous system processes, Chapter 3 examines movement execution as a function of the peripheral neuromuscular system, and Chapter 4 examines movement monitoring by the peripheral sensory system. Chapter 5 combines all these elements and looks at a holistic view of movement by examining movement models.

2 | Neural Mechanisms in Planning and Initiating Movement

PURPOSE, IMPORTANCE, AND OBJECTIVES OF THIS CHAPTER

The purpose of this chapter is to describe the major components, organization, and functioning of the nervous system responsible for controlling movements. In particular, emphasis is placed on the central nervous system as the system responsible for planning and initiating movement. Understanding these structures and their working qualities gives rise to understanding how skilled motor performance is carried out and, further, the instructional, training, and rehabilitation strategies that may be used to maximize nervous system control of movement.

After reading this chapter, you should be able to:

1. Describe the basic organization of the central and peripheral nervous systems contributing to movement.
2. Explain the basic functions of neurons in transmitting signals.
3. Describe the specific motor control function of each of the major components of the central nervous system, as well as describe the integration of these functions in producing effective motor planning.
4. Explain the processes of sensorimotor integration, feedforward control, and feedback control.
5. Detail the changes made in the CNS as a result of practice and physical training.

Nearly every system within our body is designed to support movement of one form or another. Standing out among these systems from a motor control standpoint are the nervous and muscular systems. In this chapter, the physiology and function of the relevant nervous system structures are examined. An exhaustive coverage of these systems is out of the scope of this text, but rather, emphasis is placed on the nervous system components responsible for the four components of carrying out and learning goal-directed movement: planning, initiating, executing, and monitoring. The planning and initiation stages are entirely central nervous system processes, whereas execution and monitoring are largely the role of the peripheral nervous system and the neuromuscular system. This chapter focuses on the role of the central nervous system in planning and initiating movement and begins by looking briefly at the basic qualities and organization of the nervous system.

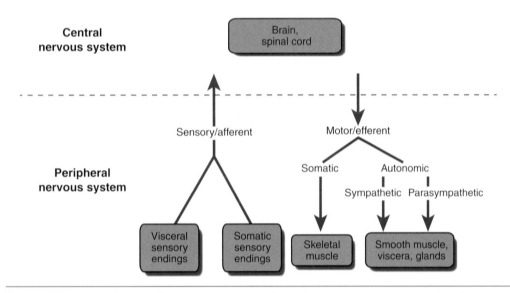

Figure 2.1 • Organization of the nervous system. The study of motor control emphasizes the somatic (voluntary) motor and sensory aspects of the PNS and the CNS.

ORGANIZATION OF THE NERVOUS SYSTEM

The human nervous system can be divided into the **central nervous system** (CNS) and the **peripheral nervous system** (PNS) (Fig. 2.1). The CNS includes the brain and spinal cord and is the integration and command center for the entire nervous system. The PNS can be divided into sections based on different criteria. When divided by the *direction of information*, the PNS can be divided into **sensory** and **motor** divisions. Sensory (or **afferent**) division sends signals from the periphery to CNS. Motor (or **efferent**) division sends signals from CNS to effector organs, namely, the muscles. The PNS can also be divided based *on involuntary versus voluntary* control systems. The voluntary system, also called the **somatic system**, is defined as that controlling voluntary motor behavior. The involuntary system, also called the **autonomic nervous system**, regulates visceral and bodily processes at the subconscious level, including heart rate, ventilation, digestion, and other systems involving smooth muscle and glands. The autonomic system can be further divided into the **sympathetic** and **parasympathetic** divisions. Though the autonomic systems do play a supporting role in motor behavior, we only consider them in brief.

NEURON FUNCTION

At the heart of the nervous system are **neurons**, the nerve cells. Neuron cell bodies house typical cellular organelles, but the key working features of neurons are the cell processes, namely, **dendrites** and the **axon**. Dendrites branch from the cell body acting as receptive sites for signals from other neurons. The dendrites conduct impulses from synapses to the cell body. The axon carries electrical impulses in the form of an action potential (AP) away from the cell body and out to synapses on its distal end.

Sensory (afferent) neurons make up the sensory division of the PNS. At the distal end of a long branching dendrite are attached receptors to detect stimuli. These receptors are out in the body tissues and send signals to the sensory neuron cell body. From the cell body, the signal is sent out the axon to make connections in the spinal cord. **Motor (efferent) neurons** in the PNS have their cell bodies and dendrites in the spinal cord and connect to muscle fibers at the distal end of the axon. These motor neurons are specifically referred to as lower motor neurons to distinguish them from upper motor neurons

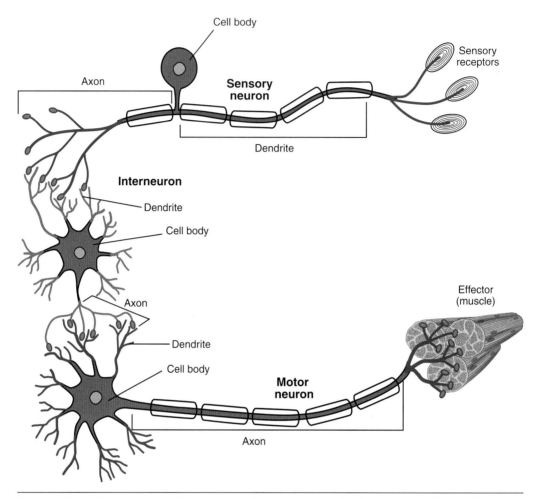

Figure 2.2 • Motor, sensory, and interneurons. Sensory neurons arise from sensory endings and converge onto the spinal cord where they make connections with interneurons, motor neurons, and other sensory neurons. Lower motor neurons are shown originating from the spinal interneurons and exiting out of the spinal cord to the muscles. Not shown are upper motor neurons descending out of the brain and connecting to interneurons and lower motor neurons.

arising from the brain and descending down the spinal cord. A single lower motor neuron and all the muscle fibers it innervates is called a **motor unit**. **Interneurons** lie between motor and sensory neurons, linking the sensory and motor divisions. The typical arrangement of sensory and motor neurons, and interneurons, is shown in Figure 2.2.

A cluster of neuron fibers enclosed within a connective tissue sheath is called a **nerve**. Nerves may contain only afferent or efferent fibers, but typical spinal nerves contain both afferent and efferent fibers.

Communication among Neurons

Neurons communicate information among each other and to muscles in the form of a bioelectrical signal called an **action potential (AP)**. The AP does not degrade as it travels down an axon or as it travels from one neuron to another neuron or from neuron to effector organ, like muscles or glands. The AP is spread by way of connections called **synapses**. Synapses may transmit the AP directly through electrical connections (electrical synapse) or by the release of chemicals (chemical synapse). Chemical synapses are much more common and dominate the motor control networks, so we will only consider them. The more synapses along a neuron chain, the slower the transmission of the signal; monosynaptic paths have one synapse, and polysynaptic pathways have more than one synapse. The neuron on the transmitting or "upstream" end of a synapse is called the presynaptic neuron, and the receiving or "downstream" neuron is called the postsynaptic neuron.

Very rarely does one neuron make just a single connection with another neuron. In the brain and spinal cord, a single neuron may form multiple synapses with another neuron, and a neuron may make connections with hundreds or thousands of other neurons, resulting in thousands upon thousands of synaptic connections on any given neuron. When an AP reaches the synapse at the end of the axon, a chemical neurotransmitter is released from the presynaptic side, which then floats across the synapse and binds to the postsynaptic neuron. This neurotransmitter on the postsynaptic neuron creates an electrical potential called an excitatory postsynaptic potential (EPSP), but this does not mean that an AP will be automatically generated. Forming an AP in even a single neuron is a complex process involving many AP inputs from many different neurons and the overall number of APs bombarding the neuron.

In chemical synapses, the AP is propagated by sending chemicals from the presynaptic side to the postsynaptic side. When the AP in the presynaptic neuron reaches the end of the axon (axon terminal) where the synapse is located, it causes small containers called synaptic vesicles to release a neurotransmitter. The neurotransmitter, such as acetylcholine (ACh), floats across the synaptic cleft (the actual space between the neurons) to bind to the postsynaptic membrane. The neurotransmitter causes depolarizing currents in the postsynaptic neuron.

APs are generated in a neuron based on the amount of electrical impulses coming into that neuron. Dendrites on the cell body receive depolarizing stimuli from other neurons that synapse on them. These stimuli cause the postsynaptic neuron cell membrane to **depolarize** in a graded fashion, and these depolarizing currents travel to the axon hillock. At the hillock, the graded potentials will sum, and if the total current is strong enough, an AP will be created. The amount of current needed to create an AP is considered the **threshold** level. The more APs acting on a postsynaptic neuron at a given time enable more summation of the graded depolarizations, and thus, a greater likelihood of forming an AP.

Depolarizing stimuli on the postsynaptic side can be excitatory (**excitatory postsynaptic potentials or EPSPs**) or inhibitory (**inhibitory postsynaptic potentials or IPSPs**). The summing of the EPSPs can occur over time (**temporal summation**) from a single presynaptic input or from several different inputs (**spatial summation**). Thus, to generate an AP in the postsynaptic neuron, there can be summation of rapid firing EPSPs from the presynaptic neurons or summation of many different EPSPs from different presynaptic neurons. Of course, there can be a combination of both temporal and spatial summation. Also, some of the depolarizations will be inhibitory (IPSPs), which stop the formation of EPSPs, essentially reducing the amount of graded depolarizations summing at the hillock and effectively reducing the likelihood of an AP. Thus, generation of an AP is dependent not only on temporal and spatial summation but also on the ratio of excitatory to inhibitory inputs.

A general schematic depicting formation of an AP is illustrated in Figure 2.3. Consider a single motor neuron whose cell body is in the spinal cord and axon terminates on a muscle fiber. The inputs, both inhibitory and excitatory, come from other motor neurons, sensory afferents, interneurons, and direct connections from the brain. To "fire" this neuron (and subsequently activate the muscle), the neuron membrane potential must change to reach a threshold level. To do so, the CNS controls a precise combination of spatial inputs, temporal inputs, and the ratio of EPSPs to IPSPs. If they summate sufficiently to reach a threshold level of neuronal excitability, the postsynaptic neuron will generate an AP, but an insufficient number may result in no AP and thus the bioelectric signal dies out. If the postsynaptic neuron is excited by incoming APs, but not quite enough to generate an AP, it may be in a **facilitated** state. In this state, the postsynaptic neuron is ready to fire, like a sprinter at the starting block, and needs just a bit more AP inputs to fire. Conversely, if IPSPs are bombarding the postsynaptic neuron, it becomes more difficult to generate an AP and is said to be **inhibited**.

Chemical synapses have numerous advantages over electrical synapses in that the CNS can control them to a much larger extent. Threshold levels, temporal and spatial summation, and the multitude of synaptic connections on each neuron (including pre- and postsynaptic) enable the CNS to set the responsiveness of neurons and neural pathways, filter out unwanted background noise, and route and

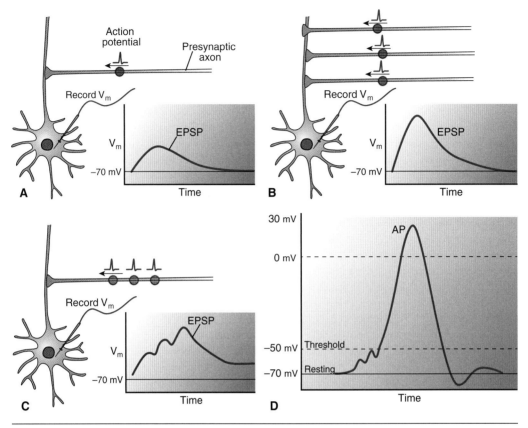

Figure 2.3 • Generation of the action potential. **A.** A single presynaptic AP arrives at a postsynaptic neuron and triggers an EPSP, but this is not large enough to reach a threshold level and create an AP in the postsynaptic side. **B.** Spatial summation of EPSPs: When two or more presynaptic inputs from different neurons arrive at the same time, their individual EPSPs add together to generate a large depolarizing current. **C.** Temporal summation of EPSPs: When the same presynaptic fiber fires APs in quick succession, the individual EPSPs add together. **D.** If the summating EPSPs reach a threshold level, an AP will be generated. If the EPSPs do not reach threshold, the neuron may stay in a facilitated state. Not shown are IPSPs that can block the summating effects of the EPSPs or lower the resting membrane potential to put the neuron in a state of inhibition.

reroute signals to any number of targets. Chemical synapses enable the CNS and PNS a degree of plasticity to change and adapt to needs and circumstances. The importance of this plasticity in motor learning and control cannot be overstated. It is here, in these pathways and subtle changes in synaptic functioning, that learning is carried out. In fact, all of learning and training should be considered to impact the nervous system first, followed then by changes in movement performance.

■ Thinking It Through 2.1   Why Inhibit?

It may seem strange that a neuron would inhibit the action of another neuron, that is, purposefully attempt to stop the transmission of an AP. After all, if the brain did not want a signal to be transmitted, would it simply not send a signal in the first place? Can you think of reasons why there are neurons that inhibit other neurons, that is, why does neural inhibition exist? For a quick review of your answer, check out the Farlex Online Encyclopedia: http://encyclopedia.farlex.com/inhibition,+neural or a more detailed answer on Scholarpedia: http://www.scholarpedia.org/article/Neural_inhibition

MOTOR CONTROL IN THE CENTRAL NERVOUS SYSTEM

The CNS is responsible for the planning and initiating of motor skills. Planning requires a broad spectrum of functions, including data gathering, motivating and intention setting, retrieving memories, organizing, decision making, evaluating and judging, and predicting outcomes. Planning also draws upon comparisons to previously learned behaviors and makes considerable use of sensory feedback. The concept of CNS planning within a motor action context is synonymous with the terms *action preparation* and *movement preparation* used by some authors, but we use the term CNS planning to distinguish this process from movement preparatory actions such as warming up or "psyching up."

Initiating refers to the process of taking the plan and sending it down and out of the CNS. This seemingly simple task of initiation requires that the plan be encoded into a precise pattern of electrical signals within thousands of motor neurons such that when the plan reaches the muscles an effective movement is carried out. Both the plan and initiation phases must take into account that as the signal descends from the CNS to the PNS changes are made along the way.

Neither planning nor initiating can be pinpointed to a specific area of the brain, but rather, they are distributed across many areas. Fundamentally, the brain can be divided into four areas: the cerebrum, the diencephalon, the cerebellum, and the brain stem (Fig. 2.4). Along with the spinal cord these areas make up the CNS (Fig. 2.5). It is important to understand that each of these areas house specific areas devoted to motor functions and nonmotor functions, but a large amount of interconnectedness between the motor and nonmotor areas reveals considerable complexity of movement planning and initiating that cannot be pinpointed to select areas of the brain.

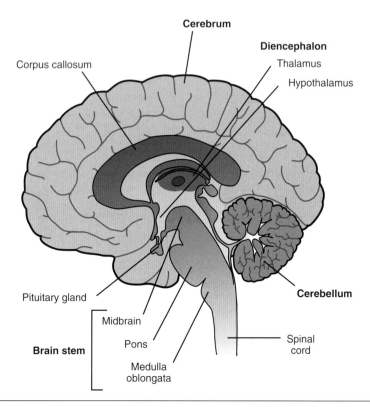

Figure 2.4 • The primary organizational structure of the brain, showing the cerebrum, the diencephalon, the brain stem, and the cerebellum. Also shown is the pituitary gland that receives direct instructions from the brain to release numerous hormones into the bloodstream, and the corpus callosum that is the major tract of fibers connecting the left side of the brain with the right side.

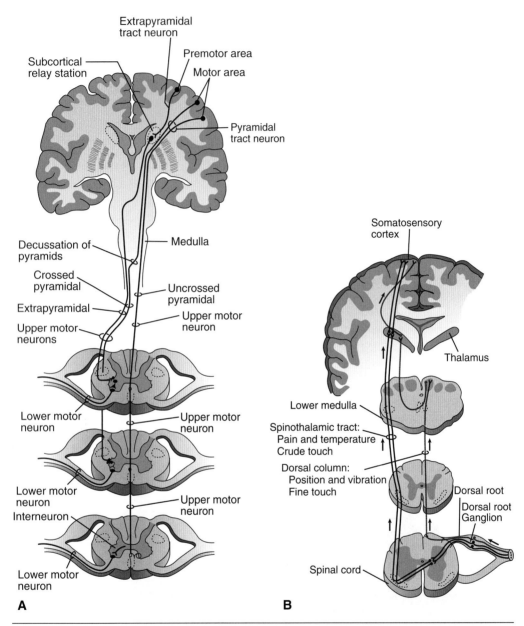

Figure 2.5 • The basic motor control organization of the CNS. **A.** Motor commands originate in the higher brain centers and descend through lower brain centers and the spinal cord, eventually exiting the spinal cord to the muscles. Most motor neurons descend through the pyramidal tract and cross over (decussate) to the opposite side, but other neurons do not cross over and some originate from other areas of the cortex and descend through extrapyramidal tracts. **B.** Sensory signals originate in the periphery and ascend through the spinal cord to various centers of the brain, but most somatosensory signals end up in the somatosensory cortex. Due to the numerous types of sensory endings and the need to process this information across a wide spectrum of brain resources, the sensory pathways are more variable than typical motor neuron pathways. This schematic illustrates that some receptor sensory neurons decussate in the spinal cord and others in the medulla. Not shown is that some sensory fibers terminate in the cerebellum or basal ganglia areas.

The Cerebrum

The cerebrum is made up of two cerebral hemispheres, which can be further divided into an outer or superficial area called the cerebral cortex and a deep area underneath the cortex. The cerebrum houses the conscious mind, stores learned experiences, and receives sensory information. Together with these processes, the entire cortex acts to organize, plan, and initiate purposeful, adaptable, and complex movements, making it the area of highest level of movement control. The left and right cerebral cortexes can be anatomically and functionally mapped based on lobes and Brodmann areas (Fig. 2.6). Cerebral lobes are anatomical divisions of the cerebral hemispheres that include the frontal lobe (anterior), parietal lobe (top of brain), occipital (dorsal) aspect of brain, and temporal lobes (lateral sides). These lobes house the **Brodmann areas**, which are groups of brain cells with similar structure, and because of that, similar function. These functional areas range from speech to cognition to emotion to motor function. Brodmann areas that regulate conscious thought and executive decision making are mostly located in the frontal lobe; hearing, taste, and facial recognition in the temporal lobes; motor and sensory function in the frontal and parietal lobes, and visual processing in the occipital lobe. The Brodmann areas most directly related to the production of movement are those areas that include the motor cortex, somatosensory cortex, visual cortex, and association cortexes.

From the motor cortex, a group of neurons called pyramidal cells originate and form the pyramidal tract (see Fig. 2.5). The pyramidal tract neurons are called upper motor neurons and they are the major motor-controlling tract of neurons that descend from the brain to the spinal cord. These neurons, along with upper motor neurons in extrapyramidal tracts, make direct connections in the spinal cord with lower motor neurons that go out to the muscles. The upper motor neurons also make connections with other neurons in the brain and spinal cord. Thus, not all of the neurons that will eventually connect to and activate the muscles originate in the same areas of the brain, or even in the highest areas of the brain. Within the

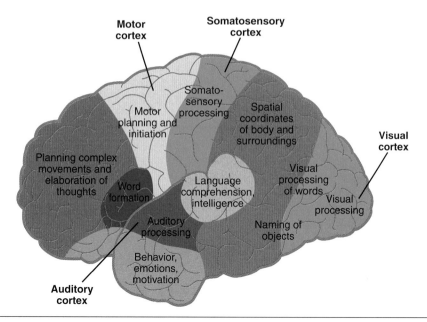

Figure 2.6 • A general mapping of brain areas and function. The outside labels point to specifically identified cortical areas—the motor cortex, somatosensory cortex, auditory cortex, and visual cortex. The interior labels identify functional tasks carried out across these and other cortical areas. The motor areas extend from the parietal to frontal lobes, the somatosensory areas are in the parietal lobes, and the visual cortex is in the occipital lobe. Not specifically labeled are the association cortexes, which are adjacent to the visual, somatosensory, and motor cortexes.

motor cortex are distinct separate motor areas, namely, the premotor area and the supplementary motor area, each of which may have separate functional duties in the regulation and initiation of movement.

The somatosensory cortex receives sensory information from the body regarding movement (proprioception) and touch, whereas the visual cortex is responsible solely for processing visual information. Visual processing is very complex and includes interpretation of movement (e.g., direction, speed), color and shading, and pattern recognition. Processing of visual information is so demanding that some of it is farmed out to other areas of the brain, in particular the identification of objects ("what") sent along a ventral stream (pathway) to the temporal areas and the localization of objects ("where") sent along a dorsal stream to parietal regions of the brain. Auditory processing has a limited direct effect on motor commands, but does play an important role some actions, such as a startle response to loud noises.

The association cortexes or areas take up more space than the other cortical regions, highlighting their importance. These areas are distributed near sensory cortical areas to help process sensory information and in the frontal lobe area to help in movement planning. Specifically, they process information concerning the perception of the external world around us and the internal bodily environment, ascribing meaning to what is going on around us and enabling us to interact with the world in meaningful ways. The highest order functions occur here, including cognition, language, reasoning, and abstract thought.

Areas of the motor cortex and sensory cortex that correspond to body regions are arranged in a specific fashion. The topographical map of this arrangement is called the **homunculus**, and a quick look gives a strong indication of the priority the brain gives to certain body parts (Fig. 2.7). Muscles of the hands and face, though small in mass and number, have the largest representation in the brain. The large amount of brain tissue devoted to motor and sensory function of the hands and face enables the brain to precisely control these muscles for communication and expression of emotion.

Concepts in Action

Brain Differences

Like the physical differences that characterize different people, the brains of individuals also vary. Could these differences provide reasons for individuals to practice or train differently? Gender differences provide a good look at this question. Research over the past 20 years has pointed to a number of gender differences in brain structure that are purported to contribute to behavioral differences. Though controversy exists over these data (Fine, 2010), the most recent and best information reveals the developmental changes of boy and girl brains differ dramatically, and it is this change, not the brain structures per se, that leads to men–women differences in behavior (Raznahan et al., 2010). Raznahan et al. (2010) maintain that these developmental differences during early childhood and adolescence could account for the much higher prevalence of risky and aggressive behavior in boys and differences in cognition and visuospatial ability between boys and girls. Other authors have noted clear differences in language, emotional control, and even handwriting that have been attributed to hormone differences. These findings are consistent with reports of differences in motor skill performance between boys and girls (Sanders, 2011; Toole & Kretzschmar, 1993). Some scientists and educators have used these data to prompt the use of single gender educational settings in which the teaching strategies can target the specific ways boys and girls learn and interact (Sax, 2006), and preliminary reports indicate benefits in learning and behavior in single-gender versus coed classes (Riordan et al., 2008). Riordan and colleagues' extensive evaluation and review demonstrated that single sex classrooms often performed better than coed classes in academic accomplishments and socioemotional achievement, despite few substantive changes in curriculum. Clearly, this may have implications for male and female coaches with opposite gender athletes. Coaches in these settings should make note of important gender differences.

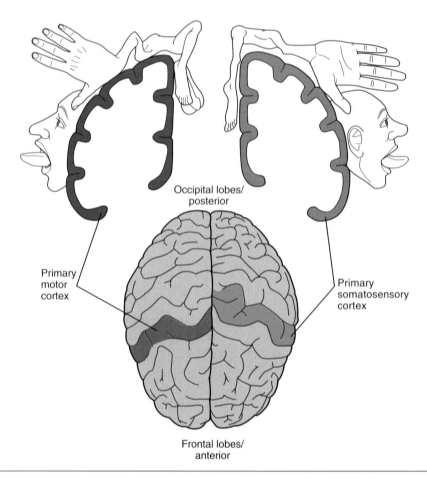

Figure 2.7 • A homunculus is a specific map of a cortex region corresponding to a body part. In this image, the homunculi of motor and somatosensory cortexes are shown. The size of the body part image is indicative of the topographical space given to serve those parts, both for motor output and sensory input.

The motor cortex needs considerable help from other regions to plan and initiate coordinated movements. The motor cortex integrates information from other brain centers and is responsible for initiating, or sending out, the majority of motor plan commands. These commands are sent out through upper motor neuron tracts, but they may be modified at many points along the way.

Deep in the cerebrum are pockets of neuron cell bodies called the basal ganglia. These information processing areas are involved with initiation, stopping, and intensity of motor outflow, in addition to regulating learned acts of posture and equilibrium. Also deep in the cerebrum are communication linkage areas, such as the corpus callosum. The corpus callosum links the left and right sides, allowing communication between the sides of the brain.

The Diencephalon

The diencephalon sits on top of the brain stem directly between the cerebrum and the brain stem. It comprises the thalamus, hypothalamus, subthalamus, and epithalamus (includes the pineal gland). The thalamus processes information flowing between the brain stem and the cerebrum. In particular, most of the sensory information arising from visual and somatic receptors goes through the thalamus, where it is filtered, processed, and relayed to other destinations. The thalamus also serves to relay information

SIDE**NOTE**	**MEASURING THE BRAIN**

Over a 100 years ago, our understanding of how the brain worked came largely from examining persons with brain injuries, including open head wounds. Many attempts were made in the early years to noninvasively investigate the brain, but it was not until the 1920s when electroencephalography (EEG) was invented that noninvasive and safe monitoring of the brain was possible. EEG detects brain electrical activity and is still a valuable tool in evaluating brain activity, but newer imaging techniques developed beginning in the 1970s, such as positron emission tomography (PET), computerized axial tomography (CT or CAT), and magnetic resonance imaging (MRI), have dramatically improved our ability to image and understand the brain at work. A PET scan requires a radioactive tracer to be inserted into the body through a biologically active molecule, and a detection device monitors the movement and breakdown of the tracer. A CT scan is essentially an x-ray fired at different angles, and a 3-D reconstruction of the image is made by computer. An MRI scan uses powerful electromagnets to line up hydrogen atoms in the body. A radio signal is then sent into the tissues and bounced back off the aligned atoms, providing an image of the tissue. Motor control research has made great strides since the 1990s with functional MRI (fMRI) that allows brain imaging during active movements, enabling researchers to directly associate motor and nonmotor activities with areas of brain activity.

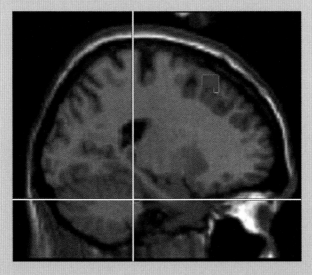

This sagittal plane view of an fMRI scan of the brain during motor activity is able to demonstrate changes in brain activation during motor activities. This computer color-enhanced view shows areas of the motor cortex and cerebellum active during arm and hand motor skills. (Image reprinted from Doyon, J., et al. (2009). Contributions of the basal ganglia and functionally related brain structures to motor learning. *Behavioural Brain Research, 199*(1), 61–75, with permission from Elsevier.)

among the motor cortex, basal ganglia, and cerebellum. The entire diencephalon regulates the autonomic nervous system, control hormonal secretion and general endocrine function, and plays a large role in limbic system functioning (see below).

The Cerebellum and Brain Stem

The cerebellum sits at the base of the brain and is involved in the planning and organizing of smooth, coordinated movements. This may be especially true for very rapid movements. Commands from the motor cortex regarding an intended movement are sent to the cerebellum and are processed and compared to incoming PNS sensory information. It is here the cerebellum fine tunes the movement for timing and precision. This updated information is then fed back to the motor cortex so that movement plans can be updated.

The brain stem sits beneath the diencephalon and is the junction of the brain and spinal cord. It is made up of the midbrain, pons, and medulla oblongata. These structures act as a passageway for all fibers between the spinal cord and the cerebrum, processing, filtering, and routing the signals like a switchboard through various nuclei structures. A complex neural network across the entire brain stem, called the reticular formation, receives and integrates information from all regions of the brain and sensory information from the body. From these structures come programmed, automatic movement behaviors like locomotion and posture, control of muscle tone, and autonomic function like regulation of breathing and heart rate. In the medulla, about 75% of the motor neurons from the pyramidal tract cross over to the other side. This crossover, called decussation, gives rise to the right side of the brain controlling the left side of the body and the left side of the brain controlling the right side of the body. Similar percentages of ascending sensory neuron also decussate, mostly in the medulla, but also in the spinal cord.

The Spinal Cord

The spinal cord is the CNS component linking to the PNS (Fig. 2.8). The outer portion of the spinal cord is mostly groups of axons sending sensory signals up and motor signals down the spinal column, and the interior portion is where signals are processed and routed through massive networks of synaptic connections. The spinal cord can be mapped like the homunculus of the cortex, with motor and sensory tracts belonging to certain muscles being located in specific areas. It was once thought that the spinal cord was simply responsible for making connections between the CNS and PNS, but it is now recognized that a great deal of information processing also occurs in the spinal cord. Not only does the spinal cord tune or modify descending supraspinal motor commands before these commands are

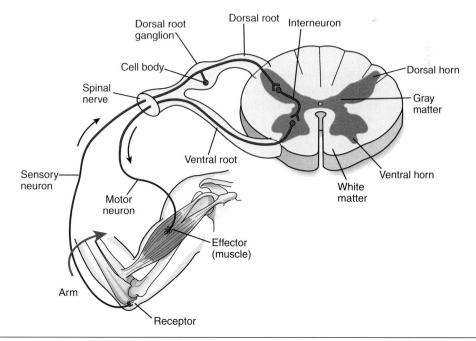

Figure 2.8 • Organization in the spinal cord. Sensory information from the PNS enters into the dorsal side (dorsal horn) of the spinal cord and motor commands exit out the ventral horn. White matter consists of myelinated axons from the ascending and descending tracts of neurons. Gray matter consists of cell bodies and houses the synaptic connections among neurons. The ganglion houses the cell bodies of the sensory neurons outside of the spinal cord, which differ from the motor neuron cell bodies which are in the spinal cord.

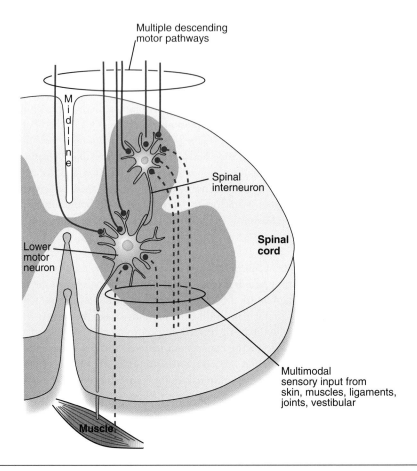

Figure 2.9 • Simplified schematic of multimodal sensory input and sensorimotor integration in the spinal cord. The convergence of sensory (*dashed lines*) and motor (*solid lines*) inputs onto the spinal interneurons and the lower motor neuron reflect sensorimotor integration. Much of the convergence occurs on inhibitory interneurons. The multimodal sensory inputs may arise from many different tissues and receptors. Not shown are presynaptic connections.

routed out to lower motor neurons, but the spinal cord directly organizes and initiates motor functions through reflexes and specialized neuronal circuits. In particular, the spinal cord likely houses complex neuronal circuits called pattern generators that produce rhythmic motor actions. When set in motion, these pattern generators create relatively complex yet stereotyped actions such as walking.

Through complex interneuron networks the descending motor signals converge with incoming sensory signals arriving from multiple sensory sources, called **multimodal sensory input** (Fig. 2.9). The convergence of sensory and motor signals, called **sensorimotor integration**, occurs in the spinal cord and in supraspinal centers. Eventually, a final converging of signals is made onto the lower motor neurons of the motor units, making these motor units the **final common pathway** for all nervous system motor activity.

A MODEL OF CNS ORGANIZATION FOR MOVEMENT

The exact neural mechanisms and events to plan and initiate a motor action, and further to learn skilled motor actions, are highly complex and have proved difficult to measure. These processes have been theorized based on brain recordings, assessment of persons with brain damage, and circumstantial data, and from these data has emerged consensus on some functions. Voluntary movement follows a chain of events, but each link in the chain connected to numerous other links. Movement must first begin with the will to move, which may begin somewhere in cortical or subcortical areas. The intention to move is a topic of considerable physiological and philosophical debate, but at this point, it seems that the **limbic system** plays some role. The limbic system is a widespread and interconnected network of regions that includes memory, emotional control, motivation, hormonal regulation, and instinctual processes like sexual drive and feeding. The limbic system is connected to movement and sensation control centers through the thalamus and indirectly through other centers.

Planning of the movement is thought to begin in the association cortex, basal ganglia, and cerebellum (Fig. 2.10). In all three of these areas, the movement plan information is gathered together and refined. This plan takes into account the movement goal and a wide range of the situational circumstances. Information from numerable sources is used, including memory, emotional state, and sensory information regarding movements just completed and similar movements from long ago. It is well recognized that the movement plan includes a prediction of the movement outcome and takes into

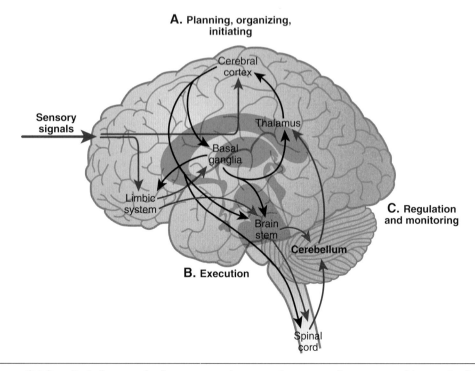

Figure 2.10 • Basic framework of motor control command structures for posture and locomotion based on work from Takakusaki and Okumura (2008). This model includes (*A*) planning/organizing/initiating, (*B*) execution, and (*C*) regulation and monitoring. The planning and initiating originate from emotional areas in the limbic system (*gray lines*) or cognitive/volitional centers in the cortex (*black lines*). Emotional plans, which may include fight or flight decisions, may be sent directly to the brain stem and out the spinal cord or sent to the basal ganglia where they are eventually routed to cortical regions for further modification. These and cortex-derived plans are modified and regulated as they are routed in and out of the basal ganglia, thalamus, and cerebellum, and are eventually initiated out the brain stem and spinal cord. Regulation pathways (*orange*) require feedback from all sensory systems, including information on the external world and internal bodily environment. The execution process is a function of the lower motor neurons and muscles. (Adapted from Takakusaki, K., & Okumura, T. (2008). Neurobiological basis of controlling posture and locomotion. *Advanced Robotics*, *22*(15), 1629–1663, Taylor & Francis, Ltd. reprinted by permission of the publisher [Taylor & Francis Ltd, http://www.tandf.co.uk/journals].)

account the inherent variability in the movement execution. The plan is relayed to the motor cortex through the thalamus. The motor cortex further plans and refines the movement and then initiates the movement plan by sending signals down the pyramidal and extrapyramidal tracts to the spinal cord.

In the spinal cord, the upper motor neurons originating in the brain connect to the lower motor neurons of the PNS. At the spinal cord level, more processing of the signal occurs, particularly the integration of the motor commands with sensory information arising from the sensory division of the PNS. This sensorimotor integration occurs in the spinal interneurons and eventually the final commands emerge onto the motor neurons heading out to the muscles. These lower motor neurons represent the start of the motor execution process of the nervous system.

Movement planning and initiation in the brain uses both feedforward and feedback control. **Feedforward control** are those commands that originate in the major brain structures and proceed relatively unabated to their target (e.g., muscles); in particular, they are minimally influenced by sensory feedback arising from the muscles and other body structures. This type of control system is otherwise known as open loop control and may provide what are called centrally preprogrammed movements. **Feedback control** systems, also known as closed loop control, are largely influenced by sensory feedback that regulates and changes the nature of the feedforward commands. In some cases, such as reflexes, feedback may initiate and regulate the entire movement process. In goal-directed movements, feedback is always influencing movement control processes in both the brain and spinal cord. The differences, then, between feedforward and feedback control lie in the origins of the the control signals and the amount of control.

Schematic models of the CNS command and feedback pathways are illustrated in Figure 2.11. Feedforward motor commands are seen to arise in the motor cortex and will eventually make their way down the spinal cord and to the motor neurons controlling muscles. Along the way, considerable feedback from sensory systems is used by higher centers to evaluate the plan and serve as a basis for modification. In some cases, the feedback may directly overrule the feedforward command. Motor command is not only sent down to the body, but also is sent internally to higher brain centers in a process called efference copy. **Efference copy** enables the brain to have a record of the command and enables the brain to

SIDE**NOTE**	**EXPERIMENTS IN FEEDBACK AND FEEDFORWARD COMMANDS**

Examples of feedforward and feedback are nicely illustrated in work from the 1970s and 1980s on rapid arm movements. In a typical experiment, the subjects were asked to perform maximally fast elbow flexion or extension movements of about 45- to 60-degree range of motion and stop abruptly at a target. This action produces a stereotypical pattern of EMG activity showing a large burst of agonist activity to propel the limb followed by a burst of antagonist activity to stop the limb at the target. In subjects with no sensory information arising from the moving arm (due to disease or experimental manipulation), the movement proceeds with the characteristic EMG pattern even if the movement is perturbed, showing that sensory feedback is not necessary to complete the movement (Hallett et al., 1975; Sanes & Jennings, 1984). In other studies, the movement was blocked soon after the movement began, but the characteristic agonist and antagonist burst of activity still occurred (Wadman et al., 1979). If the movement was slow, or if the perturbation occurred late, then the EMG patterns revealed signs of rapid adaptation to the perturbation, revealing feedback-mediated corrections. These results demonstrate that feedforward central commands can be sufficient to carry out a movement without sensory feedback influence, particularly in very fast movements or the initial phase of a movement when feedback corrections are too slow to be of use. Given enough time, however, subjects with intact nervous systems display changes to the EMG pattern as a consequence of sensory feedback arising from perturbed movements.

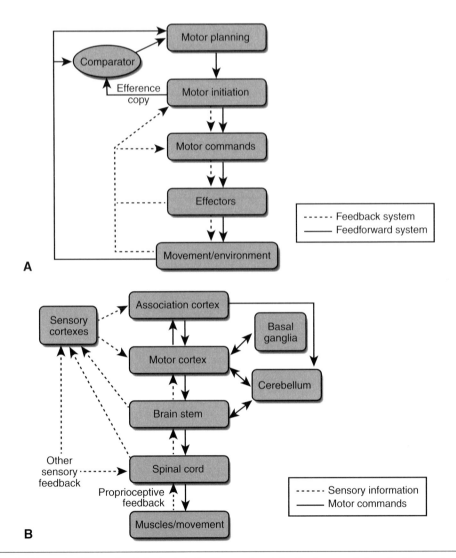

Figure 2.11 • A. Schematic of the brain's feedforward and feedback control. In a feedforward system, the descending commands (*dark arrows*) go directly to their intended targets with minimal or no feedback correction. Feedback is supplied from sensory endings, but this information is not used to modify the motor commands that have already been sent. Instead, in a feedforward system the feedback is only sent back up to higher centers (brain) and used to plan and compare the predicted movement outcomes (through efference copy) with the actual feedback outcomes. In a feedback system (*dashed lines*), the feedback arising from muscles and environmental stimuli is fed back to the initiated or ongoing motor commands to alter them directly. **B.** An anatomical schematic of the command structure from the highest brain centers to the muscles. *Dashed lines* represent sensory feedback and *solid lines* represent descending motor commands and planning commands.

predict the movement results and the expected nature of sensory feedback. If the outcome of movement and the sensory feedback are not as expected, that is, there is a mismatch, the brain goes to work to figure out what went wrong and determine a better motor command or a better prediction plan.

So why is this all important to an exercise science practitioner? An understanding of the fundamental processes in planning and initiating skill motor behaviors leads to two practical conclusions. The first is that the formation of motor skills is a highly complex and adaptable act that moment to moment draws upon a diverse array of brain functions. This tells us that no motor plan is really the same, not even those repeated again and again. Circumstances and situations greatly influence what movement is selected and how that movement is planned and initiated. Therefore, practice and training aimed at improving skilled motor performance should take into account and take advantage of the inherent variability in motor planning brought about by different circumstances and situations. The second conclusion is that because the brains of individuals are different, individuals plan and initiate motor skills differently, implying that practice and training is best when designed for individuals.

CNS ADAPTATIONS TO PRACTICE AND TRAINING

If the mind and body are truly connected, then there should be direct evidence that they influence one another, in particular the influence of practice and training on CNS structures. Indeed, it has been demonstrated by fMRI and other imaging techniques that numerous changes occur in the CNS as a result of practice that reflect learned behaviors, and as a result of rigorous physical training that reflects both learned behaviors and physiologically induced changes. In this section, we examine CNS changes under both circumstances, and then look at fatigue in the CNS during exercise.

CNS and Practice: Adaptations to Learning

Examinations of CNS adaptations to motor skill practice have generally used simple motor skills and practice sessions specifically aimed at improving skill coordination and efficiency. In contrast to training as discussed in the next section, the practice sessions are not associated with high physiological effort, and changes to muscle physiology, cardiovascular function, or other physiological changes that accompany rigorous exercise are not expected. Thus, any changes noted are ascribed solely to learning in the CNS. Learning a motor task after hours or days of practice is associated with a number of brain-related changes as seen on brain scans. Precise changes are hard to pinpoint due to different stages of learning, type of practice, and nature of the motor skill itself, but there are general observations that the brain become more active in some areas and less active in other areas (Classen et al., 1998; Kelly & Garavan, 2005; Smith et al., 1999), even during resting states (Ma et al., 2011).

Generally, after days or weeks of motor skill practice, less brain area is active during performance of the task. It is thought that this reflects some level of automaticity and freeing up of resources as the brain becomes more efficient in task execution. Conversely, it has also been found in some cases that more brain areas are active after learning, particularly areas of interconnectivity, which is thought to reflect use of previously unused resources in order to maximize movement capability (Ma et al., 2011; Petersen et al., 1998). In their review, Duchateau and Enoka (2002) noted that after intense and focused motor skill training, areas of the motor cortex and sensorimotor cortex corresponding to the practiced muscles may get bigger or more excitable. More brain areas active during a well-learned movement may reflect that the motor skill is being planned and executed in fundamentally different ways than in the initial learning. Similarly, observations of different brain areas being used could reflect different strategies in planning and execution (Lacourse et al., 2005; Petersen et al., 1998). It is important to note that how one practices, for instance, practice organization, may lead to different brain adaptations (Lin et al., 2011).

Changes in areas of activation reflect changes in neuronal structure in both the brain and spinal cord. More synaptic connections, more neurotransmitter receptor sites, and more efficient neurotransmitter receptor sites are formed, and the most efficient neural pathways are found and used to a greater extent than other pathways. These changes reveal that the brain is quite plastic. It can change its morphological structure (e.g., new synapses), and even the somatotopic map of motor and sensory areas (the Brodmann areas and perhaps the homunculus) can be altered (Carroll et al., 2001; Classen et al., 1998; Jäncke et al., 2000; Karni et al., 1998; Petersen et al., 1998; Smith et al., 1999).

■ Thinking It Through 2.2 Brain Plasticity

Current research indicates that the brain is much more adaptable, or plastic, than once believed. Dramatic examples of this plasticity can be found following amputation in humans and animals, particularly within the somatosensory cortex. For example, the sensory cortical region corresponding to the missing limb of an amputee may get "taken over" by neighboring sensory regions. This takeover and topographical reorganization may result in strange sensations, such as the feeling in a phantom limb when touched in the face (Ramachandran et al., 2010). Rapid plasticity and topographical reorganization may be due to reawakened synapses, and long-term changes due to dendritic sprouting and new pathways being developed. Visual cortex remapping has also been seen following a stroke affecting neuronal projections to areas of the visual cortex (Dilks et al., 2007). Dilks et al. investigated an individual who suffered a stroke that caused visual information to be stopped on route to one area of the visual cortex. After the stroke, the patient still had normal vision except for a small blind spot. After several months, however, the patient's vision became distorted in an elongated manner as the visual cortex was being remapped in a manner that caused an overrepresentation of neurons processing vertical information. Prominent brain plasticity researcher Michael Merzenich maintains that plasticity remains even into old age and that older individuals can use positive brain changes to overcome losses in sensation, cognition, memory, motor control, and affect using the right training paradigms (Mahncke et al., 2006).

With this in mind, how do you think exercise and motor skill training can play a role in brain plasticity for elders? Access the Mahncke et al. (2006) and Cotman et al. (2007) articles and compare your thoughts with these authors.

CNS and Training: Physiological and Psychological Adaptations to Exercise

Rigorous physical training, including aerobic, anaerobic, and strength training, potentially may induce changes in the CNS due to a combination of motor learning processes and forced physiological adaptations. These changes may induce psychological changes in behavior and cognition, such as improved mood states and better cognition in elders.

Exercise—primarily aerobic exercise—is often recommended as a mental health wellness strategy. An abundant amount of research supports this recommendation, with evidence that mood can be enhanced, anxiety reduced, self-efficacy and positive affect improved, self-esteem improved, mild depressive symptoms reduced, and possibly a reduction in physiological reactivity to psychological stressors. These exercise effects can be experienced from an acute exercise bout or following chronic exercise. However, despite what seems to be a compelling amount of research and anecdotal evidence, these findings are not universal nor are they without problems. Much of the data are beset by methodological issues, like expectation effects, gender-related changes, issues regarding the exercise environment, and publication bias. For example, researcher Thomas Plante (Plante, 1999; Plante et al., 2000) has shown that many people feel better *before* exercise, suggesting expectancy effects and not some exercise-induced psychophysiological adaptations.

Researchers have yet to uncover if mood state alterations are rooted in biological adaptations. It is known that the brain's neurochemical system is highly active during exercise, but their exact roles in mediating behaviors are unknown. At this point, the best explanation for the effects of exercise on mood is a complex biopsychosocial model, that is, that a confluence of physiological processes, and social and psychological issues contribute to mood state and mental health outcomes.

Exercise is also recommended as a cognitive health strategy. A large number of individual reports showing improvement in cognitive function, memory, and learning, or delayed loss in executive function, in fit or exercising elders supports this view (e.g., see reviews Colcombe et al., 2004; Kramer et al., 2002). Others, however, caution that there is limited evidence, albeit promising, for exercise as a treatment for individuals with CNS deficits (McDonnell et al., 2011).

Most reports highlight the benefit of aerobic fitness or training, but recent evidence indicates that strength training may also have benefits for psychological health as well (Voss et al., 2011). Though Voss et al. (2011) have recently reviewed the role of exercise and cognition across the lifespan and reported encouraging findings, they also pointed out that much work needs to be done in this field.

Regardless of the uncertainty over cognitive outcomes due to exercise, there are clear and demonstrable neurobiological effects in elders who exercise, or are fit, or who maintain motor skill proficiency. According to reviews by Cotman et al. (2007) and Davenport et al. (2012), human and animal models suggest many brain-related changes, including cell proliferation, increased blood flow, alterations in brain chemistry, neurotransmitters, receptors, synapses, capillarization, an overall slowing of brain tissue loss, and changes in brain activation areas (Fig. 2.12). Even with these data, it is difficult to come to definitive conclusions about the role of exercise and cognition function in elders. Outcome data are supported by brain imaging data, but there are psychosocial and self-selection interactions that come into play.

Exercise has long been promoted to improve academic performance in school children, and indeed, most data suggest a positive relationship between physical activity and academic performance. The evidence, though, is generally weak, short term only, and without a strong causal link. For example, is the exercise effect a neurobiological cause, or is it self-efficacy, or is it psychosocial, or some aspect of concentration? Hillman et al. (2011) have suggested that neuroelectric changes in children's brains resulting from acute or chronic exercise could account for better cognitive processing. Yet, it is still difficult to tease out these influences, in part because the sociocultural and socioeconomic interactions are large. The effect of exercise on learning disabilities like ADHD and dyslexia is highly controversial, and is without a great deal of supporting data.

Heavy strength training may increase the amount of "neural drive" to the muscles, in part due to increased descending commands from supraspinal centers and increased motor neuron excitability, or reduced presynaptic inhibition in the spinal cord (Aagaard, 2003; Duchateau & Enoka, 2002). Balance training may reduce spinal reflex excitability, decrease cortical involvement, and increase subcortical

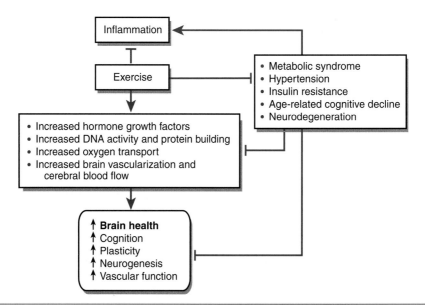

Figure 2.12 • A model of neurological protective mechanisms arising from exercise based on Cotman et al. (2007) and Davenport et al. (2012). In this model, exercise produces a number of hormonal growth factors to stimulate neuronal and other tissue growth. In addition, genes are stimulated to create proteins for tissue growth and repair. Thus, exercise over the long term leads to better neural health and function. At the same time, the negative consequences of various diseases and dysfunction, including inflammation, are blunted by exercise.

Concepts in Action

Using Cross-Transfer to Maintain Strength in Immobilized Limb

Limb immobilization, such as during casting or splinting, results in rapid disuse muscle atrophy and loss of strength and function in the immobilized limb. Using cross-transfer to maintain strength in the immobilized limb would seem to be a way to overcome this problem, but overcoming atrophy would seem more difficult. Two recent studies (Farthing et al., 2011; Magnus et al., 2010) have looked at the effects of unilateral strength training on an immobilized limb. Both research teams found that compared to control groups strength in the untrained limb was maintained over a 3- to 4-week period, but results of muscle size changes were ambiguous. Magnus and his group found hypertrophy in the untrained upper arm, but Farthing et al. found atrophy in the untrained forearm. These differences may lie in the specific muscles being trained and the nature of the training, but that is as far as speculation allows at this time. Nevertheless, Hendy et al. (2012) maintain that unilateral strength training to elicit cross-transfer effects is a valid technique in the rehabilitation of athletes and injured workers, and may hold promise as in the training of individuals with paralysis from stroke or trauma.

involvement (Taube et al., 2008). Among the most compelling evidence for CNS changes with strength training involve the phenomenon of cross-transfer. Cross-transfer (also called cross-education) occurs when unilateral strength training in one arm results in strength gains in the unexercised arm. Some authors have reported up to 47% and 135% increases in strength in the untrained limb (Farthing et al., 2007; Hortobagyi et al., 1997). Researchers have hypothesized several reasons for this effect, but at this time, the strongest data support a greater ability to activate areas in the motor cortex, which then enables stronger drive to activate the muscles (Farthing et al., 2007; Lee et al., 2009). Farthing et al. (2007) reported that after unilateral strength training of the right arm, the right side of the brain corresponding to specific sensory and motor cortex areas became more active during contractions of the untrained left arm. What this means is that training the right arm resulted not only in changes corresponding to the contralateral (left) side of the brain, but also resulted in changes in the ipsilateral (right) side of the brain that could be used when exercising the left arm. These data thus reveal that learning in one hemisphere is communicated or "spilled over" to the opposite hemisphere, in a process called motor irradiation (Hendy et al., 2012).

Central Fatigue

Fatigue is defined as an inability to produce the required or expected force or work, though the behavioral expressions of fatigue often do not correlate with the physiological indices. It is well known that in a tiring muscle physiological and biochemical mechanisms are associated with fatigue, such as depletion of ATP and energy substrates, and the accumulation of lactate and other metabolic byproducts that impair cellular function. Researchers have shown that muscles are not the only site of fatigue but that the central and peripheral nervous systems may also falter. For example, there is speculation that excessive work leading to muscle fatigue may disrupt performance (e.g., balance performance) because of alterations to proprioceptive mechanisms (Johnston et al., 1998). There is strong evidence that long-term fatiguing exercise (e.g., triathlon) reduces reflex sensitivity, such as weakening the stretch reflex response and making it difficult to elicit. This could be due to the removal of facilitation from muscle spindles afferents, or presynaptic inhibition of the reflex circuitry (Avela et al., 1999). Alternately, it could be that sensory endings in the muscle (mostly chemoreceptors and nociceptors) respond to a buildup of metabolic waste and may have powerful effects on inhibitory interneurons connecting to motor neurons in the spinal cord. There is also some speculation that sensory signals arising from muscles and visceroreceptors signaling pain or metabolic waste buildup may cause inhibitory effects in both the spinal cord and brain (Peltier et al., 2005). Other evidence indicates that some sensory areas receiving fatigue-based information may inhibit the motor cortex in sending out motor commands (Tanaka et al., 2011).

A number of authors have recently put forth evidence that glycogen depletion and faltering neurotransmitter regulation during fatiguing exercise are culprits in CNS fatigue (Roelands et al., 2011; Matsui et al., 2011). It is thought that fatiguing conditions lead to a loss in central drive, perhaps from lowered oxygen levels. It has been hypothesized that nonmotor areas in the brain begin integrating signals differently, which may alter sensations and behavioral states, and some evidence points to disruptions in neurochemical systems, including serotonin (5HT), acetylcholine, dopamine, and tryptophan (Yamamoto & Newsholme, 2000). Researchers have noted that central fatigue is not only associated with exercise, but may be a contributor to conditions like chronic fatigue syndrome (Castell et al., 1999; Kent-Braun et al., 1993) and multiple sclerosis (Chang et al., 2011).

| SIDE**NOTE** | **MEASURING CENTRAL FATIGUE** |

There is a lot of speculation about the causes of central fatigue, but its existence is not in question. The most common way to identify central fatigue is by use of electrical stimulation superimposed onto a maximal voluntary isometric contraction (MVIC). In a typical experiment (e.g., Kent-Braun & Le Blanc, 1996), a subject exerts an MVIC under nonfatigued conditions and maximal force is recorded. The subject then performs the MVIC again, at which time, a large jolt of electrical stimulation is applied in an attempt to recruit any muscle fibers that may not be activated under voluntary effort alone. If additional force is recorded during the stimulation, it reveals that the voluntary effort and the CNS are not fully activating the muscle. The ratio of MVIC force to MVIC + stimulation force is called the central activation ratio (CAR). Under normal circumstances in trained persons the CAR is near 1.0, indicating that voluntary effort can recruit the muscle fully. However, during high levels of fatigue, when the maximal force being exerted drops considerably, most researchers are able to increase the force output by superimposing a large amount of electrical stimulation, reducing the CAR to <1.0. These data suggest that not all of force failure is due to the muscle, but to the inability of the CNS to drive the muscle.

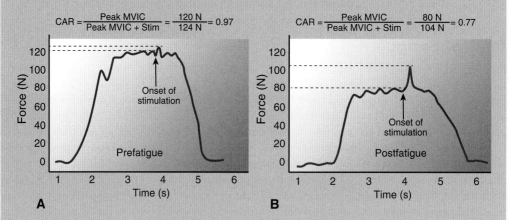

$$CAR = \frac{Peak\ MVIC}{Peak\ MVIC + Stim} = \frac{120\ N}{124\ N} = 0.97 \qquad CAR = \frac{Peak\ MVIC}{Peak\ MVIC + Stim} = \frac{80\ N}{104\ N} = 0.77$$

Force curves demonstrating central fatigue by superimposing electrical stimulation on top of a maximal voluntary isometric contraction. **A.** Nonfatigued condition illustrating a minimal addition of force with stimulation, indicating near maximal voluntary activation. **B.** MVIC after an extensive number of fatiguing contractions. The large spike in force with electrical stimulation reveals that fatigue is occurring in central drive to the muscles as well as the muscle itself.

Ongoing findings regarding central fatigue may have profound effects for rehabilitation, occupational motor performance, and sport performance, most notably in the area of nutrition and ergogenic aids. In particular, animal studies give promising results for using serotonin, tryptophan, and related amino acids in delaying central fatigue in exercise settings, chronic fatigue patients, postoperative stress, and other stressful situations (Castell et al., 1999; Newsholme & Blomstrand, 2006). Unfortunately, studies with humans have yet to provide good evidence that using these nutritional supplements are effective, but manipulating the delivery of the amino acids to the brain remain problematic (Meeusen & Watson, 2007).

SUMMARY

The CNS is responsible for planning and initiation of movement. Carrying out the movement plan is the responsibility of the peripheral neuromuscular system. The highest centers of the CNS, namely, the motor, sensory, and association cortexes, subcortical areas, and the cerebellum, are responsible for movement planning functions including data gathering, goal setting, organizing, and decision making. The motor cortex is the primary structure involved in initiating movement. Lower brain centers such as the brain stem route and refine motor and sensory signals and are responsible for autonomic movement behaviors. Within the brain, information is feedforwarded to initiate actions, but feedback is constantly used to update and refine commands. This feedback is compared to the brain's internal model of the expected movement and is then used in the refining and learning of better movement. The spinal cord is the connection point between the planning and initiating of the CNS and the execution and monitoring functions of the PNS and neuromuscular system.

Movement training, either through practice or exercise, has a real and measurable effect on the CNS. Morphological changes, neurochemical changes, and topographical changes highlight the considerable plasticity exhibited in the human brain that comes about from both generalized exercise training and specific practice. Though the neurophysiological changes are measurable, changes in cognitive function and mood are harder to pinpoint, in part due to many confounding factors.

The application of this information is that exercise and practice must be thought of as nervous system training as much as body training. Psychophysiological outcomes are specific to the practice and training variables, and thus practice and training should be directed toward the desired outcomes.

STUDY QUESTIONS

1. Describe the organization of the nervous system and its classification systems.
2. Describe the differences between sensory, motor, and interneurons.
3. Define facilitation and inhibition and describe the process leading to each.
4. Identify the key areas of the brain involved with planning movement. Discuss the processes involved in planning and what brain structures may be involved in each of these processes. Discuss how feedback and feedforward commands are used in this context.
5. Identify the key areas of the brain involved in movement initiation; be sure to identify the pathway from brain to spinal cord. Discuss what is involved with initiating movement.
6. Define Brodmann areas, homunculus, sensorimotor integration, and final common pathway.
7. What functions occur in the spinal cord?
8. What is the limbic system and why is it so important in the planning of movement?
9. What is efference copy and what role does it play in planning movement?
10. Describe two practical applications that arise from knowledge of the planning and initiation of movement.

11. List the anatomical and morphological changes occurring in the CNS as a result of training and practice. Distinguish between practice-related effects and training-related effects.
12. Describe central fatigue.

References

Aagaard, P. (2003). Training-induced changes in neural function. *Exercise and Sport Sciences Reviews*, *31*(2), 61–67.

Avela, J. J., Kyrolainen, H. H., & Komi, P. V. (1999). Altered reflex sensitivity after repeated and prolonged passive muscle stretching. *Journal of Applied Physiology*, *86*(4), 1283–1291.

Carroll, T. J., Riek, S. S., & Carson, R. G. (2001). Corticospinal responses to motor training revealed by transcranial magnetic stimulation. *Exercise and Sport Sciences Reviews*, *29*(2), 54–59.

Carroll, T., Selvanayagam, V., Riek, S., & Semmler, J. (2011). Neural adaptations to strength training: Moving beyond transcranial magnetic stimulation and reflex studies. *Acta Physiologica*, *202*(2), 119–140.

Castell, L., Yamamoto, T., Phoenix, J., & Newsholme, E. (1999). The role of tryptophan in fatigue in different conditions of stress. *Advances in Experimental Medicine and Biology*, *467*, 697–704.

Chang, Y., Hsu, M., Chen, S., Lin, C., & Wong, A. (2011). Decreased central fatigue in multiple sclerosis patients after 8 weeks of surface functional electrical stimulation. *Journal of Rehabilitation Research and Development*, *48*(5), 555–564.

Classen, J., Liepert, J., Wise, S., Hallett, M., & Cohen, L. (1998). Rapid plasticity of human cortical movement representation induced by practice. *Journal of Neurophysiology*, *79*(2), 1117–1123.

Colcombe, S., Kramer, A., McAuley, E., Erickson, K., & Scalf, P. (2004). Neurocognitive aging and cardiovascular fitness: Recent findings and future directions. *Journal of Molecular Neuroscience*, *24*(1), 9–14.

Cotman, C., Berchtold, N., & Christie, L. (2007). Exercise builds brain health: Key roles of growth factor cascades and inflammation. *Trends in Neurosciences*, *30*(9), 464–472.

Davenport, M., Hogan, D., Eskes, G., Longman, R., & Poulin, M. (2012). Cerebrovascular reserve: The link between fitness and cognitive function? *Exercise and Sport Sciences Reviews*, *40*(3), 153–158.

Dilks, D., Serences, J., Rosenau, B., Yantis, S., & McCloskey, M. (2007). Human adult cortical reorganization and consequent visual distortion. *Journal of Neuroscience*, *27*(36), 9585–9594.

Duchateau, J. J., & Enoka, R. M. (2002). Neural adaptations with chronic activity patterns in able-bodied humans. *American Journal of Physical Medicine & Rehabilitation*, *81*(11 Suppl), S17–S27.

Farthing, J., Borowsky, R., Chilibeck, P., Binsted, G., & Sarty, G. (2007). Neurophysiological adaptations associated with cross-education of strength. *Brain Topography*, *20*(2), 77–88.

Farthing, J., Krentz, J., Magnus, C., Barss, T., Lanovaz, J., Cummine, J., et al. (2011). Changes in functional magnetic resonance imaging cortical activation with cross education to an immobilized limb. *Medicine and Science in Sports and Exercise*, *43*(8), 1394–1405.

Fine, C. (2010). From scanner to sound bite: Issues in interpreting and reporting sex differences in the brain. *Current Directions in Psychological Science*, *19*(5), 280–283.

Hallett, M., Shahani, B., & Young, R. (1975). EMG analysis of stereotyped voluntary movements in man. *Journal of Neurology, Neurosurgery, and Psychiatry*, *38*(12), 1154–1162.

Hendy, A., Spittle, M., & Kidgell, D. (2012). Cross education and immobilisation: Mechanisms and implications for injury rehabilitation. *Journal of Science and Medicine in Sport*, *15*(2), 94–101.

Hillman, C., Kamijo, K., & Scudder, M. (2011). A review of chronic and acute physical activity participation on neuroelectric measures of brain health and cognition during childhood. *Preventive Medicine*, *52*(Suppl 1), S21–S28.

Hortobágyi, T., Lambert, N., & Hill, J. (1997). Greater cross education following training with muscle lengthening than shortening. *Medicine and Science in Sports and Exercise*, *29*(1), 107–112.

Jäncke, L., Shah, N., & Peters, M. (2000). Cortical activations in primary and secondary motor areas for complex bimanual movements in professional pianists. *Cognitive Brain Research*, *10*(1–2), 177–183.

Johnston, R. B., Howard, M. E., Cawley, P. W., & Losse, G. M. (1998). Effect of lower extremity muscular fatigue on motor control performance. *Medicine and Science in Sports and Exercise*, *30*(12), 1703–1707.

Karni, A., Meyer, G., Rey-Hipolito, C., Jezzard, P., Adams, M., Turner, R., et al. (1998). The acquisition of skilled motor performance: Fast and slow experience-driven changes in primary motor cortex. *Proceedings of the National Academy of Sciences*, *95*(3), 861–868.

Kelly, A. M., & Garavan, H. (2005). Human functional neuroimaging of brain changes associated with practice. *Cerebral Cortex*, *15*, 1089–1102.

Kent-Braun, J., & Le Blanc, R. (1996). Quantitation of central activation failure during maximal voluntary contractions in humans. *Muscle & Nerve*, *19*(7), 861–869.

Kent-Braun, J., Sharma, K., Weiner, M., Massie, B., & Miller, R. (1993). Central basis of muscle fatigue in chronic fatigue syndrome. *Neurology*, *43*(1), 125–131.

Kramer, A., Colcombe, S., Erickson, K., Belopolsky, A., McAuley, E., Cohen, N., et al. (2002). Effects of aerobic fitness training on human cortical function: A proposal. *Journal of Molecular Neuroscience*, *19*(1–2), 227–231.

Lacourse, M., Orr, E., Cramer, S., & Cohen, M. (2005). Brain activation during execution and motor imagery of novel and skilled sequential hand movements. *Neuroimage*, *27*(3), 505–519.

Lee, M., Gandevia, S., & Carroll, T. (2009). Unilateral strength training increases voluntary activation of the opposite untrained limb. *Clinical Neurophysiology*, *120*(4), 802–808.

Lin, C., Knowlton, B., Chiang, M., Iacoboni, M., Udompholkul, P., & Wu, A. (2011). Brain-behavior correlates of optimizing learning through interleaved practice. *Neuroimage*, *56*(3), 1758–1772.

Ma, L., Narayana, S., Robin, D., Fox, P., & Xiong, J. (2011). Changes occur in resting state network of motor system during 4 weeks of motor skill learning. *Neuroimage*, *58*(1), 226–233.

Magnus, C., Barss, T., Lanovaz, J., & Farthing, J. (2010). Effects of cross-education on the muscle after a period of unilateral limb immobilization using a shoulder sling and swathe. *Journal of Applied Physiology*, *109*(6), 1887–1894.

Mahncke, H., Bronstone, A., & Merzenich, M. (2006). Brain plasticity and functional losses in the aged: Scientific bases for a novel intervention. *Progress in Brain Research*, *157*, 81–109.

Matsui, T., Soya, S., Okamoto, M., Ichitani, Y., Kawanaka, K., & Soya, H. (2011). Brain glycogen decreases during prolonged exercise. *Journal of Physiology*, *589*(Pt 13), 3383–3393.

McDonnell, M., Smith, A., & Mackintosh, S. (2011). Aerobic exercise to improve cognitive function in adults with neurological disorders: A systematic review. *Archives of Physical Medicine and Rehabilitation*, *92*(7), 1044–1052.

Meeusen, R., & Watson, P. (2007). Amino acids and the brain: Do they play a role in "central fatigue"? *International Journal of Sport Nutrition and Exercise Metabolism*, *17*(Suppl), S37–S46.

Newsholme, E., & Blomstrand, E. (2006). Branched-chain amino acids and central fatigue. *Journal of Nutrition*, *136*(1 Suppl), 274S–276S.

Peltier, S. J., LaConte, S. M., Niyazov, D. M., Liu, J. Z., Sahgal, V., Yue, G. H., et al. (2005). Reductions in interhemispheric motor cortex functional connectivity after muscle fatigue. *Brain Research*, *1057*, 10–16.

Petersen, S., van Mier, H., Fiez, J., & Raichle, M. (1998). The effects of practice on the functional anatomy of task performance. *Proceedings of the National Academy of Sciences*, *95*(3), 853–860.

Plante, T. (1999). Could the perception of fitness account for many of the mental and physical health benefits of exercise? *Advances in Mind-Body Medicine*, *15*(4), 291–295.

Plante, T. G., Coscarelli, L. L., Caputo, D. D., & Oppezzo, M. M. (2000). Perceived fitness predicts daily coping better than physical activity or aerobic fitness. *International Journal of Stress Management*, *7*(3), 181–192.

Ramachandran, V., Brang, D., & McGeoch, P. (2010). Dynamic reorganization of referred sensations by movements of phantom limbs. *Neuroreport*, *21*(10), 727–730.

Raznahan, A., Lee, Y., Stidd, R., Long, R., Greenstein, D., Clasen, L., et al. (2010). Longitudinally mapping the influence of sex and androgen signaling on the dynamics of human cortical maturation in adolescence. *Proceedings of the National Academy of Sciences*, *107*(39), 16988–16993.

Riordan, C., Faddis, B. J., Beam, M., Seager, A., Tanney, A., DiBiase, R., et al.; Office of Planning, Evaluation and Policy Development Department of Education. (2008). Early Implementation of Public Single-Sex Schools: Perceptions and Characteristics. *US Department of Education* [serial online]. August 1, 2008.

Roelands, B., Klass, M., Levenez, M., Fontenelle, V., Duchateau, J., & Meeusen, R. (2011). Neurotransmitter modulation and supraspinal fatigue. *British Journal of Sports Medicine*, *45*(15), A12.

Sanders, G. (2011). Sex differences in coincidence-anticipation timing (CAT): A review. *Perceptual and Motor Skills*, *112*(1), 61–90.

Sanes, J., & Jennings, V. (1984). Centrally programmed patterns of muscle activity in voluntary motor behavior of humans. *Experimental Brain Research*, *54*(1), 23–32.

Sax, L. (2006). *Why gender matters: What parents and teachers need to know about the emerging science of sex differences*. New York: Broadway Books.

Smith, M., McEvoy, L., & Gevins, A. (1999). Neurophysiological indices of strategy development and skill acquisition. *Brain Research. Cognitive Brain Research*, *7*(3), 389–404.

Tanaka, M., Shigihara, Y., & Watanabe, Y. (2011). Central inhibition regulates motor output during physical fatigue. *Brain Research, 1412*, 37–43.

Taube, W., Gruber, M., & Gollhofer, A. (2008). Spinal and supraspinal adaptations associated with balance training and their functional relevance. *Acta Physiologica*, *193*(2), 101–116.

Toole, T. T., & Kretzschmar, J. C. (1993). Gender differences in motor performance in early childhood and later adulthood. *Women in Sport and Physical Activity Journal*, *2*(1), 41–71.

Voss, M., Nagamatsu, L., Liu-Ambrose, T., & Kramer, A. (2011). Exercise, brain, and cognition across the life span. *Journal of Applied Physiology*, *111*(5), 1505–1513.

Wadman, W. J., Denier van der Gon, J. J., Geuze, R. H., & Mol, C. R. (1979). Control of fast goal-directed arm movements. *Journal of Human Movement Studies*, *5*(1), 3–17.

Yamamoto, T., & Newsholme, E. (2000). Diminished central fatigue by inhibition of the L-system transporter for the uptake of tryptophan. *Brain Research Bulletin*, *52*(1), 35–38.

3 | Peripheral Neuromuscular Mechanisms in Executing Movement

PURPOSE, IMPORTANCE, AND OBJECTIVES OF THIS CHAPTER

The purpose of this chapter is to describe the primary neuromuscular structures responsible for movement and how they work to coordinate efficient motor skill execution. Emphasis is placed on the different ways the motor unit is controlled by the nervous system and on the properties of skeletal muscle that execute movement. Understanding these structures and their working qualities gives rise to understanding how skilled motor performance is carried out and, further, the instructional, training, and rehabilitation strategies that may be used to maximize nervous system control of movement.

After reading this chapter, you should be able to:

1. Describe the basic physiology and organization of the motor unit.
2. Describe the properties and characteristics of motor units and how they influence motor unit behavior.
3. Detail the three ways the nervous system regulates the motor unit to regulate force output.
4. Describe and distinguish between intramuscular and intermuscular coordination.
5. Determine how training may influence adaptations of motor unit behavior.
6. Detail the properties of skeletal muscle and what the nervous system does to control these properties.
7. Describe the force–velocity and length–tension relationships and how they come into play during movement.
8. Describe the training-related influences on muscle mechanical properties and evaluate the potential changes in movement quality that may result.

Eventually, the plan of action that was created and initiated in the brain makes its way out to the peripheral nervous system (PNS) and the specific neuromuscular structures responsible for executing the movement plan. The structure responsible for the final execution is the **motor unit (MU)**. A motor unit is defined as a lower motor neuron and all the muscle fibers it innervates. It is here where the movement plan, translated from a set of nervous system electrical pulses, is turned into a precise pattern of skeletal muscle actions, and subsequently, mechanical output of force and movement. The final movement outcome is also dependent on the properties of the muscle and biomechanical systems that moderate how muscle contractions are coordinated into force and direction and speed of movement. The relationship between the neural control of movement and the mechanical output of muscle is termed **neuromuscular mechanics**, or simply **neuromechanics**. In this chapter, we first focus on the motor unit and muscle action, and, secondly, look at the neuromechanical properties of muscle.

THE MOTOR UNIT

The final common pathways of all central nervous system (CNS) motor commands are the motor neurons of the motor units (Fig. 3.1). The axons of each of these motor neurons branch off into many axon collaterals and each of these collaterals attaches to a muscle fiber via a synapse called neuromuscular junction. The motor unit is the smallest unit of movement controlled by the CNS. A **motor unit pool** (or motoneuron pool) is a grouping of all motor units that activate a particular muscle or muscle group.

Each motor neuron can excite from 15 to 2,000 muscle fibers depending on the particular muscle (Gath & Stålberg, 1981; Santo Neto et al., 1998). The **innervation ratio** is the ratio of one neuron to the number of muscle fibers it innervates. Muscles used for finer control have smaller innervation ratios and gross movement muscles tend to have larger innervation ratios. For instance, small intrinsic hand muscles may have about 130 motor neurons and an average innervation ratio of about 1:110 (Santo Neto et al., 1998), and intrinsic laryngeal muscles may have a ratio of about 1:10 (Santo Neto & Marques, 2008). Large muscles such as the vastus lateralis (VL) or gastrocnemius may have innervation ratio of about 1:1,500 to 1:2,000 (Enoka, 1995; Rich et al., 1998).

All muscle fibers within a motor unit are of the same type (e.g., fast twitch, slow twitch) and they are spread out and intermingled with muscle fibers of other motor units in the same region: medial, lateral, deep, or superficial (Enoka, 1995). In addition, most muscle fibers do not extend the length of

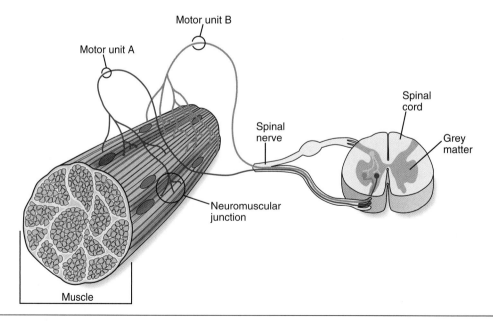

Figure 3.1 • Organization of motor units. Motor unit A has a smaller innervation ratio than motor unit B. Note that the muscle fibers are distributed throughout deep and superficial aspects of the muscle.

the entire muscle, and thus, muscle fibers congregate in distal or proximal regions in the muscle. Motor units of a particular type may group in areas, for example, fast twitch muscle fibers may group on the superficial aspect of the muscle or more near the distal insertion area (Knight & Kamen, 2005). These areas of motor unit groupings form separate compartments within the muscle that can be independently controlled as "task groups" (Bawa, 2002).

■ Thinking It Through 3.1 Neuron Type and Muscle Fiber Numbers

Because most slow twitch motor units have small innervation ratios, it takes a lot more of these units to create a bulk of muscle mass compared to fast twitch motor units. In fact, a typical soleus muscle may have about 70% slow twitch muscle fibers but have about 93% of the motor neuron pool to activate those slow twitch fibers. Similarly, a triceps brachii muscle may only have about 30% slow twitch muscle fibers, but 75% of the motor neuron pool is required to activate those slow twitch fibers (Enoka & Fuglevand, 2001). There are important clinical implications of these data, particularly for the elderly and those with various neuromuscular diseases. The aging process appears to cause a reduction in fast twitch muscle fibers, and many diseases attack fast twitch neurons preferentially. With this in mind, and using the data and comments by Enoka and Fuglevand (2001), consider which muscle groups may be more affected by aging and most neuromuscular diseases, and consequently, the types of movements most affected.

Motor Unit Characteristics

Motor unit sizes are classically defined as large to small based on the size of their neurons (Mendell, 2005), though researchers have also functionally defined motor unit size based on the number of attached muscle fibers (e.g., Santo Neto et al., 1998) (Table 3.1). Generally, small motor units also have few muscle fibers and large motor units have many muscle fibers. The motor unit size definition is largely comparative as there is no precise axon size or innervation ratio separating small from large motor units. Small and large motor units also tend to have certain other characteristics that are important for their function. These characteristics, as detailed below, are activation energy requirements, muscle fiber type, and precision of control.

The larger-diameter neurons of large motor units require more stimulation energy to reach threshold levels, and consequently, they take longer to be activated (Mendell, 2005). These units are alternately known as high-threshold motor units. Small motor units also tend to have slow twitch muscle fibers (type I, aerobic, or fatigue resistant), large motor units tend to have fast twitch (type IIB or IIX,

TABLE 3.1	Motor Unit Properties and Characteristics		
	Small	**Medium**	**Large**
Neuron/axon size	Small	Medium	Large
Number of muscle fibers	Few	Medium	Many
Type of muscle fiber	Slow twitch	Either/intermediate	Fast twitch
Energy needed for activation	Least	Moderate	Most
Recruitment order	First	Second	Third
Function	Endurance precision	Mixed	Force/ power

anaerobic, or fast fatigable), and intermediate-size motor units may have type I or an intermediate fiber type like type IIA (Lieber, 2002; Mendell, 2005). Note that while the trend is for slow twitch units to have small innervation ratios and fast twitch units to have large innervation ratios, such is not always the case and may vary between genders and among muscles. For example, a large motor unit with fast twitch fibers in the hand may have a relatively small innervation ratio compared to a large motor unit in the rectus femoris muscle. Small innervation ratios permit finer or more discrete control of muscle force.

Principles of Motor Unit Behavior

The brain can selectively activate just one motor unit or thousands upon thousands, making motor unit activation a serious degrees of freedom problem. There are various "rules" that govern the firing of a motor unit that lessen this problem. Primary among these rules are the all-or-none principle and the size principle of recruitment.

The **all-or-none principle** refers to the activation of muscle fibers within each motor unit. All muscle fibers within a motor unit contract or none contract in response to the neuron's action potential. The **size principle of recruitment** states that motor units are recruited in order from small units to large units. This principle also applies to derecruitment, in which motor units are derecruited in order from large to small. The reason for the orderly recruitment is largely due to the neuron size and the stimulation energy needed to reach threshold. As stated above, larger neurons need more energy, and in addition, may have other morphological characteristics that delay their recruitment, such as number of dendrites, axon diameter, tissue electrical resistance, neurotransmitter receptor sensitivity, and distribution of synapses on dendrites and cell body.

The size principle is a robust physiological mechanism. Recruitment order inconsistencies have been noted but are generally thought to be largely explained by task-specific activation of some motor units that make it appear that motor units activate out of order (Chalmers, 2008; Duchateau & Enoka, 2011). For example, some motor units in multifunction muscles may participate in one of the muscle's actions, but not another, or some motor units may only be recruited during eccentric contractions versus concentric contractions.

Concepts in Action

Electromyography and Mechanomyography

The neuron action potential initiates electrical activity to spread across the muscle fibers which begins the contraction process. This muscle electrical activity, called the muscle (or motor) action potential, can be detected with electrodes in a technique known as **electromyography** (EMG). Electrodes can be inserted into the muscle (indwelling) or placed on the skin surface above the muscle (surface EMG). Depending on how the EMG is set up, a single muscle action potential or the combined sum of a number of muscle action potentials can be detected. When muscle action potentials sum together within the detection and recording equipment, the result is called the interference pattern. **Mechanomyography** (MMG) is a more recent development in measuring muscle activity. MMG uses special piezoelectric vibration sensors placed on the skin surface to detect minute vibrations during contractions; more vibration is associated with more sarcomeres contracting.

EMG has been in use for many decades to assess four general categories of muscle function. The first is muscle timing, such as when the muscle is on or off. Second is relative muscle force, third is muscle fatigue, and the last is muscle pathology. With each category comes an increasing need for sophistication in equipment, computer processing, and human interpretation of the data.

continued on following page

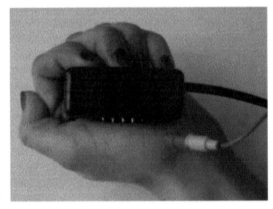

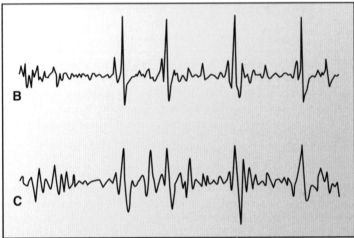

Surface and needle electrodes recording electrical activity of thumb muscles. **A.** A needle electrode inserted into thumb muscle detects muscle action potentials from a limited area within the muscle tissue, while a special multielectrode array detects from the surface of the same muscle. **B.** EMG recordings from the needle electrode. Many of the spikes seen in the EMG signal may be from individual motor units. **C.** EMG recordings from the surface electrodes illustrate more electrical activity is detected and recorded, resulting in an interference pattern. (Reprinted from Hogrel, J.-Y. (2005). Clinical Applications of surface electromyography in neuromuscular disorders. *Clinical Neurophysiology, 35*(2), 59–71, 61, with permission from Elsevier.)

CONTROLLING FORCE OUTPUT BY MOTOR UNIT BEHAVIOR

Motor units are activated for one fundamental purpose, and that is to control the force of muscle contractions. Motor units are activated to control small amounts of force within an individual muscle and whole limb and body movements. The nervous system regulates three basic factors to control force output: (1) **recruitment** of motor units, (2) **rate coding** of motor units, and (3) **coordination** of motor units and muscles.

Motor Unit Recruitment

Muscle force output can be changed by increasing or decreasing the number of active motor units, which effectively increases or decreases the amount of active muscle tissue (Fig. 3.2). This activation follows the size principle of motor unit recruitment: Small motor units are activated first followed by larger motor units. Because the larger motor units tend to be fast twitch with more muscle fibers, activating more motor units generally results in a large increase in the amount of active muscle tissue.

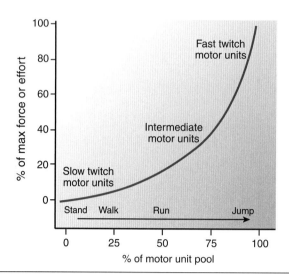

Figure 3.2 • The relationships among the degree of effort and the percentage of motor units recruited and the motor unit type. Small motor units are typically slow twitch (type I) and are recruited first. The largest motor units are normally fast twitch (type IIb or IIx) and are recruited after slow twitch motor units and intermediate type IIa units. (Adapted from Edgerton, V. R., Roy, R. R., Bodine, S. C., & Sacks, R. D. (1983). The matching of neuronal and muscular physiology. In *Frontiers of exercise biology* (pp. 51–70). Champaign, IL: Human Kinetics.)

The consequences of an orderly recruitment are greatly practical. Small motor units have fewer muscle fibers, which enables finer control of force output and therefore are better for precise movements. This is the primary reason that muscles of the hands, eyes, and face have smaller motor units. These first recruited small motor units are also the last to be derecruited during relaxation and are those most active during prolonged exercise. The fatigue-resistant characteristics of these predominately slow twitch fibers lend themselves to this type of activity.

The larger, fast twitch, motor units are not typically activated until at least 60% of maximum force output during isometric contractions. Some motor units are not activated until 85% to 90% of maximum force output, but this is dependent on the individual muscle and the speed of contraction. The adductor pollicis, for example, may have all units recruited at about 55%, whereas in the biceps brachii all units may not be recruited until about 85% (Duchateau & Enoka, 2011; Enoka, 1995). These data should not necessarily be interpreted that it is absolute force output that dictates motor unit recruitment. Rather, it is more likely that the level of effort that gives rise to recruitment, whether this effort is lifting a weight, vertical jumping, or during the end of fatiguing submaximal contractions (Carpinelli, 2008). For example, maximal effort ballistic training (high speed, low force) may result in full motor unit recruitment but with loads equivalent to only about 33% of maximal isometric force (Duchateau et al., 2006; Van Cutsem et al., 1998).

At one time, it was thought that size principle violations would occur as motor units moved in and out of rotation during fatiguing contractions. This rotation may happen with motor units of similar size or recruitment threshold, but it does not appear to happen with large and small motor units rotating with one another (Bawa et al., 2006).

Motor Unit Rate Coding

When a single action potential reaches the muscle and causes a muscle action potential, the muscle responds with a single twitch contraction immediately followed by relaxation. When repetitive action potentials reach the muscle fibers they cause the muscle to twitch repetitively. When repetitive twitches

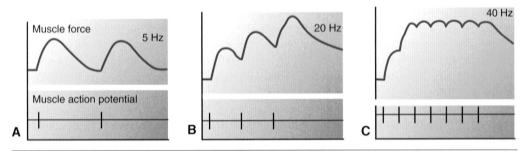

Figure 3.3 • Firing rate and force. A. Slow neuron firing rates do not permit force summation at the muscle because the muscle has time to relax between twitch contractions. B. Faster firing rates do not permit full twitch relaxation, resulting in force summation. C. At the fastest firing rates, the force summates completely. This figure depicts a state of unfused tetanus, where force has reached its maximal due to high firing rates.

follow closely after one another the muscle fibers do not have time to relax and tension begins to summate. The faster the **firing rate** of the action potentials the more tension can summate (Fig. 3.3). Regulation of the firing rate to modify force output is termed **rate coding**.

Human muscle firing rates range from a minimum of 5 to 8 Hz to a maximum of about 50 to 60 Hz for isometric contractions and up to 120 Hz for ballistic contractions (Duchateau & Enoka, 2011) (Fig. 3.4). Fast firing rates cause tension summation in two primary ways. First, with repetitive action potentials there is not enough time for calcium to be reuptaken, resulting in an abundance of calcium in the muscle cell. This leads to a maximal number of cross-bridges forming. Secondly, because there is not enough time to relax the elastic elements in the muscle, they remained stretched and thus tension is

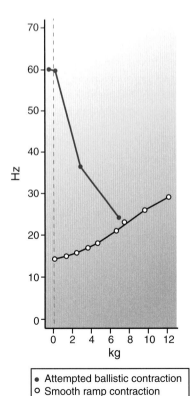

• Attempted ballistic contraction
○ Smooth ramp contraction

Figure 3.4 • This graph illustrates motor unit firing rate differences between rapid ballistic-type contractions and controlled ramp isometric contraction. The firing rate of a single motor unit, recorded from indwelling electrodes, was measured in the tibialis anterior muscle during a slowly increasing isometric contraction and an attempted maximally fast ballistic contraction. The slow isometric contraction starts with a firing rate of about 15 Hz and increases in firing rate to about 30 Hz result as a maximum of 12 kg of force is reached. The attempted ballistic contraction begins at a maximal firing rate of 60 Hz and decreases over time as force increases. (Adapted with permission from Desmedt, J., & Godaux, E. (1977). Ballistic contractions in man: Characteristic recruitment pattern of single motor units of the tibialis anterior muscle. *Journal of Physiology*, *264*(3), 673–693. Figure 4, p. 680.)

increased. If the twitches are fast enough a state of tetanus will occur. In humans, under artificial stimulation, tetanus can increase the force output of a muscle over a single twitch by 3 to 15 times (Enoka, 1995). It is questionable whether tetanus is a normal occurrence in humans, though. Like motor unit recruitment, the fastest firing rates are not seen until higher-intensity contractions. For example, Conwit et al. (1999) noted stable firing rates in the quadriceps up to 30% MVC, and steady increases until 100% MVC.

So how does the nervous system mix and match motor unit recruitment and firing rate? If more force is needed are motor units added or firing rates increased? Both happen, but exactly what happens is dependent on the particular muscle and type of movement. Small muscles, such as in the hand, may have full motor unit recruitment at 30% of maximum force, and then all additional force is due to rate coding. Larger muscles may do more rate coding early and not fully recruit all motor units until 80% to 90% of maximum effort. Classic work by Monster and Chan (1977) found that the first motor units recruited in finger muscles during slowly increasing isometric contractions rapidly increased firing rate to a plateau and then remained active for much of the contraction duration. At high force levels, numerous motor units were recruited in rapid succession, and each motor unit tended to increase its firing rate to a maximal level and then be derecruited.

Many other factors influence the interplay between recruitment and rate coding. For example, static contractions and dynamic contractions done at the same relative workload have different recruitment and rate coding behavior, and the same goes for concentric versus eccentric contractions (Enoka & Fuglevand, 2001; Kossev & Christova, 1998a,b; Søgaard et al., 1998). What this means is that at the start of the contraction, something must dictate recruitment thresholds in the involved motoneuron pools and set a pattern of rate coding and recruitment (Enoka & Fuglevand, 2001).

When new motor units are recruited, it has been speculated that the already active units slow their firing rates (by a process called disfacilitation) in order to smooth out the force increment (Broman et al., 1985), but not all scientists agree with this observation (Kamen & Du, 1999). Changes in muscle morphology during aging may also affect the way the body regulates recruitment versus firing rate (Graves et al., 2000).

Neuromuscular Coordination

Neuromuscular coordination is arguably the most important way the nervous system controls muscle force output from within-muscle force to whole-body force expressions. Coordination can be classified as intermuscular coordination or intramuscular coordination, and both are fundamental in regulating muscle force and movement precision in real life activities. **Intermuscular coordination** is defined as coordination of muscle groups and body segments, and refers to the actions of muscles and segments working together to produce efficient and purposeful movements in the context of environmental and task demands. When a skilled dance performer or an outstanding athlete is in action it is easy to recognize a coordinated movement. The movements seem smooth, graceful, powerful, and efficient. Movements may seem effortless without a lot of extraneous actions.

Concepts in Action

Variation in training

Researchers have shown that firing rates and the coordination between rate coding and recruitment vary greatly depending on circumstances. The type (e.g., isometric vs. concentric) of contraction, the attempted speed of contraction, the load being moved, and the duration of contraction all influence motor unit recruitment and firing rate and thus provide considerable rationale for training variation. Developing a well-conditioned and peak-functioning neuromuscular system requires that it be trained with different movement types and directions, and different contraction speeds, loads, and durations.

What we see and understand as a coordinated action is really a precise patterning and role-playing of different muscles. Muscles are designed for certain roles, which may change from one moment to the next. Sometimes a muscle may function as an agonist, sometimes as a stabilizer, sometimes as a neutralizer. Modifications in intermuscular coordination due to changing task demands are often seen in EMG recordings. Consider, for example, the work by Rota et al. (2012) who evaluated 10 different trunk and arm muscles during tennis forehand drives of different velocities. These authors noted that onset and offset timing and amplitudes of muscle activation differed greatly depending on the swing velocity. Among the most pronounced changes was an earlier, longer, and stronger response of the erector spinae muscle of the back during higher-velocity hits, which they attributed to a greater need to stabilize the spine against high force outputs of the arm.

Intramuscular coordination is defined as the patterning and use of motor units within a muscle to produce effective and efficient forces and movements. We have already seen how motor unit recruitment and firing rates are mixed and matched to meet the task demands. Coordinating firing rate and recruitment is one of three fundamental mechanisms in intramuscular coordination; the other two are discharge patterning and compartmental coordination.

Discharge patterning refers to specific manipulation of the firing rate to meet specific task demands. For instance, a sequence of two to three rapid action potentials (doublet or triplet) can increase the tension output greatly, and even if the firing rate returns to normal, the tension may remain high, which may lessen the metabolic cost. During ballistic contraction, a near-maximal firing rate at the start of the contraction quickly decreases over the course of the movement. Another form of discharge patterning is **muscle wisdom**. Muscle wisdom refers to the change in discharge rates during fatigue. During fatigue there tends to be a calculated slowing of a motor unit's firing rates that is not in response to physiological processes like the buildup of metabolic wastes or a decline in ATP energy. This slowing seems to be an automatic response in healthy muscle to balance force output with energy sparing. Muscle wisdom has also been ascribed to an initial high firing rate to "jump start" a contraction, and then the firing rate declines (Conwit et al., 1999). Muscle wisdom is an adaptive process that matches the neural activity to the changing conditions of the muscle, and is controlled in some fashion by the muscle itself (Kuchinad et al., 2004). **Synchronization** is another, albeit controversial, discharge patterning process. Normally, motor units tend to fire asynchronously, that is, out of timing with one another, which provides for smooth movements. However, some research data indicate that at times the activation of different units, and especially the firing rates of already active units, become synchronized to fire all at the same time (Cormie et al., 2011a,b). This "pulling together" behavior enables an explosion of force, and in particular, has been suggested to be a coordination strategy to stabilize joints under high force outputs in complex movements (see Cormie et al., 2011a,b, for reviews).

Among the more recently explored intramuscular coordination mechanisms is the control of individual parts of a muscle. **Compartmentalization** (Enoka, 1995; Richmond, 1998) refers to smaller and independently controlled groups of muscle fibers contained within a single muscle or group of muscles (e.g., quadriceps femoris). Compartmentalization may also cross over from one muscle to another, implying that a single compartment may exist between two muscles in an inter–intramuscular coordination system (Brown et al., 2007). These compartments might be based on muscle morphology (a group of slow twitch or fast twitch), or on neural recruitment (a particular part of the muscle may only be activated during certain movements, tasks, or force requirements), or on different biomechanical functions. Biomechanical compartments are well known; for example, the shoulder deltoid has long been identified as having medial, anterior, and posterior compartments (Fig. 3.5). Yet, new compartments continue to be identified, such that even the old three compartment deltoid is now recognized to have seven compartments (Wickham & Brown, 1998). Brown et al. (2007) later identified 19 compartments across the three major shoulder muscles (pectoralis m., latissimus dorsi, deltoid) and noted that compartments were coordinated across muscles and that groupings of motor units across neighboring muscles were formed as functional "task groups."

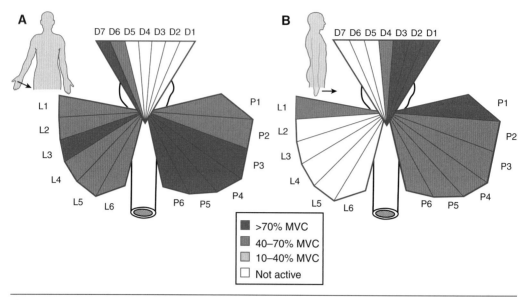

Figure 3.5 • Schematic illustration of muscle activity across various compartments of the deltoid (D1–D7), latissimus dorsi (L1–L6), and pectoralis major (P1–P6) during different tasks. These sagittal views of the muscle insertion area on the humerus reveal muscle activity during (**A**) isometric shoulder adduction and (**B**) isometric shoulder flexion during a 75% MVC contraction. The *shading* reflects the relative amount of electrical activity compared to maximal, with *darker shades* indicating higher muscle activation levels. Note that each compartment may act as a prime mover, a synergist, and even an antagonist, as in the case of compartment L1 during shoulder flexion. (Reprinted from Brown, J., Wickham, J., McAndrew, D., & Huang, X. (2007). Muscles within muscles: Coordination of 19 muscle segments within three shoulder muscles during isometric motor tasks. *Journal of Electromyography and Kinesiology*, *17*(1), 57–73, with permission from Elsevier.)

Compartments in many muscles, particularly long series–fibered muscles, may be grouped along the length of the muscle. This makes for a proximal and distal section of the muscle, and histological studies have shown proximal and distal innervation zones (Enoka, 1995). The exact role of compartments is not well known, other than that they give the nervous system more choices in coordinating muscle action to precise task demands.

■ Thinking It Through 3.2   Calf Muscle Coordination

Walter Herzog and his colleagues (e.g., Kaya et al., 2003) have done extensive studies on cats and the coordination between the cat gastrocnemius and soleus muscles. As in humans, these muscles work together to produce plantar flexion, having a common distal tendon but different origins. In both species, the gastrocnemius crosses the knee and ankle (two joint: biarticular) and soleus crosses only the ankle (single joint; monoarticular), but in cats the gastrocnemius is predominately fast twitch, whereas the soleus is slow twitch. These authors have inserted force transducers and EMG electrodes in the cat muscles and have recorded forces and electrical activity during level walking, uphill walking, and fast and slow movements. From these and other works, it has been shown that the two muscles behave differently depending on the task, such as minimal gastrocnemius activity during standing and vastly increased gastrocnemius activity and reduced soleus activity with high-speed paw shaking. Why do you think these muscles work differently, and what properties do they have that contribute to these differences? Do these findings have implications for humans? See Kaya et al. (2003, 2008) and Herzog (2000) for their views.

MOTOR UNIT BEHAVIOR ADAPTATIONS TO TRAINING

The behavior of motor units appears highly adaptable to training and practice, and forms the basis for any training-induced changes. Though caution must be urged in stating definitive adaptations (Carroll et al., 2011), the "neural factors" involved with muscle force regulation have been suggested to account for the early gains in strength during a strength training program, and fine-tuning of functional strength in experienced athletes (Cormie et al., 2011a,b; Gabriel et al., 2006; Kamen, 2004). Strength and power training have been shown to increase the maximal level of motor unit activation to 100% if not previously maximal, increase average or maximal firing rates, and bring about an earlier onset of high-threshold units without violating the size principle (Van Cutsem et al., 1998; for reviews see Cormie et al., 2011a,b; Duchateau & Enoka, 2002). Furthermore, high firing rates can be reached sooner or contractions started at a higher firing rate, more doublets produced, and possibly more synchronization (Bawa, 2002; Duchateau & Enoka, 2002, reviews). Training-induced changes may be specific to the training demands and the motor unit type. For instance, lowering of recruitment thresholds for large motor units may mostly occur in muscles that are largely slow twitch, and may depend on training speed and muscle length (Duchateau et al., 2006). Following strength training, there may be fewer motor units recruited for a given submaximal effort, suggesting higher discharge rates for active units, delayed recruitment for other units, and possibly changed intramuscular coordination (Duchateau et al., 2006). It should be noted that during immobilization or detraining the motor behavior properties are reversed from that of training (Duchateau & Enoka, 2002).

Accounting for compartmental intramuscular coordination during muscle training remains uncertain, but it can be speculated that task-specific motor unit groups adapt to specific task demands. Specific intermuscular coordination mechanisms are also likely specific to the task demands, but there do appear to be some commonalties. Ross et al. (2001) hypothesized in their review that sprint training changed the timing and sequencing of muscles to improve stride length and stride rate. Other authors have suggested that training-induced adaptations on maximal effort tasks include less agonist–antagonist cocontraction, enhanced activation of synergists and stabilizer muscles, and overall changes in timing among synergists and antagonists (Cormie et al., 2011a,b; Duchateau et al., 2006) (see Fig. 3.6). Adaptations in motor behavior also occur in low-force contractions and precise movement training; for instance, motor unit discharge rates become less variable as movement becomes more steady and controlled (Duchateau et al., 2006).

The important conclusions from these data are that the actions of motor units and muscles are situation dependent. Simply referring to textbooks and similar information sources to determine the actions of muscles provides an incomplete, if not erroneous, view of the actions of muscles. A muscle's inter- and intramuscular coordination is dependent on movement speed, force needs, the number of joints being moved, muscle length, and joint position. Further, coordination is highly dependent on the outcome purpose of the contraction, whether it is limb movement, postural stabilization, or any number of other roles muscle contraction can play (Kornecki et al., 1998).

MUSCLE PROPERTIES AND NEUROMUSCULAR MECHANICS

As we have seen in previous sections, the nervous system must take into account properties of the muscle when planning to activate the muscle. These properties include size, strength, length, elasticity, angle of pull, amount of fatigue, health or injury, morphology, and more. Not only that, but nervous system activation purposefully modifies the mechanical characteristics of the muscle–tendon complex (i.e., neuromechanics).

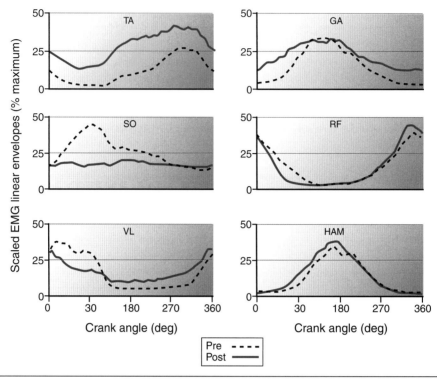

Figure 3.6 • Muscle activation changes from six different muscles before (*dashed lines*) and after (*solid lines*) 16 trials of single leg bicycle pedaling practice by novice cyclists on a computerized ergometer. Shown are smoothed EMG records during the course of an entire pedal crank revolution from the tibialis anterior (TA), soleus (SO), vastus lateralis (VL), gastrocnemius (GA), rectus femoris (RF), and hamstrings (HAM). Practice changed the coordination patterns, most noticeably by increasing the activity of the tibialis anterior and smoothing out the amount of soleus activity. (Reprinted from Hasson, C., Caldwell, G., & van Emmerik, R. (2008). Changes in muscle and joint coordination in learning to direct forces. *Human Movement Science*, *27*(4), 603, with permission of Elsevier.)

Mechanical Properties of Skeletal Muscle

Most skeletal muscles comprise a central area of muscle tissue with tendons on both ends. Connective tissue, namely, the epimysium, perimysium, and endomysium, run longitudinally throughout the muscle tissue and merge at the ends to form the tendons. Muscle tissue is an **excitable** tissue, meaning that it responds to electrical impulses. Functionally, the muscle–tendon complex has three important mechanical properties: (1) **extensibility**, its ability to stretch; (2) **elasticity**, the ability to recoil from stretch; and (3) **contractility**, the ability to shorten to produce force. Only muscle tissue has contractile properties, and it can shorten about half its resting length. Though both muscle tissue and connective tissue have extensibility and elasticity, muscle tissue has a greater range of stretch and recoil, being able to stretch about 50% of its resting length. Elongation capability is proportional to muscle length, and inversely proportional to its cross-sectional area. Extensibility and elasticity are less in the tendon tissue.

The muscle–tendon unit can be modeled to be like a mechanical device based on its properties. Figure 3.7 illustrates this model, in which the tendons and other connective tissue are springs with stretch and recoil properties, and the muscle is a force producer with shortening properties.

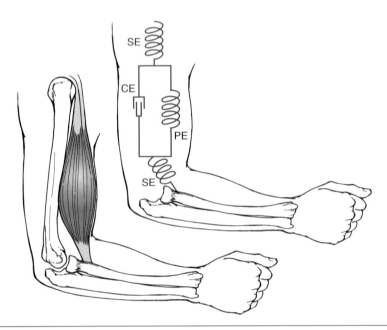

Figure 3.7 • This biceps b. muscle is modeled as a mechanical device based on its mechanical properties. The sarcomere's sliding filaments providing shortening force are the contractile elements (CE). The physiological construction of the tendons (series elastic element; SE) and other connective tissues (parallel elastic element; PE) gives these tissues spring-like properties.

The tendons are called serial elastic elements (SE), the epimysium, perimysium, and endomysium are collectively called parallel elastic elements (PE), and the muscle is the contractile element (CE). The stretch and recoil properties can vary greatly depending on shortening or lengthening velocity of the tissue, tissue length and thickness, and health of the tissue. The nervous system actively regulates the amount of stiffness, force absorption, and recoil by changing the timing and amount of muscle contraction. Changing these properties changes the flow of forces, or energy, through the body. Figure 3.8 illustrates three basic directions of force flow that are regulated by changing the mechanical properties of the muscle–tendon complex. These forces are redirected, amplified, or attenuated.

Neuromechanics and the Length–Tension Relationship

The amount of isometric force a muscle can generate and store is dependent in part on the length of the muscle. This relationship is modeled as the **length–tension curve** and includes both contractile and elastic elements. The length–tension curve thus has three parts: an active curve based on contractile elements, a passive curve based on elastic elements, and an overall curve that is the sum of adding the active and passive components.

The active portion curve is based on the amount of overlap of the actin–myosin filaments. The filaments form the sarcomere, which is the force-generating unit of the contractile element. Figure 3.9 illustrates that when the muscle is short the filaments are grossly overlapped and when the muscle is long there is not enough overlap. Too much or too little overlap results in unavailability of actin–myosin binding sites and thus fewer cross-bridge formations. Fewer cross-bridges result in

SIDENOTE | MECHANICAL WALKING

The importance of biomechanical properties such as inertia and spring-like behavior in human movement can be better grasped by the elegant experiments by Coleman and Ruina (1998). These researchers developed a two-legged, passively dynamic walking toy that could not stand on its own, but when given motive force by gravity would walk in a realistic human-like manner. This toy, constructed out of TinkerToys and shown in the photo below, engages in a fluid stepping motion as it walks down an inclined plane. The walking motion is enabled by the oscillating, spring-like behavior of the outrigger arms that cause a side to side rocking motion that lifts the legs up forward. Walking parameters, like stride length, speed, and step height, are based on the intrinsic mechanical properties of the toy, including inertia, stiffness of the joints, and elastic properties of the materials. These authors have developed more sophisticated walking models that have helped us understand the relationships between mechanical properties of our bodies and the neural control of these systems. For videos of the walker and other model robots walking, see videos at: http://ruina.tam.cornell.edu/research/topics/locomotion_and_robotics/tinkertoy_walker/index.php

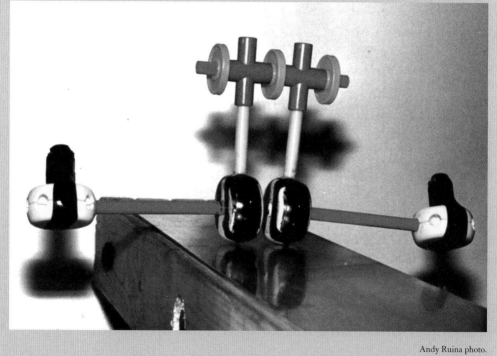

Andy Ruina photo.

less force. An optimal amount of overlap enables full cross-bridge formation and is just longer than resting length.

The passive portion of the curve is nonlinear due to the nature of the connective tissue. At longer stretches, a large amount of force can be stored in the elastic element. This passive tension is stored and provides a recoiling force when released. This recoiling force is always less than the original force needed to stretch the tissue, and the tissue often does not immediately return to its original length. The

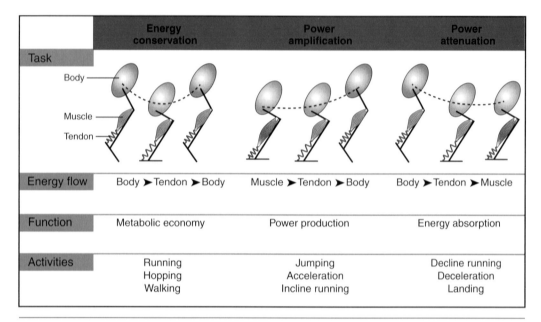

Figure 3.8 • A schematic illustrating the regulation of force flow based on regulation of mechanical stiffness. The objects in *orange* show the flow of force between body, tendon, and muscle. Energy conservation may occur when external forces (downward movement of body weight) cause a stretch in the muscle–tendon complex. These forces are conserved by being stored in the elastic elements and then released by recoil to do work. Power amplification occurs when muscles forces built up over time are transferred and stored in the tendons, and then released rapidly. Power attenuation occurs when high external forces are stored in the elastic elements and then transferred to the muscles where they are absorbed. By changing the contractile state of the muscle, the forces are dissipated, such as when softening the impact forces from a landing. (Figure reprinted with permission from Roberts, T. J., & Azizi, E. (2011). Flexible mechanisms: The diverse roles of biological springs in vertebrate movement. *Journal of Experimental Biology, 214,* 354, Figure 1.)

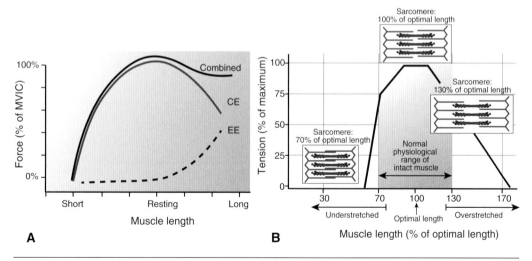

Figure 3.9 • The length–tension relationship. **A.** The CE force production capability is dependent on the muscle length. The storage and recoil force in the elastic elements is also dependent on tissue length. The CE and EE combined give the muscle its overall mechanical properties. **B.** The force-generating capacity of the CE is dependent on sarcomere length. Too much and too little overlap lead to fewer sites for actin–myosin binding, leading to less capability for force generation.

difference between the stretch force and length and the recoil force and shortening is called **hysteresis**, and affects both the connective tissue and muscle tissue. The amount of hysteresis is affected by prior movements, particularly cyclical movements such as running and cycling, flexibility training, and tissue health (Gao et al., 2011).

The separation of the contractile and elastic elements in the length–tension curve hides the complexity of this system in action. For example, a stretched muscle does not necessarily mean that the elastic and contractile elements are both stretched. Consider a high force contraction against a very heavy load. As the force is increased, the contractile element shortens and the elastic element stretches. At this point there is no movement because the shortening of the contractile element is countered by the lengthening of the elastic element. When enough contractile force is generated and transmitted to the elastic element, the load will move. As the limb begins to move, the contractile element will shorten, but the elastic tissue will likely remain elongated.

■ Thinking It Through 3.3   Maintaining Muscle Length

If a muscle could stay at its optimal resting length it could maximize force producing capability and efficiency. Can a muscle, though, stay at optimal length even though it must shorten to produce movement, and shortens as the limb moves? In the figure below are length–tension curves of the medial gastrocnemius (MG) muscle during jumping and walking and the vastus lateralis (VL) muscle during pedaling. Note that even during movements with full ranges of motion the gastrocnemius muscle stays in a length–tension relationship that enables high force capability. In contrast, the VL lengthens greatly, which sharply reduces its force generating capability. Why is this? What differs between these two muscles that could contribute to these differences? For help see Fukunaga et al. (2002).

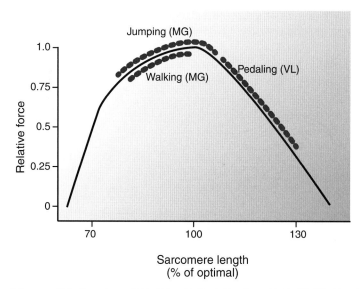

(Adapted from Fukunaga, T. T., Kawakami, Y. Y., Kubo, K. K., & Kanehisa, H. H. (2002). Muscle and tendon interaction during human movements. *Exercise and Sport Sciences Reviews, 30*(3), 106–110.)

Movements like walking, vertical jumping, and squatting take advantage of the favorable length–tension relationship properties afforded by multijoint muscles. These movements are called **concurrent movements**. In a concurrent movement, a multijoint muscle is contractile shortening on one joint to move a load, and at another joint is being stretched. This enables the muscle tissue to minimize changes in length. The minimal change in length occurs during the important force-producing part of the movement, implying that the nervous system must control the muscle activation level and movement of the surrounding joints to maintain the favorable length–tension curve.

Sometimes, the arrangement of multijoint muscles leads to a length–tension disadvantage. Most biarticular (or multiarticular) muscles are not long enough to permit full range of motion (ROM) at the same time of both joints. For example, flexing the hip and extending the knee at the same time are a result of rectus femoris shortening at both joints. This shortening is rapid and pronounced, causing the rectus femoris length and shortening velocity to quickly get into the unfavorable areas of the length–tension–velocity curve. At the same time, the hamstrings are lengthening at both joints, thus the elastic tension rises rapidly and may reach a point where full ROM of hip flexion and knee extension is prohibited (and sometimes painful!). This type of movement is referred to as **countercurrent**.

Neuromechanics and the Force–Velocity Relationship

In a concentric contraction, the muscle loses force-generating capabilities as the speed of shortening increases. This is due to inefficient coupling of the actin–myosin crossbridges and greater fluid viscosity at higher speeds. The cross-bridges need time to connect, and with less time available, fewer cross-bridges will form. The relationship between contraction velocity and force output forms the **force–velocity curve** (Fig. 3.10). In the illustration, note that at maximal shortening speeds the force output is very low, and at zero shortening speed (isometric) and during lengthening contractions (eccentric) maximum force is produced. The shape of the eccentric portion of the force velocity curve is highly variable depending on factors such as training status and muscle tested and is not elaborated further. It is clear that a high shortening velocity is an inefficient use of the contractile machinery. Under normal circumstances, the nervous system tries to avoid these movements and does so in the same way it controls the length–tension curve.

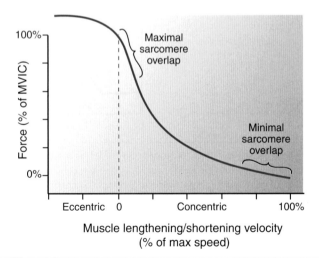

Figure 3.10 • The force–velocity curve. At high shortening speeds the actin and myosin filaments have trouble connecting and the overall coupling process is too slow to enable effective cross-bridge formation. During eccentric actions, the force produced is larger.

NEUROMECHANICS AND THE STRETCH–SHORTEN CYCLE

If a muscle is stretched rapidly prior to concentric contraction then it can produce more force. This phenomenon is called an eccentric–concentric contraction or a stretch–shorten movement and is readily seen in a windup or a countermovement action. Many common activities like running, jumping, and throwing are movements of this type. It takes advantage of a phenomenon called the

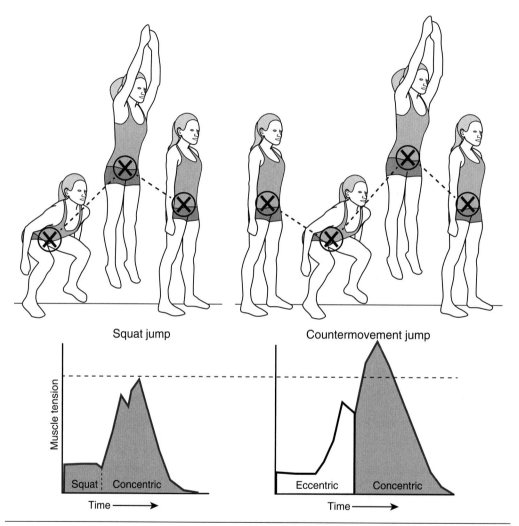

Figure 3.11 • SSC activity during two types of jumps. On the left is a squat jump, in which the jumper begins in an isometric squat position and proceeds with an explosive concentric action. On the right is a countermovement jump that begins with a downward movement (eccentric) followed by a rapid reversal concentric action. By the time the concentric contraction begins in a countermovement jump, a considerable amount of force has already been developed. This added contraction time may be up to 50% longer without simultaneously causing excessive muscle shortening. The velocity of eccentric stretch and the quickness of the eccentric to concentric reversal are both vital to the effectiveness of the movement and contribute to the rate of tension development. In general, faster eccentric velocities and faster reversal times create more explosive movements, but excessively fast eccentric velocities may overwhelm the system and result in slow reversals and ineffective stretch–shorten movements. Optimizing the stretch–shorten movement requires a balance between eccentric velocity and reversal time.

| SIDE**NOTE** | **WHAT IS MUSCLE MEMORY?** |

"Muscle memory" is a term often used in lay circles but has no precise scientific meaning. Sometimes, the term is erroneously used to mean motor memory, which is remembering how to perform motor skills even after long periods of no practice (see Chapter 7). Among weight lifters, muscle memory is used to refer to the ability of previously trained muscle to rapidly regain its hypertrophied state following periods in injury, detraining, or atrophy. This ability of muscle to rapidly rehypertrophy is probably due to the prior establishment of DNA signaling pathways and additional cellular nuclei that contribute to the ability to synthesize new proteins.

stretch–shorten cycle (SSC). Exactly why the force can be increased is not fully known, and several theories have been proposed. The theories behind the SSC include (1) release of stored elastic energy, (2) the preload effect, (3) excitation of reflex mechanisms, and (4) making available more time for contraction. Regardless of the mechanism, this method is most effective if the countermovement is not passive but is an active eccentric contraction, that is, the muscle being stretched is being activated at the same time.

The most commonly cited reason for SSC enhancement is that it takes advantage of the stored elastic energy to enable more forceful contractions. The amount of stored energy is based largely on stretch velocity, and somewhat on the length of the stretch. The faster the velocity, the more stored energy, and the quicker the transition from stretch to shorten (or eccentric to concentric), the more stored energy is released (Fig. 3.11). The stretch–shorten may make available more chemical energy (i.e., ATP) in a phenomenon called the preload effect. This is simply the fact that the contraction starts at a higher level of force (due to the eccentric contraction), and this spares available chemical energy. There is not much empirical evidence to support this theory.

The stretch portion of the SSC may cause the stretch reflex to occur, thus facilitating the muscle to contract stronger and with a faster rate of tension development. By doing this, not only is the power of the contraction increased but the eccentric to concentric contraction coupling time is reduced, which increases the storage and use of elastic energy. There is some experimental evidence for this effect, but it is not a consistent finding. Likely, the most important factor in the SSC is that the eccentric contraction of a muscle prior to its concentric phase enables the muscle to contract for a longer period of time, thereby providing sufficient time to build force.

EXERCISE TRAINING AND NEUROMECHANICS

Some exercise training modes have a direct impact on the muscle mechanical system. Flexibility training (stretching), in particular, is specifically designed to reduce the elastic stiffness of the muscle–tendon complex. Hypertrophied musculotendinous tissue also affects stiffness, but not to the same extent. The implications of these training-induced changes are described below.

Flexibility Training and Neuromechanics

Flexibility exercises as typically done are intended to increase joint ROM. A single stretching exercise session may lead to transient increases in ROM, and a long-term program may result in chronic increase in ROM. An increased joint ROM may result from (1) decreased stiffness of the muscle–tendon complex, (2) a longer muscle–tendon complex, (3) more pain tolerance to stretching, or (4) relaxation of the contractile element. Surprisingly, very little is known about what actually happens in humans.

Animal studies reveal that the effects of long-term stretching may increase muscle length by adding sarcomeres and/or add length to the tendon (Noonan et al., 1993; Taylor et al., 1990). In humans: there is some evidence for decreased stiffness of the muscle–tendon unit that may be a result of more compliant muscle–tendon properties and a reduction in neural excitability. Depending on the nature of stretching, such as cyclic versus static, the hysteresis properties of the muscle–tendon unit may change (Kubo et al., 2002; Magnusson et al., 1998). The involvement of neural systems in flexibility training, including proprioceptive neuromuscular facilitation (PNF), is largely speculative (Guissard & Duchateau, 2006). Some investigators have provided good evidence that the improvement in chronic ROM from a stretching program may be due to an increased pain tolerance to stretch and has little to do with changes in the muscle itself (e.g., Magnusson et al., 1996). Increased pain tolerance may be a purely psychological adaptation or could be due to changes in sensory outflow from the muscle. Weppler and Magnusson (2010) have proposed solid rationale that a reduction in sensory outflow and a reduction in pain signaling are the primary reasons.

The acute effects of stretching may be to alter the viscoelastic properties of the muscle to become more compliant. Changes in the inherent stiffness or elasticity, though, are relatively short-lived (<10 minutes) even with highly intense stretching protocols (Magnusson et al., 1998, 2000). The lack of a definitive mechanism for stretching effects, coupled with evidence for rather transient effects, raises the question of the usefulness of stretching exercises. Indeed, a large amount of research over the past 15 years has demonstrated that stretching before strength and power performance reduces performance. It has been speculated that increased musculotendinous viscoelasticity following an acute stretching bout reduces the transmission of force through the system. A compliant musculotendinous system is suggested to absorb and dissipate force rather than transmit it. In addition, a compliant system alters the production of force because of changes in the length–tension–velocity conditions.

However, many of these studies are difficult to translate to real-world situations because the stretching duration and intensity far exceed what is normally done, and the subsequent exercise trials follow much too soon. In short, a session of normal intensity or duration of static or dynamic stretching may have little effect on endurance, strength, or power performance (Behm & Chaouachi, 2011).

Data regarding stretching and injury prevention are more difficult to gather (Schilling & Stone, 2000; Stojanovic & Ostojic, 2011). Extensive literature reviews have largely concluded that there is little evidence to suggest that stretching before or after exercise has an effect on exercise-related injuries or muscle soreness (Gleim & McHugh, 1997; Herbert et al., 2011; Small et al., 2008), though there may be a hint that some stretching may reduce some muscle–tendon injuries (Small et al., 2008; Stojanovic & Ostojic, 2011). Reexamination of previous data led Woods et al. (2007) to suggest that acute stretching does have positive effect on reducing muscle–tendon injuries during exercise. Apart from exercise injury, stretching is used as a therapeutic tool to improve symptoms in a variety of musculoskeletal disorders (Bovend'Eerdt et al., 2008; da Costa & Vieira, 2008). Perhaps most of all, it is a tool to maintain muscle health and is an important component of exercise leading to better health outcomes and quality of life, particularly in aging populations (Kell et al., 2001).

Strength, Plyometric Training, and Neuromechanics

Tissue stiffness is dependent on the morphological and histochemical makeup of the tissue fibers, health of the tissue, the length of the tissue, and the thickness of the tissue. Typical stretching exercises as described above may alter the morphological tissue characteristics or the length of the tissue to increase compliance. Hypertrophied muscle and tendon tissue, such as the result of a resistance training program, increases stiffness by increasing tissue thickness and perhaps tissue density. Hypertrophied muscles may also result in the muscle fascicles becoming more angled, thus changing the angle of force application that may not be in parallel with the tissue fibers (Seynnes et al., 2007).

Plyometric training is rigorous training targeting the SSC. In its basic form, plyometrics are a form of high-effort power training emphasizing a forceful eccentric phase of the SSC movement followed by an explosive rapid reversal of the concentric phase of movement. Traditionally, plyometric training involves jump training, including "depth jumps" and "box jumps," with loads only supplied by body weight and varied based on the height of box jumped down from. More recently, upper body exercises such as explosive stretch–shorten pushups have been added to plyometric training regimens. A version of plyometrics, called ballistic training, emphasizes maximal speed of the concentric phase of movement during light-load weight lifting exercises.

Plyometric and ballistic training are designed to change the shape of the force–velocity curve at the high velocity end in order to improve leg and arm movement speed, jump height, and explosive power in general. It is thought by training at this end of the force–velocity curve it is possible to increase tissue stiffness, maximize elastic energy recoil, and develop neural coordination mechanisms that maximize rapid contractions and effectively coordinate a rapid reversal in a muscle acting first as an antagonist and then as an agonist. Indeed, direct and circumstantial evidence point to changes in muscle architecture, increased neural drive, increased muscle tendon stiffness, improved intermuscular coordination, and an overall improvement in the SSC performance with plyometric training (Markovic & Mikulic, 2010). Improvements in stretch–shorten performance center on an improved stretch tolerance to high velocities, which in turn, enable a more rapid and complete transfer of force from the tissue to mechanical work, as is illustrated in Figure 3.8.

From a functional standpoint, there is abundance support that plyometric and ballistic training can improve muscle power and jump height (Cormie et al., 2011a,b; Ziv & Lidor, 2010), though running speed gains are hard to consistently realize across different populations. Plyometric jump training improves running and jumping in children and may improve kicking, agility, and balance (Johnson et al., 2011). Overall, the benefits gained by this type of training are numerous and can be realized in many different populations from young to old, and from athlete to nonathlete.

OTHER MUSCULOSKELETAL PROPERTIES INFLUENCING NERVOUS SYSTEM CONTROL

The nervous system takes into account mechanical factors such as muscle length, velocity, and stretch. It also takes into account the fiber-type distribution, anatomical arrangement of the muscle fibers (e.g., long and straight fusiform vs. angled pennate), muscle size and fiber length, tendon length and thickness, and biomechanical musculoskeletal characteristics. The influence of these characteristics on movement production is in Table 3.2.

Muscles contract in order to produce force, but that force may be used in numerous ways other than to move a body part. How that force can and will be used is largely dependent on the purpose of movement and is a key outcome of coordination strategies. Muscles directly involved in producing the desired movement are **agonists**. Agonists can be either prime movers or **synergists**. **Antagonist** muscles oppose the action of the agonists. Other muscles have an indirect, but vital role in movement. **Fixators** and **stabilizers** usually contract statically to stabilize a body part against the pull of contracting muscles. Many of these muscles are categorized as postural muscles. **Neutralizers** act to prevent an undesired action of one of the agonists. It is important to understand that at any given moment the same muscle may act as an agonist, stabilizer, neutralizer, or even antagonist. Agonist and antagonist muscles may work together as synergists. All of these roles—to move, to stabilize, to neutralize, to oppose—require the muscle to contract in a different manner and require a different coordination scheme.

For example, antagonist muscles must be controlled alongside the agonist, either by inhibition or cocontraction. It is generally desirable to have the antagonists inhibited (relaxed) during agonist action. This allows the agonist muscle to exert a full amount of joint torque and increases overall metabolic efficiency. Although antagonist quietness during agonist action appears to be desirable,

TABLE 3.2	Musculoskeletal Design Factors Influencing Muscle Output
Tendon length and thickness	Long tendon increases the range of muscle and increases dampening and energy storage. Thicker tendons are stiffer and more resistant to stretch, and thus tend to transmit force quicker and with less force storage.
Muscle insertion moment arms	Long moment arm enables more force. Short moment enables increased speed and ROM.
Fiber type	Fast twitch enables fast and powerful contractions, and slow twitch provides fatigue resistance.
Muscle fiber area	Large muscle cross-sectional area enables increased force production.
Muscle fiber length and fiber arrangement	Long fibers provide increased speed and increased ROM. Oblique or pennate muscle fibers may provide force vectors different from longitudinal muscles.

oftentimes, the contraction of the antagonists during agonist action (**cocontraction**) is necessary. Cocontraction can help stabilize the joint, especially during very rapid or very forceful agonist contractions.

SUMMARY

Movement execution is a function of the peripheral neuromuscular system, namely, the motor unit. Executing even a simple motor skill requires coordinating the behavior of each single motor unit among hundreds or thousands of motor units. Motor units are most commonly classified by size of their neurons, with smaller motor units also being associated with slow twitch muscle fibers and smaller innervation ratios. These units are also recruited first, are fatigue resistant, and are used for finer force control. Several rules govern the actions of motor units; the most prominent are the size principle of recruitment and the all-or-none principle. Motor units and overall muscle force output are regulated by motor unit recruitment, rate coding, and intramuscular and intermuscular coordination. Intramuscular coordination is based on regulating recruitment and firing rate, altering discharge patterning, and compartmentalization.

The mechanical properties of the muscle tendon complex, including its contractile characteristics, elasticity, and extensibility, are important factors in how the nervous system controls muscle force output and movements. The nervous system must take these properties into account, and even purposefully modify them, to produce efficient and effective movements.

Understanding the movement execution process is important to understanding how training and practice can be manipulated to induce changes. Whether for rehabilitation or maximizing athletic performance, practice and training must take into account specific task requirements so that the neuromuscular system can organize itself to produce task-specific coordination patterns that subsequently result in task-specific neurophysiological adaptations. These adaptations include faster firing rates, changes in recruitment and firing rate manipulation, and vast changes in inter and intramuscular coordination. Simply exercising muscles based on movements the muscle is capable of making will not produce highly coordinated actions or necessarily even develop the muscles in manners they were intended to work.

STUDY QUESTIONS

1. Define motor unit, and describe the defining difference between a large motor unit and a small motor unit.
2. There are several physiological features associated with small motor units. (a) What are they, and (b) How are they important in the size principle of motor unit recruitment? Contrast these to large motor units.
3. There are three general ways to change muscle force using neural factors, that is, to vary the force output at any given joint. What are they? Explain in detail, including the three mechanisms of intramuscular coordination. Give examples of intermuscular coordination.
4. Provide a reason(s) for lifting very heavy weights, as opposed to lighter weights, as a method to build strength.
5. Define and describe the criteria by which muscles are compartmentalized.
6. It is generally noted that during isometric contractions the level of muscle activation, as shown by EMG, rises much faster than the level of force. That is, as force rises in a steady linear manner during a forceful contraction, the amplitude of the corresponding EMG from the muscle begins to rise rapidly and in an exponential manner when the force output gets high. Can you explain why? Conduct a literature search on a scientific database to find support for your answer.
7. How may training change motor unit behavior and neuromuscular mechanics?
8. What are the reasons that stretch–shorten movement enable the production of more muscle force than concentric contractions alone? How may plyometric training enhance this effect?
9. Discuss the potential benefits and problems with stretching exercises.
10. How may tendon and muscle size, length, and orientation influence the control of movement?

Bibliography

Bawa, P. P. (2002). Neural control of motor output: Can training change it? *Exercise and Sport Sciences Reviews*, 30(2), 59–63.

Bawa, P., Pang, M. Y., Olesen, K. A., & Calancie, B. (2006). Rotation of motoneurons during prolonged isometric contractions in humans. *Journal of Neurophysiology*, 96, 1135–1140.

Behm, D., & Chaouachi, A. (2011). A review of the acute effects of static and dynamic stretching on performance. *European Journal of Applied Physiology*, 111(11), 2633–2651.

Bovend'Eerdt, T., Newman, M., Barker, K., Dawes, H., Minelli, C., & Wade, D. (2008). The effects of stretching in spasticity: A systematic review. *Archives of Physical Medicine and Rehabilitation*, 89(7), 1395–1406.

Broman, H., De Luca, C., & Mambrito, B. (1985). Motor unit recruitment and firing rates interaction in the control of human muscles. *Brain Research*, 337(2), 311–319.

Brown, J., Wickham, J., McAndrew, D., & Huang, X. (2007). Muscles within muscles: Coordination of 19 muscle segments within three shoulder muscles during isometric motor tasks. *Journal of Electromyography and Kinesiology*, 17(1), 57–73.

Carpinelli, R. N. (2008). The size principle and a critical analysis of the unsubstantiated heavier-is-better recommendation for resistance training. *Journal of Exercise Science and Fitness*, 6(2), 67–86.

Carroll, T., Selvanayagam, V., Riek, S., & Semmler, J. (2011). Neural adaptations to strength training: Moving beyond transcranial magnetic stimulation and reflex studies. *Acta Physiologica*, 202(2), 119–140.

Chalmers, G. (2008). Can fast-twitch muscle fibres be selectively recruited during lengthening contractions? Review and applications to sport movements. *Sports Biomechanics*, 7(1), 137–157.

Coleman, M., & Ruina, A. (1998). An uncontrolled toy that can walk but cannot stand still (Tinkertoy walker). *Physical Review Letters*, 80(16), 3658–3661.

Conwit, R., Stashuk, D., Tracy, B., McHugh, M., Brown, W., & Metter, E. (1999). The relationship of motor unit size, firing rate and force. *Clinical Neurophysiology*, 110(7), 1270–1275.

Cormie, P., McCuigan, M. R., & Newton, R. U. (2011a). Developing maximal neuromuscular power: Part 1—biological basis of maximal power production. *Sports Medicine*, 41(1), 17–38.

Cormie, P., McGuigan, M., & Newton, R. (2011b). Developing maximal neuromuscular power: Part 2— training considerations for improving maximal power production. *Sports Medicine*, *41*(2), 125–146.

da Costa, B., & Vieira, E. (2008). Stretching to reduce work-related musculoskeletal disorders: A systematic review. *Journal of Rehabilitation Medicine*, *40*(5), 321–328.

Desmedt, J. E., & Godaux, E. (1977). Ballistic contractions in man: Characteristic recruitment pattern of single motor units of the tibialis anterior muscle. *Journal of Physiology*, *264*, 673–693.

Duchateau, J. J., & Enoka, R. M. (2002). Neural adaptations with chronic activity patterns in able-bodied humans. *American Journal of Physical Medicine & Rehabilitation*, *81*(11 Suppl), S17–S27.

Duchateau, J., & Enoka, R. (2011). Human motor unit recordings: Origins and insight into the integrated motor system. *Brain Research*, *1409*, 42–61.

Duchateau, J., Semmler, J., & Enoka, R. (2006). Training adaptations in the behavior of human motor units. *Journal of Applied Physiology*, *101*(6), 1766–1775.

Edgerton, V. R., Roy, R. R., Bodine, S. C., & Sacks, R. D. (1983). The matching of neuronal and muscular physiology. In K. T. Borer, D. W. Edington and T. P. White (Eds.), *Frontiers of exercise biology* (pp. 51–70). Champaign, IL: Human Kinetics.

Enoka, R. (1995). Morphological features and activation patterns of motor units. *Journal of Clinical Neurophysiology*, *12*(6), 538–559.

Enoka, R., & Fuglevand, A. (2001). Motor unit physiology: Some unresolved issues. *Muscle & Nerve*, *24*(1), 4–17.

Fukunaga, T. T., Kawakami, Y. Y., Kubo, K. K., & Kanehisa, H. H. (2002). Muscle and tendon interaction during human movements. *Exercise and Sport Sciences Reviews*, *30*(3), 106–110.

Gabriel, D. A., Kamen, G., & Frost, G. (2006). Neural adaptations to resistive exercise: Mechanisms and recommendations for training practices. *Sports Medicine*, *36*(2), 133–149.

Gao, F., Ren, Y., Roth, E., Harvey, R., & Zhang, L. (2011). Effects of repeated ankle stretching on calf muscle-tendon and ankle biomechanical properties in stroke survivors. *Clinical Biomechanics*, *26*(5), 516–522.

Gath, I., & Stålberg, E. (1981). In situ measurement of the innervation ratio of motor units in human muscles. *Experimental Brain Research*, *43*(3–4), 377–382.

Gleim, G. W., & McHugh, M. P. (1997). Flexibility and its effects on sports injury and performance. *Sports Medicine*, *24*(5), 289–299.

Graves, A., Kornatz, K., & Enoka, R. (2000). Older adults use a unique strategy to lift inertial loads with the elbow flexor muscles. *Journal of Neurophysiology*, *83*(4), 2030–2039.

Guissard, N., & Duchateau, J. (2006). Neural aspects of muscle stretching. *Exercise and Sport Sciences Reviews*, *34*(4), 154–158.

Hasson, C., Caldwell, G., & van Emmerik, R. (2008). Changes in muscle and joint coordination in learning to direct forces. *Human Movement Science*, *27*(4), 590–609.

Herbert, R., de Noronha, M., & Kamper, S. (2011). Stretching to prevent or reduce muscle soreness after exercise. *Cochrane Database of Systematic Reviews (Online)*, (7), CD004577.

Herzog, W. (2000). Muscle properties and coordination during voluntary movement. *Journal of Sports Sciences*, *18*(3), 141–152.

Johnson, B., Salzberg, C., & Stevenson, D. (2011). A systematic review: Plyometric training programs for young children. *Journal of Strength and Conditioning Research*, *25*(9), 2623–2633.

Kamen, G. G. (2004). Neural issues in the control of muscular strength. *Research Quarterly for Exercise and Sport*, *75*(1), 3–8.

Kamen, G., & Du, D. (1999). Independence of motor unit recruitment and rate modulation during precision force control. *Neuroscience*, *88*(2), 643–653.

Kaya, M., Leonard, T., & Herzog, W. (2003). Coordination of medial gastrocnemius and soleus forces during cat locomotion. *Journal of Experimental Biology*, *206*(Pt 20), 3645–3655.

Kaya, M., Leonard, T., & Herzog, W. (2008). Premature deactivation of soleus during the propulsive phase of cat jumping. *Journal of the Royal Society*, *5*(21), 415–426.

Kell, R. T., Bell, G. G., & Quinney, A. A. (2001). Musculoskeletal fitness, health outcomes and quality of life. *Sports Medicine*, *31*(12), 863–873.

Knight, C., & Kamen, G. (2005). Superficial motor units are larger than deeper motor units in human vastus lateralis muscle. *Muscle & Nerve*, *31*(4), 475–480.

Kornecki, S., Janura, A., & Piotrowska, A. (1988). Stabilizing functions of muscles and their electromyographic shares. In S. Kornecki (Ed.) *Studies and monographs no. 55, the problem of muscular synergism.* Proceedings of the XIth International Biomechanics Seminar, pp. 23–33.

Kossev, A., & Christova, P. (1998a). Discharge pattern of human motor units during dynamic concentric and eccentric contractions. *Electroencephalography and Clinical Neurophysiology, 109*(3), 245–255.

Kossev, A., & Christova, P. (1998b). Motor unit recruitment and discharge behavior in movements and isometric contractions. *Muscle & Nerve, 21*(3), 413–415.

Kubo, K., Kanehisa, H., & Fukunaga, T. (2002). Effect of stretching training on the viscoelastic properties of human tendon structures in vivo. *Journal of Applied Physiology, 92*(2), 595–601.

Kuchinad, R., Ivanova, T., & Garland, S. (2004). Modulation of motor unit discharge rate and H-reflex amplitude during submaximal fatigue of the human soleus muscle. *Experimental Brain Research, 158*(3), 345–355.

Lieber, R. L. (2002). *Skeletal muscle structure and function. Implications for rehabilitation and sports medicine* (2nd ed.). Baltimore, MD: Lippincott Williams & Wilkins.

Magnusson, S. P., Aagaard, P. P., & Nielson, J. J. (2000). Passive energy return after repeated stretches of the hamstring muscle-tendon unit. *Medicine and Science in Sports and Exercise, 32*(6), 1160–1164.

Magnusson, S. P., Aagard, P. P., Simonsen, E. E., & Bojsen-Moller, F. F. (1998). A biomechanical evaluation of cyclic and static stretch in human skeletal muscle. *International Journal of Sports Medicine, 19*(5), 310–316.

Magnusson, S., Simonsen, E., Aagaard, P., Sørensen, H., & Kjaer, M. (1996). A mechanism for altered flexibility in human skeletal muscle. *Journal of Physiology, 497*(Pt 1), 291–298.

Markovic, G., & Mikulic, P. (2010). Neuro-musculoskeletal and performance adaptations to lower-extremity plyometric training. *Sports Medicine, 40*(10), 859–895.

Mendell, L. (2005). The size principle: A rule describing the recruitment of motoneurons. *Journal of Neurophysiology, 93*(6), 3024–3026.

Monster, A. W., & Chan, H. (1977). Isometric force production by motor units of extensor digitorum communis muscle in man. *Journal of Neurophysiology, 40*, 1432–1443.

Noonan, T. J., Best, T. M., Seaber, A. V., & Garrett, W. E. (1993). Thermal effects on skeletal muscle tensile behavior. *American Journal of Sports Medicine, 21*(4), 517–522.

Rich, C., O'Brien, G., & Cafarelli, E. (1998). Probabilities associated with counting average motor unit firing rates in active human muscle. *Canadian Journal of Applied Physiology, 23*(1), 87–94.

Richmond, F. J. (1998). Elements of style in neuromuscular architecture. *American Zoologist, 38*, 729–742.

Ross, A. A., Leveritt, M. M., & Riek, S. S. (2001). Neural influences on sprint running: Training adaptations and acute responses. *Sports Medicine, 31*(6), 409–425.

Rota, S., Hautier, C., Creveaux, T., Champely, S., Guillot, A., & Rogowski, I. (2012). Relationship between muscle coordination and forehand drive velocity in tennis. *Journal of Electromyography and Kinesiology, 22*(2), 294–300.

Santo Neto, H., de Carvalho, V., & Marques, M. (1998). Estimation of the number and size of human flexor digiti minimi muscle motor units using histological methods. *Muscle & Nerve, 21*(1), 112–114.

Santo Neto, H., & Marques, M. (2008). Estimation of the number and size of motor units in intrinsic laryngeal muscles using morphometric methods. *Clinical Anatomy, 21*(4), 301–306.

Schilling, B. K., & Stone, M. H. (2000). Stretching: Acute effects on strength and power performance. *Strength and Conditioning Journal, 22*(1), 44–47.

Seynnes, O. R., de Boer, M. M., & Narici, M. V. (2007). Early skeletal muscle hypertrophy and architectural changes in response to high-intensity resistance training. *Journal of Applied Physiology, 102*(1), 368–373.

Small, K., Mc Naughton, L., & Matthews, M. (2008). A systematic review into the efficacy of static stretching as part of a warm-up for the prevention of exercise-related injury. *Research in Sports Medicine, 16*(3), 213–231.

Søgaard, K., Christensen, H., Fallentin, N., Mizuno, M., Quistorff, B., & Sjøgaard, G. (1998). Motor unit activation patterns during concentric wrist flexion in humans with different muscle fibre composition. *European Journal of Applied Physiology and Occupational Physiology, 78*(5), 411–416.

Stojanovic, M., & Ostojic, S. (2011). Stretching and injury prevention in football: Current perspectives. *Research in Sports Medicine, 19*(2), 73–91.

Taylor, D. C., Dalton, J. D., Seaber, A. V., & Garrett, W. E. (1990). Viscoelastic properties of muscle-tendon units. The biomechanical effects of stretching. *American Journal of Sports Medicine*, *18*(3), 300–309.

Van Cutsem, M., Duchateau, J., & Hainaut, K. (1998). Changes in single motor unit behaviour contribute to the increase in contraction speed after dynamic training in humans. *Journal of Physiology*, *513*(Pt 1), 295–305.

Weppler, C., & Magnusson, S. (2010). Increasing muscle extensibility: A matter of increasing length or modifying sensation? *Physical Therapy*, *90*(3), 438–449.

Wickham, J., & Brown, J. (1998). Muscles within muscles: The neuromotor control of intra-muscular segments. *European Journal of Applied Physiology and Occupational Physiology*, *78*(3), 219–225.

Woods, K., Bishop, P., & Jones, E. (2007). Warm-up and stretching in the prevention of muscular injury. *Sports Medicine*, *37*(12), 1089–1099.

Ziv, G., & Lidor, R. (2010). Vertical jump in female and male volleyball players: A review of observational and experimental studies. *Scandinavian Journal of Medicine & Science in Sports*, *20*(4), 556–567.

4 | Peripheral Sensory Systems in Monitoring Movement

PURPOSE, IMPORTANCE, AND OBJECTIVES OF THIS CHAPTER

The purpose of this chapter is to understand the primary peripheral sensory and sensorimotor systems responsible for monitoring movements and how, in doing so, they initiate reflex actions and send movement information back to the central nervous system. Emphasis is placed on proprioceptive and visual sensory systems. Knowing how these systems work provides an understanding of the nature of the information the brain uses to plan and initiate skilled motor actions, as well as the information the brain uses as a basis for learning. Understanding reflex mechanisms and how they fit into skilled motor actions provides a basis for practice and training and adds to our understanding of how the brain deals with excessive degrees of freedom in movement.

After reading this chapter, you should be able to:

1. Describe the basic physiology and organization of the sensory system.
2. Classify receptors based on location and type.
3. Identify different types of proprioceptors and their specific functions.
4. Describe simple and complex reflexes and how they contribute to goal-directed movement.
5. Describe the important and unique roles played by vision in the production of skilled movement.
6. Describe the differences between focal and ambient vision and the roles each plays in feedforward and feedback control of movement.
7. Understand why reflex responses and sensory feedback to the CNS are situation dependent.

Movement planning, initiation, and execution cannot run smoothly or effectively unless information regarding the actual movement is relayed back to the central nervous system (CNS). Without this information, the CNS cannot monitor ongoing movements for the purpose of making adjustments or evaluate movement effectiveness after the fact for the purpose of learning and future movement planning. The sensory division of the peripheral nervous system (PNS) is responsible for this movement monitoring and relaying information back to the CNS. In addition, this sensory system is also responsible for initiating reflex movements that do not require participation from the brain. **Reflexes** are stereotyped and repeatable actions in the periphery that are caused by stimulation of sensory receptors in the PNS that transmit the signal to the CNS, which then routes the signal back out to the periphery to cause the action. By definition, reflexes occur without conscious involvement and are thus not considered goal-directed movements or motor skills. However, reflex actions of one form or another provide basic movement components from which many motor skills develop. In this chapter, we look at the process of monitoring of motor skills by the peripheral sensory systems and the initiation of reflex actions in sensorimotor systems. Specifically examined are proprioceptive systems and visual systems.

SENSORY SYSTEMS AND RECEPTORS

In contrast to motor neurons that have muscle at their distal ends, sensory neurons have a sensory ending, or receptor, at their distal end and feed information back to the CNS. Receptors are special organelles designed to detect stimuli from the environment and translate that stimuli into electrical signals the nervous system can understand. It is only through sensory endings that we become aware of the world around us and the world within our own body.

Receptors come in many forms and can be classified according to several classification schemes. Two main classification schemes are location and type of stimulus detected. Receptor location can be broadly classified as within the viscera and blood vessels (**interoreceptors** or **visceroreceptors**), close to the outer surface of the body (**exteroreceptors**), or within the musculoskeletal system (**proprioceptors**). Visceroreceptors feed information back to the CNS regarding basic physiological processes, such as core temperature, acid balance, and smooth muscle movement. Because of their location, exterorecep-tors provide information on the outside world, including tactile sensation (touch, pain, temperature) in the skin, and vision, hearing, taste, and smell. Proprioceptors are located in muscles, joints, ligaments, and tendons and detect stimuli related to body movement and the actions and condition of the tissues housing the receptors. Traditionally, visceroreceptors, skin receptors, and proprioceptors together have been grouped as **somatoreceptors**, but data have emerged that visceroreceptors are processed differ-ently than the others (Craig, 2003). For this reason, we use the terms somatoreceptors and somatosensa-tion to refer only to proprioception and sensation arising from the skin and joint receptors.

Visceroreceptors and somatoreceptors provide ongoing information to the CNS regarding the ongoing physiological functioning and health of our bodies, including pain. Because of this informa-tion, we are afforded both conscious and subconscious awareness of our bodies. Body awareness has two components, viscero-awareness and somatosensory awareness (also called **kinesthesia**) and both have implications for exercise and motor performance. The role of kinesthesia, in particular, in motor performance is discussed throughout this text as it is the awareness of body and limb positioning and movement in space (see SideNote on next page).

Receptors detect numerous types of stimuli and are classified based on these stimuli. Thermore-ceptors (temperature), chemoreceptors (chemical and pH), baroreceptors (fluid pressure), photorecep-tors (light), olfactory receptors (smell), taste receptors, auditory receptors (sound), mechanoreceptors (mechanical disturbances), and nociceptor (pain) are located throughout the body. **Proprioceptors** are specific types of mechanoreceptors designed to detect movement within the musculoskeletal system and, as such, play a vast role in motor behavior. Included in this category are special receptors in the labyrinth of the inner ear, called labyrinthine or vestibular receptors, designed to monitor and maintain posture and balance. All sensory endings provide feedback to the CNS, and most have other functions as well. Many play a role in maintaining tissue homeostasis, modifying the output of other receptors (particularly the muscle spindle), and participating directly or indirectly in reflex arcs (Hogervorst & Brand, 1998).

SIDE**NOTE**	**BODY AWARENESS AND WELLNESS**

Under normal circumstances, we only become consciously aware of our internal physiology when our sensory feedback goes outside of a normal range. This conscious body awareness in the form of viscero-awareness may be a high heart rate during exercise, excessive body temperature when sick, or a full bladder. This enables us to be aware of those processes when they need attending to, rather than a moment to moment barrage of sensory signals. Some people, though, have too much conscious and even subconscious viscero-awareness. This may result in an obsession over health and contribute to a number of negative outcomes, including somatoform disorders. Somato-form disorders are a category of conditions characterized by complaints of bodily pains and dys-function without concrete medical explanations. Though these are considered mental illnesses, they are accompanied in many cases by real physiological dysfunction and contribute to eating disor-ders and body image problems that are prevalent among adolescents and young adults, includ-ing athletes. The cause of this disordered body awareness may be due to overamplified sensory signals, exaggerated and faulty perception, or a constant self-focus on oneself (Houtveen et al., 2003; Rietveld & Houtveen, 2004). One's behavioral state may contribute to disordered aware-ness, and conversely, amplified sensory signals may contribute to one's behavioral state. Barrett et al. (2004), for instance, reported that one's sensitivity to detecting his or her own heartbeat was associated with the experience of emotion, supporting statements from others that somatosensory and viscerosensory information influences overall cognitive processing (Berntson et al., 2003). So, when one has "gut feelings," one really does.

PROPRIOCEPTION AND REFLEXES

Proprioceptors are somatoreceptors feeding information to the CNS on bodily movement, including the amount and direction of movement, rate of movement change, and forces. This information is pro-cessed by the CNS and gives rise to kinesthesia, the conscious and subconscious awareness of body and limb positioning and movement in space. Proprioception and kinesthesia are not the same and should not be confused. In addition to providing movement feedback, proprioceptors directly or indirectly initiate skeletal muscle reflex actions, and because of their locations, some provide information regard-ing tissue homeostasis to the CNS.

Proprioceptors are located in muscles, tendons, ligaments, skin, and numerous other tissues, particularly tissues surrounding joints (Fig. 4.1). Each of these tissues can contain different types of proprioceptors, each proprioceptor supplying a different amount and type of information. Some pro-prioceptors have nerve endings contained within bulbous tissue corpuscles, surrounding tissues masses, or are free endings intertwined among tissue. The type of stimulus and how a sensory ending responds to that stimulus are dependent on the organization of the tissue and nerve endings. Some endings may respond to rapid stretch, some to slow sustained pressure, some to shear forces, and some to direct pressure.

When a proprioceptor is disturbed by a mechanical stimulus, it forms action potentials that are sent along its sensory neuron to the spinal cord. The pattern and firing rate of these action potentials are directly related to the strength and nature of the stimuli. Receptor **sensitivity** is the ability of a receptor to detect or discriminate a stimulus. Low sensitivity means that it takes a large stimulus to elicit a response from the receptor, or that small changes in stimulus strength are not detected. Receptor **acuity** is similar to sensitivity but generally refers to groups of receptors working together. Many recep-tors packed densely together, each with a small **receptive field**, enable a finer discrimination of stimuli than fewer receptors with larger receptive fields.

SIDE**NOTE**	**BODY AWARENESS AND ATHLETES**

Students in exercise and sport sciences often think that athletes and others proficient in motor skill performance must have a keen sense of their bodies, whether kinesthetic awareness, viscero-awareness, or both. Despite constantly working with their bodies, there is no evidence for chronically better viscero-awareness in athletes that may contribute to better wellness. There is a small bit of evidence that elite athletes reduce aversive or unpleasant viscerosensory information in the brain during exertion and are less affected by that sensory information than less trained individuals (Paulus et al., 2012).

In a similar manner, evidence of better kinesthesia in athletes is mixed. Sometimes, athletes have been found to have better kinesthesia (Lephart et al., 1996), but most non–sport-specific tests generally show no differences between athletes and controls (Freeman & Broderick, 1996). In some cases, higher-performing athletes have been shown to have poorer kinesthesia (Starosta et al., 1989) or, in the case of baseball players, have worse kinesthesia in their pitching arm (Allegrucci et al., 1995). In sum, the notion of athletes being "in-tune" with their bodies really cannot be entirely justified by the available research evidence.

Most proprioceptors play a role in movement via reflex activation. Each somatic reflex has a sensory ending to detect a stimulus, a sensory neuron to transmit the signal, an integrating center like the spinal cord to encode and relay the signal, a motor neuron to transmit the signal to the effector organ, and an effector organ. The effector organ is, of course, muscle. It is important to note that not all reflexes are designed to cause a muscle contraction; in fact, some reflexes are designed to inhibit the target muscles. The simplest reflex pathway, the stretch reflex, provides a basic illustration on how reflexes work (Fig. 4.2).

Though sensory endings in nearly every type of tissue can provide some level of movement information, there are four types of proprioceptors that are most important. These are muscle spindles, Golgi tendon organs (GTOs), joint kinesthetic receptors, and the vestibular apparatus.

The Muscle Spindle

Muscle spindles are relatively large receptors located throughout a muscle, though generally concentrated in the muscle belly. The function of the muscle spindle is to detect muscle stretch and contraction characteristics in order to provide muscle function feedback to the CNS and to initiate a **stretch reflex**. Both of these functions are critical in the production of coordinated movement. The complexity of the spindle allows it to be sensitive to rapid stretch and long slow sustained stretches, stretch velocity, static position, and perhaps stretch force. What makes the spindle different from other sensory organs other than the eye is the ability of the CNS to control spindle function. The spindle has tiny muscle fibers in it, called **intrafusal fibers**, which the CNS can control by small motor neurons called **gamma motor neurons** (Fig. 4.3). By contracting or relaxing these intrafusal fibers, the CNS can change the property of the muscle spindle to make it more sensitive to stretch (contracting the intrafusal fibers) or less sensitive to stretch (relaxing the intrafusal fibers). This is known as gamma bias or setting the reflex gain.

The typical muscle spindle has two types of sensory endings, called flow spray endings (type II) and annulospiral endings (type Ia and Ib), that wrap around and within the intrafusal fibers. When the intrafusal fibers contract or lengthen the sensory endings are stimulated. Because the type Ia, Ib, and II sensory endings are located in different areas on the intrafusal fibers, and because each ending is of a different configuration, each sensory ending responds to different types of mechanical

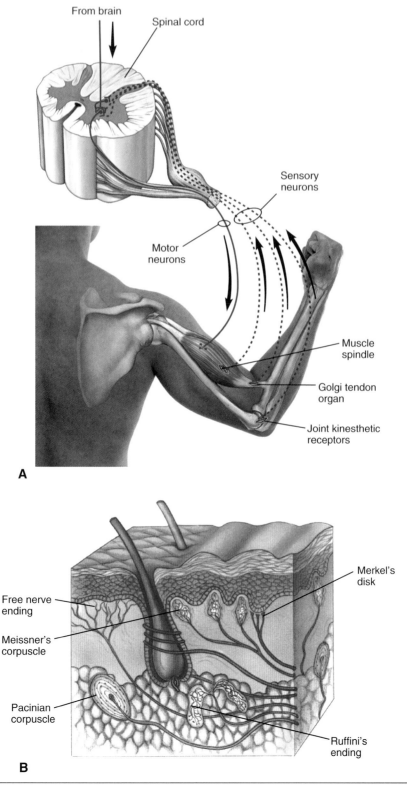

From brain

Spinal cord

Sensory
neurons

Motor
neurons

Muscle
spindle

Golgi tendon
organ

Joint kinesthetic
receptors

A

Merkel's
disk

Free nerve
ending

Meissner's
corpuscle

Pacinian
corpuscle

Ruffini's
ending

B

Figure 4.1 • A. Key proprioceptors and their approximate locations in the muscle and tissues surrounding the joint. Not shown are receptors in the skin. **B.** Types of mechanoreceptors, shown here in the skin, but may be present in ligaments, joint capsule, joint cartilage, and other structures. Each of these receptors, from corpuscles to disks to free endings, responds differently to stimuli, providing different information regarding movement.

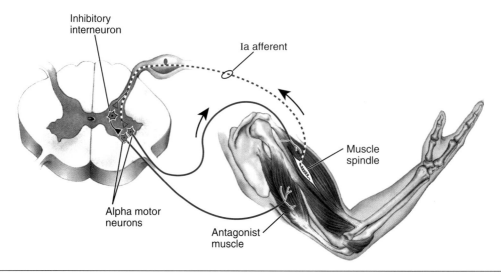

Figure 4.2 • The basic reflex arc illustrated by the stretch reflex. The arc includes a sensory ending (here a muscle spindle), a sensory neuron, a central information processing area (spinal cord), a motor neuron, and an effector organ (muscle). In the diagram, a rapid stretch to the biceps brachii muscle would result in a stretch to the muscle spindle, which would eventually cause a contraction of the homonymous muscle. A reflex circuit may activate other pathways as well; in the illustration, an inhibitory interneuron is excited to cause inhibition to the antagonist muscle (reciprocal inhibition). Reflex arcs from most receptors do not result in overt contraction, but instead may result in a facilitated or inhibited muscle that may be located near or far from the sensory organ.

stimulation and have different sensitivities. The type Ia afferents are the most sensitive and generally provide the most amount of ongoing information, but the other endings also provide information on short and long stretches, rate of stretch, and static length. The muscle spindle can respond to lengthening of the muscle tissue when the muscle is passively stretched, but it also responds when the muscle tissue is shortened by contraction. The ability of the spindle to do this is because the CNS contracts the intrafusal fibers along with the rest of the muscle (extrafusal muscle fibers), thereby maintaining stretch within the spindle itself (see Fig. 4.3 E). Understanding the function of a muscle spindle during different types of contractions is challenging and not always well understood. It is sufficient at this point to note that the interaction among CNS control of the intrafusal fibers, the movement of the surrounding muscles, and the stretch within the muscle spindle itself, enables the brain to monitor and accurately interpret what is going on in the muscle during eccentric, isometric, and concentric contractions, and passive stretch.

■ Thinking It Through 4.1 Controlling Sway

Even during quiet stance people sway forward and back and side to side. This sway appears to be partially regulated by the muscle spindles controlling the amount of contractile stiffness in the leg muscles. When the eyes are closed the amount of sway increases. This increased sway is partially a result of the brain relaxing the intrafusal fibers in the spindle, which makes them much less responsive to stretch. Why would the brain do this? Try to answer on your own, then read through the text for insights to this phenomenon.

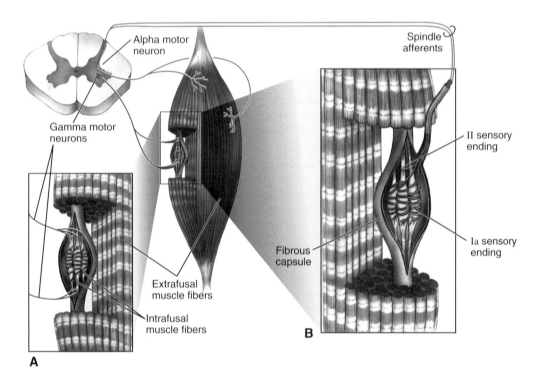

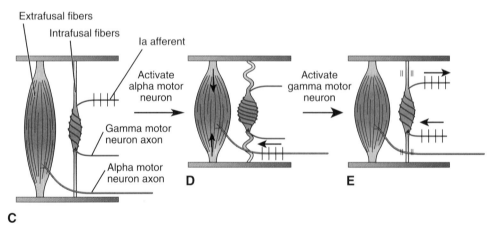

Figure 4.3 • The muscle spindle and its function. **A.** The exploded view of the spindle illustrates the motor innervations of the intrafusal fibers by gamma motor neurons. Note how the intrafusal contractile elements are located at the distal ends of the intrafusal fiber complex. **B.** This view shows the different sensory endings, type Ia and II, that arise from the spindle. The locations and structures of these endings cause them to respond differently depending on the nature of the stretch stimuli. **C.** The muscle under passive stretch causes a stretch to the spindle, resulting in afferent discharge. In this illustration, the passive stretch results in a large discharge from the Ia afferent. **D.** During an active contraction the extrafusal muscle fibers shorten, which would cause the spindle intrafusal fibers to go slack and result in no afferent discharge. This would render the spindle useless. **E.** However, the spindle does not go slack because the intrafusal fibers are contracted via gamma motor neurons alongside the contraction of the extrafusal fibers. Notice that the contraction of the intrafusal fibers, being on the distal ends of the intrafusal complex, causes the middle portion of the complex to stretch out. This stretch activates the sensory endings.

Functions of the Stretch Reflex

When the muscle spindle is activated, either by passive stretch or active contraction, it feeds information back to the spinal cord. In the spinal cord, the sensory signal is routed via monosynaptic connections to the motor units of the homonymous muscle. These signals facilitate the motor units, and if strong enough, cause a stretch reflex response in the homonymous muscle. The facilitation and reflex actions initiated by the muscle spindle are not as simple as most reflex arc diagrams illustrate. Muscle spindle activity is ongoing and plays a direct or indirect role in nearly every movement we make. Some movements, like those involving the stretch–shorten cycle, may make direct use of a strong and rapid stretch reflex response, otherwise known as a phasic response. Other movements, such as postural stabilization, make use of tonic reflex activity, which are moderate and continual reflex actions. In some movements the spindle reflex activity must be inhibited. During most stretch reflex actions, synergist muscles are also facilitated and antagonist muscles are inhibited through a process called **reciprocal inhibition**. On the contralateral limb, there may be an opposite effect on the agonists (inhibited) and antagonists (facilitated), or even distal effects. For example, spindle activity in the soleus may inhibit activity of the quadriceps. This is a complex neural circuit involving many type of interneurons, but it is likely initiated by the standard stretch reflex (Iles & Pardoe, 1999).

The strength of the spindle afferent discharge and any subsequent reflex actions are mediated by many peripheral and central factors. Peripheral muscle factors including the prior amount and type of muscle activity (called **activation history**) and muscle length are just a few factors that influence the mechanical and neural properties of the spindle and thus how it responds to stretch and contraction. At the spinal cord, a complex neural circuitry is used to control the expression of the reflex and reciprocal inhibition. For example, if the ankle dorsiflexors are fatigued then the strength of reciprocal inhibition arising from dorsiflexor spindle activity is increased, making it more difficult to produce a strong contraction of the soleus and gastrocnemius (Sato et al., 1999). Different tasks may alter the amount of reciprocal inhibition, such as hopping producing larger amounts of reciprocal inhibition in the soleus induced by a contraction of the tibialis anterior compared to walking and standing, even when the strength of tibialis anterior contraction is the same (Lavoie et al., 1997).

Prior training, experience, and health may result in different patterns of spindle response. Elders and young adults often have very different reflex responses (Chalmers & Knutzen, 2000). Hoffman and Koceja (1995) showed that stretch reflex gain is modulated by other afferent inputs, such as visual and somatosensory receptors. In particular, with no vision or with unstable support surfaces, the spindle reflex gain is often reduced. With no vision and with unstable surfaces, the authors maintained that supraspinal inputs presynaptically inhibited the stretch reflexes in order to have more central control over posture. An alternative explanation is that the brain enables more cutaneous inputs from the feet to inhibit the reflex.

The overarching point is that the stretch reflex is far more complex than the simple knee jerk reflex. Muscle spindles are constantly at work, and the strength of the reflex action (including reciprocal inhibition) relies on many factors other than the amount of stretch or amount of contraction of the agonist muscle. The reflex characteristics, including proximal and distal facilitatory and inhibitory effects, are influenced by other reflex circuits and controlled by supraspinal centers to match the needs of the task.

THE GOLGI TENDON ORGAN AND REFLEX

Golgi tendon organs (GTOs) are free sensory endings intertwined within tendon fascicles. During stretch to the tendon, the sensory endings distort in a manner consistent with the stretch. Tendons, as opposed to muscle tissue, are very resistant to stretch and require a large amount of force to lengthen. Because of this, the tendon organ is said to act like a force detector more so than a movement or length detector.

Concepts in Action

Controlling the Expression of a Reflex

Control of reflex behavior by the brain to meet specific needs is evident in a very simple experiment. With a partner, evaluate the stiffness of the biceps and triceps brachii muscles during a couple of different contractions. First, sit at a sturdy table anchored to the floor with one hand under the table (palm up) and elbow bent to about 90 degrees. Attempt to lift the table by an elbow flexion action and have your partner palpate your biceps muscle during this action. Now, during this action attempt to contract the triceps muscle while still attempting to lift the table. Have your partner palpate and evaluate the level of contractile stiffness in both muscles. Repeat the experiment except this time push down on the table with a triceps extension movement. Attempt to contract the biceps and palpate both muscles. You should have found that the agonist muscle in either case was highly stiff whereas attempting to contract the antagonist muscle was difficult and was not stiff. This experiment reveals reciprocal inhibition of the agonist muscle inhibiting the antagonist, but does this happen all the time? Now, bend your elbow to about 90 degrees and forcibly contract both biceps and triceps to stiffen your elbow joint. Have your partner palpate for stiffness. They will notice that both muscles are highly stiff, which leads one to wonder if reciprocal inhibition is working. In all these scenarios, the elbow is bent to 90 degrees and an isometric contraction is being performed. The difference is that in the last contraction the biceps and triceps muscles are not acting as agonist–antagonist muscles, but rather, they are acting as synergists. The intent of the first two contractions was to move the table; in the last contraction, the intent was to stabilize the elbow joint. Because of the movement purpose, the muscles act in different roles, and the brain regulates reflex activity. The take-home point here is the intention of a movement with an outcome purpose in mind dictates how the brain will set up the movement.

Neuronal circuitry and early experimental evidence generally reinforces the belief that stimulation of the tendon organ via contraction of the muscle or external forces results in inhibition of the homonymous muscle and its synergists, and facilitates contraction of the antagonist muscle and its synergists. Notice that this **Golgi tendon reflex**, also known as the inverse stretch reflex, does not result in a contraction of the effector organ, and in fact, is said to limit contraction force in order to protect the muscle and joints.

In a review by Chalmers (2002), he concluded that Golgi tendon organ effects are much more complex than initially believed, having both inhibitory and facilitatory effects depending on the movement behavior, contraction type, stretch type (e.g., active vs. passive), and type of muscle involved, such as flexors versus extensors. That the tendon organ can have opposite influences, even on the same muscle, demonstrates **supraspinal** influence over reflex activity. For example, it appears that during novel and high force movements, especially with untrained persons, the tendon organ inhibitory actions override the spindle reflexes to keep the musculoskeletal framework within safety limits. As a consequence of training or experience, it appears that the tendon reflex is inhibited by supraspinal centers, enabling full facilitation by the spindles.

JOINT AND SKIN PROPRIOCEPTORS AND ACTIONS

Within joint tissues and in the skin surrounding most joints are four to five different types of receptors. Those in the joints are specifically referred to as joint kinesthetic receptors. The skin receptors are not classically considered to be proprioceptors, but they do offer movement-related information and are thus considered here to function in part as proprioceptors.

Among the receptor types are **Pacinian corpuscles** found beneath the skin and in ligaments and tendon sheaths. They are stimulated by rapid joint angle changes that put pressure on the corpuscle. **Ruffini endings** are located in the deep skin and in the collagenous fibers of the joint capsule. They respond to continual states of mechanical deformation and provide information on joint position and joint position changes. Other receptors in the skin, such as **free dendritic endings**, respond to touch and pain and can thus act as proprioceptors. In the hands and feet, cutaneous afferents couple with motor neurons controlling actions of the arm/hand and legs/feet. In fact, slight pressure to the fingers can produce relatively strong contractions of digit muscles like the thenar muscles and the flexor digitorum superficialis (McNulty et al., 1999). Receptors on the bottom of the feet contribute to postural control and neuropathic conditions that impair cutaneous sensory information from the feet may contribute to balance problems (van Deursen & Simoneau, 1999).

Except for the hands and fingers, the combined actions of the joint capsule and internal joint kinesthetic receptors often have a strong inhibitory effect on the surrounding musculature, a feature known as **arthrogenic muscle inhibition (AMI)** (Fig. 4.4). AMI is theorized to protect joints from overloading. This is especially the case if the joint already has damage and inflammation, such as the joint receptors in an injured knee inhibiting the quadriceps muscle. It is possible however, that either facilitatory or inhibitory effects may result from AMI depending on the exact nature of injury. For example, if the anterior cruciate ligament (ACL) is damaged, the hamstrings may be facilitated to help take over ACL function.

AMI has consequences for muscle function and performance. Ongoing inhibition of the quadriceps may result in weakness, motor dyscontrol, and eventually, muscle atrophy (Hopkins et al., 2001). In the shoulder, a mild stimulus to parts of the glenohumeral capsule (primarily the anterior portion and glenohumeral ligament) produces a strong and relatively long-lasting inhibition to the surrounding musculature (Voigt et al., 1998). Addressing these reflexes is a key component of any orthopedic rehabilitation program and is discussed in more detail in the final chapters of this book.

VESTIBULAR AND NECK PROPRIOCEPTORS AND RIGHTING REFLEXES

Vestibular receptors, known also as **labyrinthine receptors**, detect the movement of fluid contained in the labyrinth of the inner ear (Fig. 4.5). Fluid movement is caused by head and body movement relative to gravity, and velocity and acceleration of head movements. They act as mini gyroscopes in the head serving as major contributors helping maintain balance and equilibrium. Neck receptors are located in the joints, muscles, and ligaments of the neck and provide information on head and neck position. The neck receptors work in conjunction with the vestibular receptors to help maintain balance and equilibrium.

Reflexes initiated by vestibular and neck systems are called righting reflexes, because they help "right" one's orientation during falling or other non-upright positions. Righting involves reorienting the head, and specific patterns of leg and arm reflex activation to prevent or prepare for falling. According to Kandel et al. (2000), the **vestibulocollic** and **cervicocollic** reflexes in a forward lean will cause contraction of the dorsal neck muscles to bring the head into an upright position. **Vestibulospinal** reflexes in a forward fall or lean will cause arm extension and flexion of lower limbs, which is a response to brace for the fall (arms) and prevent or limit the fall (legs). On the other hand, **cervicospinal** reflexes in a forward head tilt will cause arm flexion, which is antagonistic to the vestibular vestibulospinal reflex. There are many other variations of these reflexes, depending on the direction of head tilt and overall positioning of the legs and trunk (Fig. 4.6). These reflexes are among the first seen in infants and are among the most suppressed or modified when learning new skills.

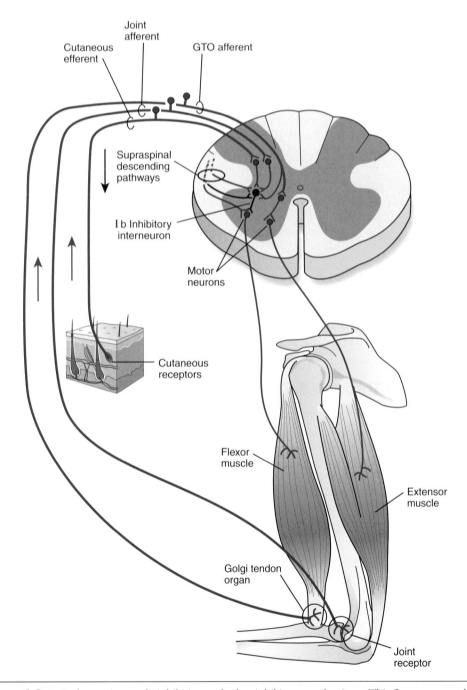

Figure 4.4 • Arthrogenic muscle inhibition and other inhibitory mechanisms. This figure, as complex as it may seem, highly simplifies the spinal reflexive circuits contributing to AMI. Sensory information arising from the tendon organ, joint receptors, and skin receptors, converge to excite spinal inhibitory interneurons. These interneurons, in turn, inhibit agonist muscle activity. Descending supraspinal commands may reinforce this inhibition or override it.

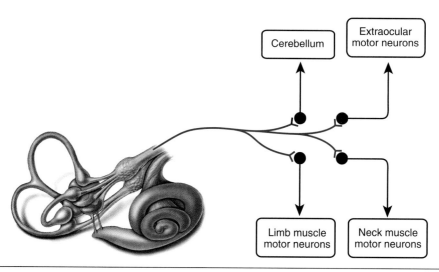

Figure 4.5 • Fluid movement in the circular structures of the labyrinthine system of the inner ear stimulates sensory endings. These endings detect rotational movements, head tilt, and acceleration in any direction. Sensory outflow from the receptors travel to the cerebellum, leg and arm motor neurons, neck motor neurons, and to the motor neurons that control extraocular muscles of the eyes.

■ Thinking It Through 4.2 The Kohnstamm Phenomenon and Neck Reflexes

In humans, righting reflexes are mostly overridden during normal activity, but sometimes, they can be brought out with a little manipulation. One way is by eliciting the postcontraction aftereffect, also called the Kohnstamm phenomenon. The Kohnstamm phenomenon is an involuntary contraction that lingers after a vigorous isometric contraction. Ongoing cortical (Duclos et al., 2007) and spinal (Mathis et al., 1996) facilitation are suggested to be the reason for the ongoing contraction. The phenomenon is most often elicited by standing with arms down at the side and pressing out (abduct) with high effort with both arms against an immovable object for about 30 seconds. This is easy to do by standing in a corner or in a narrow doorway.

To investigate cervicospinal reflexes, first elicit the Kohnstamm effect under normal circumstances. Work with several other students to get a good idea of the responses, and understand that not everyone has the same strength of response (see Ivanenko et al., 2006). Stand in a corner or doorway and press out hard with a shoulder abduction action for about 30 seconds. Then step straight ahead out of the doorway/corner and observe what happens to your arms. Do not turn your head, but look straight ahead. Wait a couple of minutes to allow the phenomenon to wear off, and do the experiment again. This time, as you step away from the doorway/corner, rotate your head sharply to the right and hold it there. Note what happens to both arms. It is necessary to test a number of people to see the variation in responses. The typical response is that the right arm will abduct higher or faster than before, and the left arm will not rise up; but if you test enough people, you will find that some may have the exact opposite effect. Can you explain the normal response, based on Figure 4.6? Can you explain why some people do not have the "normal" response?

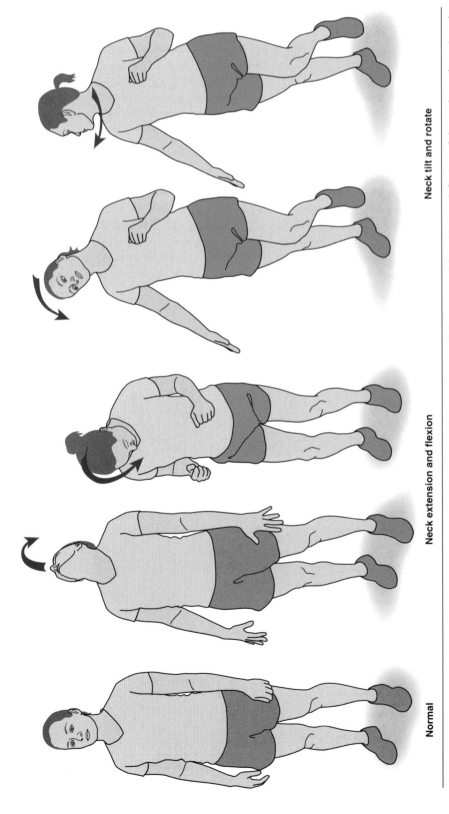

Normal   **Neck extension and flexion**   **Neck tilt and rotate**

Figure 4.6 • Neck reflex action. Backward extension of the neck produces extension of the arms and legs. Forward flexion of the neck produces just the opposite, flexion of the arms and legs. Rotation or tilting of the head to one side produces extension of the arms and legs on that side, and flexion of the limbs on the contralateral side. (Based on Tokizane, T., Murao, M., Ogata, T., & Kondo, T. (1951). Electromyographic studies on tonic neck, lumbar, and labyrinthine reflexes in normal persons. *Japanese Journal of Physiology, 2,* 130–146.)

OTHER IMPORTANT REFLEX MOVEMENTS

Receptor reflex responses rarely work alone and are generally coupled with other reflexes and automatic and voluntary movement behaviors. Consider, for instance, teeth clenching during high-strength movements. Takada et al. (2000) found that teeth clenching facilitates the reflex responses in the lower leg muscles, and reciprocal inhibition between the soleus and pretibial muscles is abolished. The sum total of this effect enables the lower leg to be highly stiffened, perhaps to stabilize the body's posture.

The actions of many sensory endings are to reinforce or inhibit other reflexes. Three well-researched reflexes, the extensor thrust reflex, the withdrawal reflex, and the crossed extensor reflex, provide notable examples of this reflex integration. In the extensor thrust reflex, pressure on somatoreceptors, particularly in the hands and feet, cause a reflex contraction, or facilitation, of extension muscles in that limb. During a pushing movement, the extensor muscles continue to be reflex facilitated, which can strengthen the extension movement. Just the opposite happens with the flexor or withdrawal reflex. This reflex is initiated primarily by nociceptors in response to a pain stimulus like a sharp poke or burn. These receptors signal proximal limb flexor muscles to contract in order to withdraw from the pain stimulus.

The crossed extensor reflex (Fig. 4.7) combines the withdrawal reflex with an extensor thrust in the contralateral limb, and only functions in weight-bearing limbs. Activation of nociceptors or

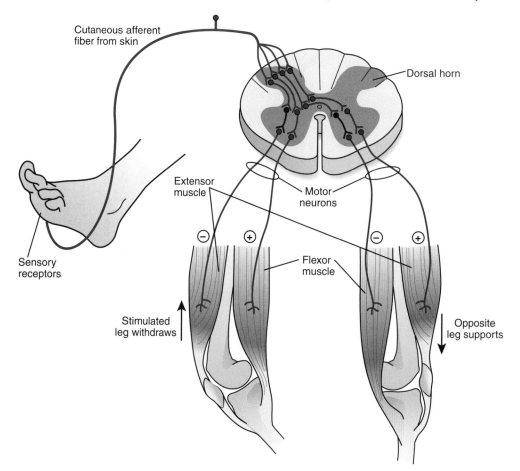

Figure 4.7 • The crossed extensor reflex. Stimulation of nociceptors in the skin of the feet exerts a strong and widespread reflex action. Flexor muscles of the stimulated leg contract to pull the leg up off the painful stimulus, while extensor muscles of the same leg are inhibited. Conversely, the opposite leg must support the full body weight and thus the extensor muscles are reflex activated.

pressure receptors causes flexion of that limb, and extension of the contralateral limb. This allows the body to maintain balance. For example, if the foot steps onto a nail, that leg would flex up and off the nail, the other leg would extend to compensate for the body weight being placed on it.

VISUAL SYSTEMS

Vision often provides the most dominant feedback information to the brain. In most cases, visual information can override any other feedback source, though there are task-specific cases when other systems, like auditory, can override vision (Burr et al., 2009). Visual feedback provides rapid information on the correctness of ongoing movements and relatively precise information on the effectiveness of movement outcomes. Vision provides two other benefits that are unmatched by other sensory systems. The first is that vision can provide the most exteroceptive information about the environment that is separate from the body itself and does not involve the body. For example, watching a distant scene unfold may have nothing to do with the individual's body, but it may influence the individual to act should they decide to do so. In such a case, vision is said to provide feedforward information because information is not being fed back to the CNS from actions within the body, but rather, provides advance knowledge on upcoming situations. Although other receptors can provide information on the immediate external environment, such as skin receptors detecting wind, temperature, and object tactile features only hearing and vision can provide such distant "out of body" information. The second feature is nervous system control over the receptor itself. The nervous system can modify muscle spindle gain, but this is nowhere near the control the nervous system has over vision function. The actual receptor—the entire eye structure—can be modified to control the light stimulus by changing pupil size, changing lens shape, moving the eyeball, and opening and closing of the eyelids.

The basic structure of the eye system is shown in Figure 4.8. Light enters though the tough outer casing called the cornea, which does have some light focusing properties. The light then proceeds through the opening called the pupil. The pupil opening is controlled by the movement of the iris, which allows more or less light into the lens. The lens focuses the light image toward the retina, which contains the actual light-sensitive receptors (photoreceptors). Two different kinds of photoreceptors, rods and cones, react differently to shades of light and dark (rods), color and acuity (cones). Distribution of rods and cones on the retina create different areas on the retina that respond to different patterns of light, for example, the high density of cones in the foveal region of the retina enable much better visual acuity when light is focused on that area. Overall, the amount of light, the focus of the light on different spots on the retina, the color of the images, and the changing gradations of light and dark provide ongoing information about object size, shape, and a myriad of other factors for object identification. This information is sent via the optic nerve to the visual cortex, which is a very large sensory processing region in the back of the brain. As mentioned in Chapter 2, visual processing is very complex and includes two distinct systems of processing of identification of objects sent along a ventral stream to temporal areas of the brain and localization of objects via the dorsal stream to parietal regions.

Focal and Ambient Vision

The construction of the retina enables the central part of the visual field to be highly acute (foveal or central vision) and the surrounding field to be less sharp (peripheral vision). Visual information detected from both systems is used and processed in two very different ways. This information can be categorized as **focal vision** and **ambient vision**, the distinction being how the brain gathers visual information and uses it. Focal vision is highly dependent on foveal vision, and is largely based on the most visually sharp information gathered from the center of the visual field (Horrey et al., 2006; Schmidt & Wrisberg, 2007). Focal vision is considered a consciously aware process controlled by voluntary processing, and is primarily used to identify objects and details in small spaces. Degraded focal vision may occur if one attempts to attend to and identify objects in peripheral vision, and when there are low light situations. For these

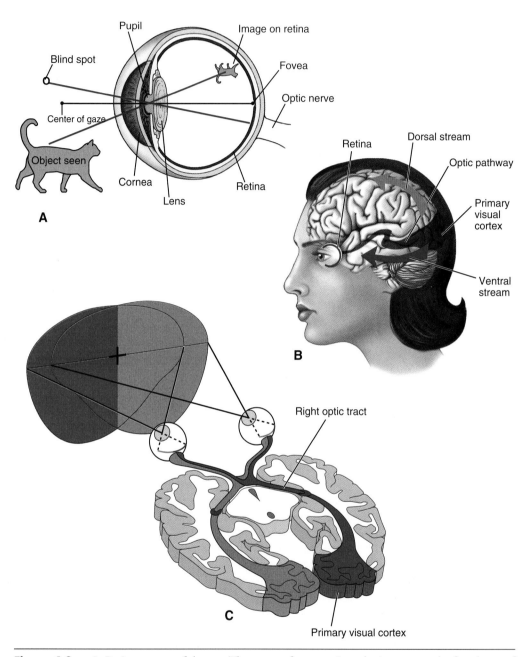

Figure 4.8 • **A.** Basic anatomy of the eye. The center of gaze projects the image onto the foveal part of the retina, where it is best focused. Outside of the foveal projection is peripheral vision. Peripheral images are projected to other parts of the retina. Voluntary control over how the eye works includes changing pupil opening size, altering lens shape, and even opening and closing the eyelids to regulate flow of light. **B.** Pathways of visual processing are shown going to the visual cortex and then out to parietal regions via the dorsal stream and to temporal regions via the ventral stream. **C.** Schematic illustrating that retinal images are sent to both left and right visual cortexes, enabling binocular visual processing for depth perception.

reasons, focal vision is dependent on eye movements, known as gaze, to maintain sharpness and light patterns. (Horrey et al., 2006). On the other hand, ambient vision is visual information implicitly gathered without conscious awareness or attention being specifically focused. Ambient visual information comes from both foveal and peripheral vision, stimulates the entire retina, and is active and useful even in low light (Schmidt & Wrisberg, 2007). Brain scans have revealed that ambient visual processing is distributed widely throughout the brain and thus likely involved in all other perceptual processing (Previc et al., 2000). Ambient vision is to gather information on the relationship between objects, distances, and motion. It is this information that provides one with knowledge of the width of a doorway as they approach it, the location and distance of a coffee mug that is set off to the side of a table.

During motor actions, both focal and ambient systems are working. Focal vision rapidly changes from one moment to the next as individuals direct their gaze from one object in the environment to another. In sport, for example, athletes view the field of play using specific strategies to recognize patterns and find and interpret information. This process, called **visual search**, gives the performer information that enables them to anticipate actions that makes for faster information processing and subsequently more efficient and more appropriate movements.

Visual search also provides a field of view from which to gather ambient visual information. As the eye moves, either from its own intrinsic movements or from motion of the head, and as objects in the environment move, the pattern of light striking the retina changes constantly. This constant influx of changing light is a feature of the ambient visual system called **optical flow**, and is thought to play a strong role in maintaining posture and balance, and provide constant information on motion (velocity, direction, time to contact) of surrounding objects and of the body within the environment. This motion information is critical in ensuring head orientation and monitoring body sway, and provides for very rapid postural corrections to maintain balance (Guerraz & Bronstein, 2008; Wade & Jones, 1997). Though focal and ambient vision occurs simultaneously, they are processed differently and their use is task specific. For instance, certain driving tasks like instrument reading and hazard response are only done effectively with focal vision, while other tasks like lane keeping can be easily done with ambient vision alone (Horrey et al., 2006).

The feedforward information provided by both focal and ambient vision holds particular relevance in motor skill performance because of time to contact information. Time to contact involves hitting targets (especially moving targets), intercepting oncoming objects (e.g., catching a ball), and general hand–eye coordination. A particular characteristic of optical flow, called **tau**, concerns the rate of change of the size of an object's image projected on the retina as the object is moving toward the eye. The rate of change is related to the velocity of the object, thus providing critical motion information and time of impending contact with the object.

Ambient vision appears critical in determining interceptive actions, but the stability and usefulness of this subconscious visual system may be dependent on the stability of the focal vision that enables the optical flow to be better interpreted. For example, focusing visual attention on a ball release or body action of an opposing pitcher coupled with tracking the ball enables a batter to anticipate speed and direction of the ball, but ambient optical flow enables the batter to more precisely and rapidly determine these flight characteristics and thus provide information to the batter when to swing the bat (Coker, 2009). The case of hitting an oncoming ball is an example of **anticipation timing**, which is when an individual begins whole-body or limb movements in accord with an external reference, often for an interceptive action.

Feedback Mechanisms of Vision

Vision provides for an abundance of feedback regarding ongoing movements and the outcomes of movement execution. As we saw above, ambient vision provides for direct postural correction and balance control. According to Schmidt and Wrisberg (2007), ambient and focal vision feedback is used

SIDE**NOTE**	**MEASURING VISUAL SEARCH**

It has only been within the past 10 to 15 years that visual search has been able to be experimentally verified in real-life situations. The development of gaze tracking devices that monitor pupil movement has advanced to eyewear style devices that are now being used for both research and training. The device shown below is being worn during driving to evaluate the gaze tracking of a driver (photos courtesy of Applied Science Laboratories, Bedford, MA). Computer software enables the gaze focal point to be projected over the entire image in view. Practitioners are using eye tracking software to train drivers, surgeons, athletes, and other professionals, although at this time the efficacy of such training has yet to be fully researched.

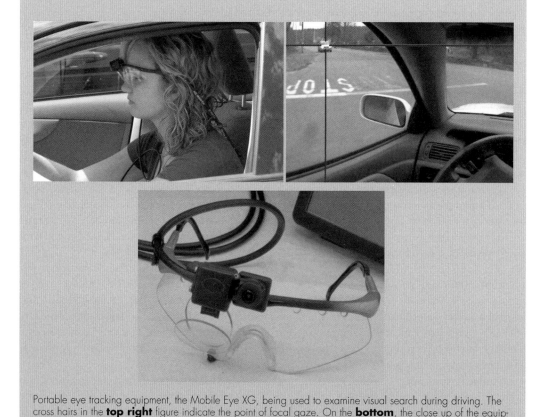

Portable eye tracking equipment, the Mobile Eye XG, being used to examine visual search during driving. The cross hairs in the **top right** figure indicate the point of focal gaze. On the **bottom**, the close up of the equipment shows a small video camera to record the entire field of view, and the special mirror and video system to record the movement of the pupil. (Images courtesy of ASL, Applied Science Laboratories, Bedford, MA.)

and evaluated differently by the brain. In their model, focal vision feedback is sent back to higher brain centers involved in planning movement, whereas ambient information is routed to brain areas involved in initiating movement and to a lesser extent, planning. Visual information is constantly integrating with other sensory information to provide a reference point of the body to the environment and ongoing self-motion calibration.

As one might expect, visual feedback of movement actions, from watching a golf ball slice off into the woods to an intense gaze of threading a needle, provides an immense amount of information from which movements can be altered for later performance or altered while ongoing. In the case of ongoing movements, such as threading the needle, visual feedback may come with a delay of 100 to 160 ms (Magill, 2006). If this delay seems long, it is because of the vast visual feedback circuits in the brain that far outnumber feedforward circuits (Shou, 2010).

We discussed above that the motion information provided by both focal and ambient vision enables feedforward information, that is, information that directly gives rise to a predictive or feedforward motor commands. This same motion information also gives continuous feedback information regarding ongoing movements. For instance, long jumpers approaching the take-off board (Lee et al., 1982) and gymnasts approaching the vault (Bradshaw, 2004) adjust each of the last few strides to hone in on hitting the take-off area in the most advantageous position. Regulation of gait timing and location is based on visual information that changes rapidly during the sprint to the board. In fact, Bradshaw (2004) believes that practicing stereotyped approach runs in gymnastics vaulting diminishes the use of visual feedback and leads to less successful vaulting performance.

SENSORY AND MOTOR INTEGRATION

Sensory receptors provide invaluable information to the CNS regarding the internal body environment and the actions of the body in the external environment. Feedback information from multiple sensory sources, proprioceptors and nonproprioceptors alike, provide multimodal information to the spinal cord and brain. Unless this vast array of information is filtered and encoded at both the spinal and supraspinal levels, it cannot be used effectively in the process of planning coordinated movement actions. **Sensory integration** is the process of filtering and encoding multiple sources of sensory information in order to better interpret and understand events.

The ability of the brain and spinal cord to integrate multimodal information to produce accurate and complete information is a highly learned process. Even the simple recognition and identification of a common object typically requires at least two modalities (e.g., touch and vision), but the ability to accurately integrate just these two sensory sources does not begin until about 8 years of age (Gori et al., 2008). In cases like this, one sensory modality "teaches" perception of the other modality, giving it richness and meaning. For instance, visual perception of a glass of water with condensation on its side provides little meaning other than size and shape. Touching and lifting the glass provide evidence of coldness, slipperiness, and weight. Visual perception subsequently interprets a pattern of water droplets on the side of the glass to reveal coldness and thus a cup filled with something cold, and even refreshing.

As we saw in Chapter 2, the CNS integrates this sensory information with motor commands in a process called sensorimotor integration. Sensorimotor integration has two overarching functions. The first is the use of motor commands and movements to enhance sensory information. Moving a hand through water provides information on the water's viscosity, resistance to movement, and ultimately, the nature of subsequent motor acts. In the cold glass example above, the motor act of lifting the glass results in useful sensory information. The second function, and most well known, is the coupling and relationship between incoming sensory information and outgoing motor actions. In healthy individuals, sensory information is paired with appropriate motor actions, such as increased muscle stiffness during walking when the support surface is seen or felt as unstable. Figure 4.9 illustrates the sensory and motor convergence in the spinal cord contributing to walking. During irregular or absent sensory information, the healthy sensorimotor system adapts by placing greater emphasis, or weighting, on some information, and less on others. An example of sensory weighting can be observed during quiet stance while manipulating visual information and tactile information from the fingers that are orienting the body to an external reference. Suddenly removing vision or tactile information leads to demonstrable changes in leg muscle activation patterns as the body tries to reconfigure the motor response to match up with the available sensory information (Sozzi et al., 2012).

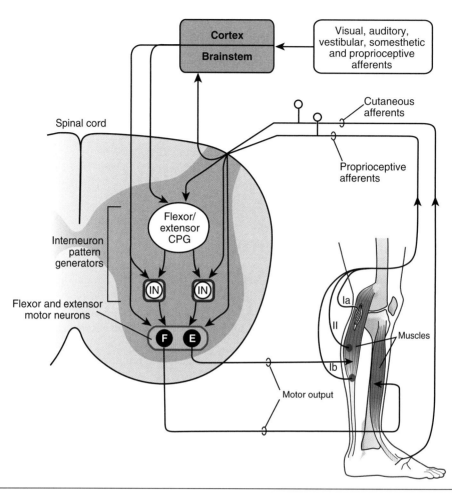

Figure 4.9 • A schematic illustration of sensorimotor interactions causing the rhythmic actions of the anterior tibialis (ankle flexor) and triceps surae (ankle extensor) muscles during walking. Motor commands originate from the motor cortex and from brain stem regions. The nature and timing of these signals are modified from ascending proprioceptive, cutaneous, vestibular, auditory, and visual sensory inputs. Some descending motor commands may directly input onto lower motor neurons, and some, most likely originating from the brain stem, may activate spinal central pattern generators (CPGs, see Chapter 5) and other spinal interneuron circuits. Sensory feedback from the moving limb and muscles (e.g., muscle spindle, foot cutaneous afferents) may influence the spinal motor commands at the spinal pattern generator level, or directly onto lower motor neurons. This influence may be to inhibit or cause facilitatory drive to neurons or pattern generators. (Adapted from Rossignol, S., Dubuc, R., & Gossard, J. (2006). Dynamic sensorimotor interactions in locomotion. *Physiological Reviews*, 86(1), 89–154. doi: 10.1152/physrev.00028.2005, Figure 1, p. 91.)

Disorders in sensorimotor integration are suggested to be important elements in disordered movements seen in patients with Parkinson's disease, Huntington's disease, and related focal dystonia neurological disorders (Abbruzzese & Berardelli, 2003). These disorders are characterized by uncontrolled muscle twitches, tics, and larger movements. Malfunctioning in filtering and screening incoming sensory information and errors in cortical interpretation of multiple sources of information, lead to sensory overflow, hyperactive reflexes, and a mismatch between incoming sensory information and outcome motor commands.

Concepts in Action

Exploiting Multimodal Sensory Information

When two (bimodal) or more (multimodal) stimuli arrive at or very near the same time, a person's reaction time can be faster than with just a single stimulus. This phenomenon, known as intersensory facilitation, is commonly observed when both auditory and visual stimuli arrive within about 100 ms of one another (Nickerson, 1973). How this happens has yet to be confirmed, but brain imaging data support the hypothesis that multiple sensory signals converge in areas of the brain and increase the overall level of neural activation (Gondon et al., 2005). It has been further suggested that the first, or accessory, signal provides information to enhance neural processing of the second stimulus, and then convergence takes place (Colonius & Arndt, 2001). Ives and Hong (2003) wondered if the superfast reaction speed during bimodal intersensory facilitation could be learned and thus take effect even during a single (unimodal) stimulus. The implication of this could be for sprinters to improve reaction time by training with multiple stimuli that would then transfer to the track or pool where only a single auditory stimulus is used. These researchers trained subjects over 4 days in a whole-body reaction time task using unimodal or bimodal stimuli. Even after 4 days of training with the bimodal superfast reaction times, reaction times slowed down to normal speed when tested with a single stimulus. These authors concluded that the multimodal sensory input was required to generate the faster neural processing, rather than being self-generated through learning.

SUMMARY

Peripheral sensory systems, namely, proprioception and vision, play a critical role in the production of motor skills by feeding information back to the CNS regarding movement and by directly initiating reflex movements that subserve voluntary movements. The monitoring of movements and subsequent feedback enables the CNS to critically evaluate its movement planning and thus serves as a basis to modify ongoing movements, plan upcoming movements, and learn to produce better movements. Not all somatosensory receptors directly cause reflex actions, but nearly all directly or indirectly influence muscle activity by inhibitory or facilitatory actions. Reflexes constantly work in the background and in many cases reinforce voluntary motor acts, but in some cases must be inhibited by supraspinal centers to enable the execution of motor skills. Though some reflexes are stable and predictable, multimodal inputs and supraspinal control over reflex activity lead to the expression of reflexes that can differ greatly from one circumstance to the next, or from one person to another.

The muscle spindle is considered the most important proprioceptor due to the strong reflex action it produces, its relatively high sensitivity to stimuli, its ability to respond to both muscle stretch and contraction, and its ability to be controlled by the CNS. Other proprioceptors, namely, the GTO, the vestibular apparatus, and joint kinesthetic receptors, play more specific roles in feedback and reflex initiation. Of all sensory systems vision plays the most dominant role. The type and amount of information provided by visual systems and the controllability of vision by the CNS are unmatched by other sensory systems. The structure of the eye enables both focal and ambient visual information, both of which play key roles in feedforward and feedback. Focal vision provides for object identification for use in feedforward control, and provides feedback used in the highest centers of information processing. Ambient vision is subconscious and enables the brain to continually monitor movement and one's place in the environment. This information is used to a great extent in tracking of objects and the timing of actions to correspond to environmental circumstances. Feedback from ambient vision is generally used much faster in movement initiation and may provide for more immediate muscle responses such as those seen in balanced corrections.

Though each of these proprioceptor types and visual systems provide a degree of stereotyped actions based on the stimuli they receive, this should not be interpreted that reflex responses or interpretation of the feedback information is stereotyped. It must be recognized that internal and environmental circumstances and situational needs may lead to very different reflex responses and use of sensory information.

STUDY QUESTIONS

1. Identify specific tissue locations where proprioceptors lie.
2. What is the difference between a stretch reflex phasic response and a tonic response?
3. What process allows the muscle spindle to continue to be effective in detecting and sending sensory information even though the muscle shortens during a contraction?
4. Consider that two different people slip and fall because of the exact same stimuli, but their leg actions are entirely different. During the fall one person extends his legs, the other person flexes her legs. Can you explain this phenomenon?
5. Following spinning movements that make one dizzy, what mechanisms cause an arm to be thrust out to gain balance?
6. How are sensory receptors classified? Explain the differences in the types of receptors within each classification.
7. A person has an injured knee joint. Even though the surrounding musculature is intact, the person cannot produce much knee extension force. Why?
8. Describe the differences between focal vision and ambient vision. Detail how each of these systems work and what kinds of information they provide.
9. Compare visual sensory systems to proprioceptive systems. How do these differ in respect to the functioning of the receptors themselves and in the information they provide?
10. What is multisensory integration and how does it play a role in sensorimotor integration? Give examples.
11. What is optic flow and how does it factor into tau, motion perception, and anticipation timing?
12. What is visual search and how does it play a role in focal vision and ambient vision?

References

Abbruzzese, G., & Berardelli, A. (2003). Sensorimotor integration in movement disorders. *Movement Disorders*, *18*(3), 231–240.

Allegrucci, M. M., Whitney, S. L., Lephart, S. M., Irrgang, J. J., & Fu, F. H. (1995). Shoulder kinesthesia in healthy unilateral athletes participating in upper extremity sports. *Journal of Orthopaedic and Sports Physical Therapy*, *21*(4), 220–226.

Barrett, L., Quigley, K. S., Bliss-Moreau, E., & Aronson, K. R. (2004). Interoceptive sensitivity and self-reports of emotional experience. *Journal of Personality and Social Psychology*, *87*(5), 684–697.

Berntson, G., Sarter, M., & Cacioppo, J. (2003). Ascending visceral regulation of cortical affective information processing. *European Journal of Neuroscience*, *18*(8), 2103–2109.

Bradshaw, E. (2004). Target-directed running in gymnastics: A preliminary exploration of vaulting. *Sports Biomechanics*, *3*(1), 125–144.

Burr, D., Banks, M., & Morrone, M. (2009). Auditory dominance over vision in the perception of interval duration. *Experimental Brain Research*, *198*(1), 49–57.

Chalmers, G. (2002). Do Golgi tendon organs really inhibit muscle activity at high force levels to save muscles from injury, and adapt with strength training? *Sports Biomechanics*, *1*(2), 239–249.

Chalmers, G., & Knutzen, K. (2000). Soleus Hoffmann-reflex modulation during walking in healthy elderly and young adults. *Journals of Gerontology. Biological Sciences and Medical Sciences*, *55*(12), B570–B579.

Coker, C. H. (2009). *Motor learning and control for practitioners*. Scottsdale, AZ: Holcomb Hathaway Publishers.

Colonius, H., & Arndt, P. (2001). A two-stage model for visual-auditory interaction in saccadic latencies. *Perception & Psychophysics*, *63*, 126–147.

Craig, A. (2003). Interoception: The sense of the physiological condition of the body. *Current Opinion in Neurobiology*, *13*(4), 500–505.

Duclos, C., Roll, R., Kavounoudias, A., & Roll, J. (2007). Cerebral correlates of the "Kohnstamm phenomenon": An fMRI study. *Neuroimage*, *34*(2), 774–783.

Freeman, M. M., & Broderick, P. P. (1996). Kinaesthetic sensitivity of adolescent male and female athletes and non-athletes. *Australian Journal of Science and Medicine in Sport*, *28*(2), 46–49.

Gondon, M., Niederhaus, B., Rösler, F., & Röder, B. (2005). Multisensory processing in the redundant-target effect: A behavioral and event-related potential study. *Perception & Psychophysics*, *67*(4), 713–726.

Gori, M., Del Viva, M., Sandini, G., & Burr, D. (2008). Young children do not integrate visual and haptic form information. *Current Biology*, *18*(9), 694–698.

Guerraz, M., & Bronstein, A. (2008). Ocular versus extraocular control of posture and equilibrium. *Clinical Neurophysiology*, *38*(6), 391–398.

Hoffman, M., & Koceja, D. (1995). The effects of vision and task complexity on Hoffmann reflex gain. *Brain Research*, *700*(1–2), 303–307.

Hogervorst, T., & Brand, R. (1998). Mechanoreceptors in joint function. *Journal of Bone and Joint Surgery*, *80*(9), 1365–1378.

Hopkins, J. T., Ingersoll, C. D., Krause, B. A., Edwards, J. E., & Cordova, M. L. (2001). Effect of knee joint effusion on quadriceps and soleus motoneuron pool excitability. *Medicine and Science in Sports and Exercise*, *33*(1), 123–126.

Horrey, W., Wickens, C., & Consalus, K. (2006). Modeling drivers' visual attention allocation while interacting with in-vehicle technologies. *Journal of Experimental Psychology. Applied*, *12*(2), 67–78.

Houtveen, J., Rietveld, S., & de Geus, E. (2003). Exaggerated perception of normal physiological responses to stress and hypercapnia in young women with numerous functional somatic symptoms. *Journal of Psychosomatic Research*, *55*(6), 481–490.

Iles, J., & Pardoe, J. (1999). Changes in transmission in the pathway of heteronymous spinal recurrent inhibition from soleus to quadriceps motor neurons during movement in man. *Brain*, *122*(Pt 9), 1757–1764.

Ivanenko, Y., Wright, W., Gurfinkel, V., Horak, F., & Cordo, P. (2006). Interaction of involuntary post-contraction activity with locomotor movements. *Experimental Brain Research*, *169*(2), 255–260.

Ives, J. C., & Hong, S. L. (2003). Fast reaction times with intersensory facilitation do not transfer to single stimulus conditions. *Journal of Sport and Exercise Psychology*, *25*(Suppl), 678.

Kandel, E. R., Schwartz, J. H., & Jessell, T. M. (Eds.). (2000). *Principles of neuroscience*. New York: McGraw-Hill.

Lavoie, B., Devanne, H., & Capaday, C. (1997). Differential control of reciprocal inhibition during walking versus postural and voluntary motor tasks in humans. *Journal of Neurophysiology*, *78*(1), 429–438.

Lee, D. N., Lishman, J., & Thomson, J. A. (1982). Regulation of gait in long jumping. *Journal of Experimental Psychology: Human Perception and Performance*, *8*(3), 448–459.

Lephart, S. M., Giraldo, J. L., Borsa, P. A., & Fu, F. H. (1996). Knee joint proprioception: A comparison between female intercollegiate gymnasts and controls. *Knee Surgery, Sports Traumatology, Arthroscopy*, *4*(2), 121–124.

Magill, R.A. (2006). *Motor learning and control: Concepts and applications*. New York: McGraw-Hill.

Mathis, J., Gurfinkel, V., & Struppler, A. (1996). Facilitation of motor evoked potentials by postcontraction response (Kohnstamm phenomenon). *Electroencephalography and Clinical Neurophysiology*, *101*(4), 289–297.

McNulty, P., Türker, K., & Macefield, V. (1999). Evidence for strong synaptic coupling between single tactile afferents and motoneurones supplying the human hand. *Journal of Physiology*, *518*(Pt 3), 883–893.

Nickerson, R. S. (1973). Intersensory facilitation of reaction time: Energy summation or preparation enhancement. *Psychological Review*, *80*, 489–509.

Paulus, M. P., Flagan, T., Simmons, A. N., Gillis, K., Kotturi, S., Thom, N., et al. (2012). Subjecting elite athletes to inspiratory breathing load reveals behavioral and neural signatures of optimal performers in extreme environments. *PLoS One*, *7*(1), doi:10.1371/journal.pone.0029394

Previc, F., Beer, J., Liotti, M., Blakemore, C., & Fox, P. (2000). Is "ambient vision" distributed in the brain? Effects of wide-field-view visual yaw motion on PET activation. *Journal of Vestibular Research: Equilibrium & Orientation, 10*(4–5), 221–225.

Rietveld, S., & Houtveen, J. (2004). Acquired sensitivity to relevant physiological activity in patients with chronic health problems. *Behaviour Research and Therapy, 42*(2), 137–153.

Sato, T., Tsuboi, T., Miyazaki, M., & Sakamoto, K. (1999). Post-tetanic potentiation of reciprocal Ia inhibition in human lower limb. *Journal of Electromyography and Kinesiology, 9*(1), 59–66.

Schmidt, R. A., & Wrisberg, C. A. (2007). *Motor learning and performance: A situation-based learning approach.* Champaign, IL: Human Kinetics.

Shou, T. (2010). The functional roles of feedback projections in the visual system. *Neuroscience Bulletin, 26*(5), 401–410.

Sozzi, S., Do, M., Monti, A., & Schieppati, M. (2012). Sensorimotor integration during stance: Processing time of active or passive addition or withdrawal of visual or haptic information. *Neuroscience, 212,* 59–76.

Starosta, W. W., Aniol-Strzyzewska, K. K., Fostiak, D. D., Jablonowska, E. E., Krzesinski, S. S., & Pawlowa-Starosta, T. T. (1989). Precision of kinesthetic sensation—element of diagnosis of performance of advanced competitors. *Biology of Sport, 6*(Suppl 3), 265–271.

Takada, Y., Miyahara, T., Tanaka, T., Ohyama, T., & Nakamura, Y. (2000). Modulation of H reflex of pretibial muscles and reciprocal Ia inhibition of soleus muscle during voluntary teeth clenching in humans. *Journal of Neurophysiology, 83*(4), 2063–2070.

van Deursen, R., & Simoneau, G. (1999). Foot and ankle sensory neuropathy, proprioception, and postural stability. *Journal of Orthopaedic and Sports Physical Therapy, 29*(12), 718–726.

Voigt, M., Jakobsen, J., & Sinkjaer, T. (1998). Non-noxious stimulation of the glenohumeral joint capsule elicits strong inhibition of active shoulder muscles in conscious human subjects. *Neuroscience Letters, 254*(2), 105–108.

Wade, M., & Jones, G. (1997). The role of vision and spatial orientation in the maintenance of posture. *Physical Therapy, 77*(6), 619–628.

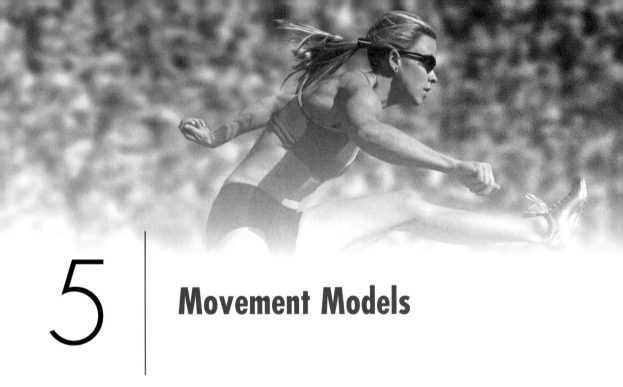

5 | Movement Models

PURPOSE, IMPORTANCE, AND OBJECTIVES OF THIS CHAPTER

The purpose of this chapter is to examine models of movement as ways to understand and explain the vast complexities of planning, initiating, executing, and monitoring movement. A comprehensive and cohesive view of the entire movement process afforded by modeling enables researchers and practitioners alike to address movement issues and problems with greater understanding and insight.

After reading this chapter, you should be able to:

1. Describe motor abundance and the degrees of freedom problem.
2. Explain the purpose of models from research and applied standpoints.
3. Compare and contrast open- and closed-loop systems and what models fit within these systems.
4. Define and explain the terms generalized motor program, central pattern generator, schema, reflex model, and internal model.
5. Explain and provide examples of synergies and coordinative structures.
6. Identify the three similarities among old and new movement models.
7. Define and explain the systems model, including the terms constraints, affordances, and perception–action coupling.

As we saw in the three previous chapters, the complexities of planning, initiating, executing, and monitoring movement are great. One of the most difficult problems in understanding human movement is the innumerable ways a movement can be made. Consider, for example, the simple act of reaching for and grasping a hot cup of tea. The brain seemingly must choose a movement pathway and speed for the hand based on movements of the wrist, elbow, and shoulder. A grip pattern and finger arrangement must be determined to hold the cup securely and without spilling the hot liquid. In doing so, the brain must balance muscle force output between agonist and antagonist muscles, choose synergist muscles, recruit certain motor units or compartments in these muscles, and provide stabilization of the trunk and shoulder. The individual must take into account environmental factors, such as the temperature and slipperiness of cup, distance of the cup, lighting, and so forth. Any number of movement solutions—called **motor redundancy**—could enable grabbing the cup of tea. Having redundancy enables a wide range of choices to meet specific task demands but also poses a problem in selection. As we have seen in previous chapters, this problem of selecting just one solution among so many is called the **degrees of freedom** problem.

In addition to the degrees of freedom problem is the question of what the nervous system is trying to control and command. In the three previous chapters, our look at the nervous and muscular systems implied a strict division of duties with higher brain centers acting as the supreme controller over motor units and muscle contractions. But if we look beyond the basic neurophysiology of motor actions, we can speculate that the brain may try to control the final position or velocity of a distal limb or control the energy cost of a movement. Perhaps, the brain is only concerned about putting forth a "go" command and letting the peripheral neuromuscular and sensory reflex systems carry out the action on their own. What the CNS does control, and how thousands of motor units and hundreds of muscles are orchestrated into producing an efficient movement, are largely unknown. However, there are a number of theories that attempt to explain in general terms the whole process of planning, initiating, executing, and monitoring movement. These theories, otherwise known as models, provide a "big picture" framework to explain how the CNS and neuromuscular systems work to make movement, and motor skills in particular. In this chapter, we take a look at different models and their contributions to our current understanding of movement organization. We then examine closely the one model that best provides a practical solution for understanding and manipulating motor control processes. This latter model, the systems model, attempts to explain movement organization not strictly from a neural or muscular standpoint, but rather, from the perspective of what factors influence the planning, initiating, executing, and monitoring of movement.

Concepts in Action

Using Models

For many students, theoretical models are abstract concepts that are useful only to researchers and not practitioners. But nothing could be further from the truth. Models provide a greater understanding and a holistic view of how many different parts fit within a larger process. Because of this, models enable individuals to see how deficits in one area impact other areas and enable prediction of performance following interventions. A notable example is the use of posture and balance models (Chapters 10 and 11) to create intervention strategies for prevention and rehabilitation of knee and ankle injuries. Changes in intervention strategies since the 1990s were developed based on new models of joint stability and balance control, and these strategies have resulted in marked reductions in injury rates for athletes following the intervention programs (e.g., Myer et al., 2011; Noyes & Barber Westin, 2012). Other models have been used to promote reductions in training loads to decrease injury prevalence without sacrificing sport performance (Gabbett & Domrow, 2007). Hoch and McKeon (2010) applied models of motor control (including those discussed in this chapter) and models of functional health to describe intervention strategies for persons with chronic musculoskeletal problems. These authors, using modeling concepts, described concrete ways of how best to change goals, design intervention tasks, and communicate effectively with patients to enhance the day-to-day living of persons suffering from chronic musculoskeletal problems. The take-home point here is that the development and use of models are not reserved for researchers but are highly useful in the hands of innovative and forward-thinking practitioners.

INTRODUCTION TO MOVEMENT MODELS

Models provide a general framework of the processes and physiological systems contributing to the formation and execution of motor acts. We use these models for two main purposes. First, the broad goal is to have a conceptual framework by which to understand how movements are formulated and executed. This enables a deeper understanding that fosters experimentation. Second, the models provide a framework for practical use. For example, with a basic framework for how movements are executed, we can devise more effective programs for rehabilitation, practice, and training. See the accompanying Concepts in Action box for more examples.

Modeling the basic workings of the motor control system has been approached from different perspectives across the domain of mathematics, computer science, physics, neuroscience, and biomechanics. Some of these models may adequately explain a rhythmic movement like walking or a discrete movement like reaching for a cup, but none can fully explain a complex movement like the dribbling footwork of a star soccer player. Moreover, serious disagreements exist among researchers on the validity of the models to even explain simple movements (e.g., Houk, 2010; Neilson & Neilson, 2010; Schmidt, 2003).

Traditional models of motor control models have been broadly described as open loop or closed loop (Fig. 5.1). Closed-loop models explain movement as an outcome of feedback-initiated reflex actions and prepatterned neural systems, neither of which requires sophisticated commands from higher brain centers. The closed-loop control models are based on feedback control systems as presented back in Chapter 2 and Figure 2.11. In contrast, open-loop models downplay the role of feedback in movement initiation and execution and suggest a strict top–down hierarchy across CNS and neuromuscular structures in planning, executing, and initiating movement. These models are derived from the feedforward control structures depicted back in Figure 2.11.

Contemporary models of motor control have built upon the traditional models, and though they do not emphasize the idea of closed-loop versus open-loop processes, they do differ in the role the CNS plays in determining the final outcome of movement. One way to view the differences in these models is by analogy to a coaching command structure. Figure 5.2A shows rigid hierarchical control in which

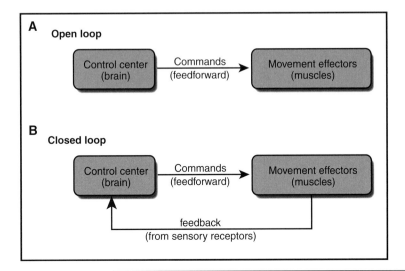

Figure 5.1 • A. A simplified open-loop or feedforward control system is shown compared to a (**B**) closed-loop or feedback control system. Except in the case of some reflexes that are purely closed loop, distinguishing a control system as purely closed or open incorrectly overlooks the fact that both systems are constantly working together.

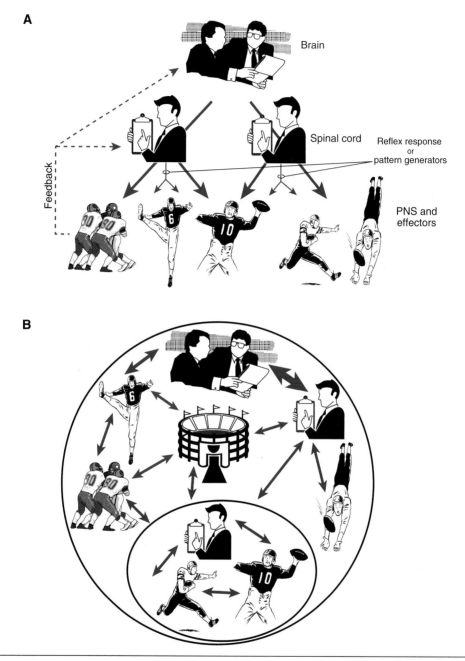

Figure 5.2 • Coaching analogy of control processes. **A.** Strict top–down hierarchy illustrated by a coaching command structure. *Heavy solid arrows* indicate strong feedforward commands. *Dashed lines* correspond to feedback, some of which goes to lower centers that make minimal adjustments (*light arrows*; reflex responses or pattern generators) on their own without permission from the top. Different players, from blockers to quarterbacks, reflect different capabilities within the muscles. **B.** The same structures exist, but each play a much more dynamic and integrative role. At the center of the diagram is the stadium, which corresponds to a movement goal within an environmental context. The *two-way arrows* correspond to simultaneous feedforward and feedback. The owners and coaches are still at the top of the list, but their command structure is less definitive in detail, relying more on the coaches and players to engage in a natural manner in which they have been trained. The circle within a circle reflects some players (effectors) working in groups as part of synergies or coordinative structures, and some lower coaches (spinal cord) making direct commands similar to a pattern generator.

the general managers and owners (higher brain centers) determine the goals and precise strategies to meet specific objectives. The owners sit high up in the owners' booth and send comprehensive instructions to coaches (lower brain centers and spinal cord) that are very specific in regard to player (effectors) actions. Different players, in terms of skill level and position played, represent different musculoskeletal resources the owners can draw upon. The instructions detail running versus passing plays, blocking patterns for the linemen, and even decoy actions of the uninvolved players. The coaches set the battle plan in motion but are under constant command from the generals and have limited autonomy to adjust plans on the field except reflexively in the case of large change in circumstances. Players carry out their assignments as commanded, with modification only under reactionary circumstances to unexpected circumstances (equivalent to reflexes). Feedback from the coaches is continually fed back to the owners for them to modify the next set of plays.

In contrast to this strict hierarchy, Figure 5.2B illustrates a different scenario in which the owners lay out a basic objective and strategy (e.g., "establish a ground game") and then let the coaches and players take action as they have been trained to do. Being closer to the action, the coaches may add strategy to meet the objectives and give basic commands to subgroups of players, such as the offensive linemen or the running backs. Each subgroup (a functional group of muscles and joints) knows how to operate by itself and needs no constant commands other than a "go" signal. Individual players within the subgroup, each with different capabilities, interact with other players and the environmental circumstances (e.g., opponents' action, weather) to meet the goals. Changing circumstances on the field cause the players to reorganize themselves with new strategies without going through the higher command structure. Constant feedback within and among subgroups results in ongoing changes in how the objectives are being met. Feedback to the owners from all sources enables the higher command structures to get a broad view on what is happening and may cause them to adjust the goals and strategies. In this view, not only are the "lower" controllers just as important as the higher centers, but also the environmental context and task goals are critical to the process.

CLOSED-LOOP, FEEDBACK-BASED, AND HETERARCHICAL MODELS

The simplest models of motor control are reflex models. These models suggest that all movement stems from chaining together of reflex actions that provide building blocks of complex behavior. In lower animals, such as mollusks and locusts, purposeful movement often works this way. Motor actions such as chewing, swallowing, reproductive acts, and "fight or flight" actions are initiated by sensory feedback and executed by reflex movements. Reflex models are based on the presence of hardwired neural circuits and produce fixed and stereotyped motor patterns.

Central Pattern Generators

Hardwired circuits can also produce more complex stereotyped movements through **central pattern generators** (CPGs). CPGs are not simply the chaining together of reflex actions but are their own innate nervous system pathways that when activated produce complex rhythmic movement patterns that can run independently of voluntary control. CPGs have been identified in lower animals and produce many repeating and rhythmic motor actions such as walking, swimming, and flying. The figure in the accompanying SideNote illustrates with very simple circuitry how the nervous system in some animals is designed to alternately activate agonist and antagonist muscles to create locomotion movements. A single command neuron, arising from the brain or sensory systems, is all that is needed to provide the impulse to set the patterning in motion (MacKay-Lyons, 2002). By definition, a CPG is neither open loop nor closed loop, but the example below on decerebrate cats demonstrates that CPGs can run entirely closed loop, which is why we have included them here.

The first solid scientific evidence for CPGs came from research on the swimming of crayfish (Hughes & Wiersma, 1960) and the flight of locusts (Wilson, 1961). Before this time, it was thought that movement was a result of either a full set of descending commands from higher brain centers or the chaining together of reflex activity (see historical review by Mulloney & Smarandache, 2010). Wilson's research on locusts, in particular, reshaped the thinking on how the nervous system was organized to produce purposeful movement. The first figure below depicts a simplified version of Wilson's experiments in which he tethered a locust in front of a miniature wind tunnel, and the bottom figure shows a simplified version of the locust CPG. In his experiments, electrodes were inserted into the locust's spinal cord and a sophisticated strobe camera apparatus (not shown) was used to record wing movements that were then linked to neuronal electrical activity. The tether was connected to a switch such that as the locust flew faster or slower it would control the wind velocity from the wind tunnel. In some experiments, whole parts of the locust were surgically removed to eliminate any sensory information, revealing that rhythmic wing movements could be produced without sensory feedback and without sophisticated brain commands.

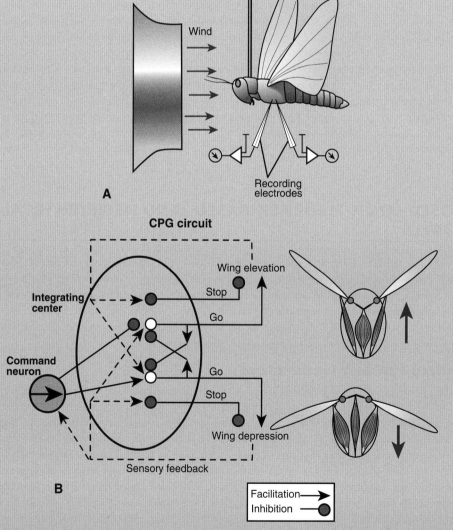

Top figure reprinted from Marder, E., & Bucher, D. (2001). Central pattern generators and the control of rhythmic movements. *Current Biology, 11*(23), R986–R996, with permission from Elsevier.

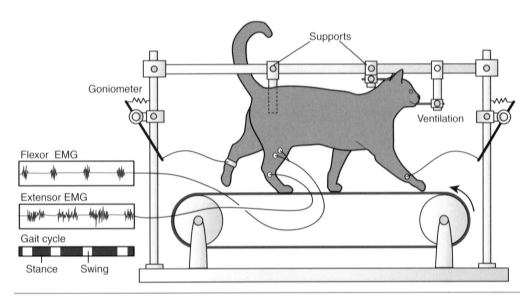

Figure 5.3 • Experiments with a "spinal cat" required lesions to be cut into the spinal cord and a special assembly to position the cat on the treadmill and to provide ventilation. EMG electrodes were implanted into the relevant leg muscles and movement sensor devices attached to the legs. Upon turning on the treadmill, the cat's legs begin an involuntary stepping pattern. Experiments such as these provided convincing evidence for CPGs for walking.

Experiments in the late 1960s in Russia on decerebrate cats (a cat with its spinal cord cut just below the brain) identified CPGs for walking in mammals (Fig. 5.3). These cats were supported over a motorized treadmill, and when the treadmill was turned on, the cats would begin a typical quadripedal walking action, even slowing and speeding in response to treadmill speed. These data confirmed that a walking pattern was contained within the spinal cord, and sensory information coming from the moving limbs was enough to set the pattern generator in action (for review see MacKay-Lyons, 2002). Not only that, but practice at treadmill walking resulted in longer and more coordinated walking, suggesting that the spinal neural circuits learn. Further experiments with animals have found that CPG circuits may be spread across the brain and spinal cord. Activation of the spinal CPGs may come from supraspinal centers or sensory feedback, but in intact animals, these systems work in tandem to drive CPGs that are adaptable to environmental circumstances.

Accumulating evidence points to humans having a form of CPG for locomotion and other rhythmic movements buried deep in other neural circuits (Dimitrijevic et al., 1998; Misiaszek, 2006; Zehr, 2005). Figure 5.4 illustrates a model of arm rhythmic movement proposed by Zehr et al. (2004). In this model, each arm has its own spinal CPG controller that can be set in motion directly by the brain or by sensory feedback. The CPGs can directly activate motor neurons to produce rhythmic movement or activate spinal interneuron reflex networks to produce movement modifications. Finally, supraspinal centers can control each level, including bypassing the CPGs altogether to individually control motor neurons. Though reflex and pattern generator models cannot explain a vast array of complex movements, they have led to basic understandings that the nervous system contains specifically designed circuits responsible for various basic movement patterns.

Heterarchical Models and Synergies

More complex closed-loop models have expanded on the simple hardwired neural systems to include more involvement of higher brain centers but still rely on feedback loops. In these complex models the higher brain centers provide basic command structures to the next lower levels, which

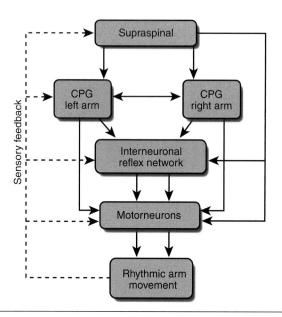

Figure 5.4 • Human CPGs are theorized to control aspects in arm rhythmic behavior such as flexion–extension arm swinging. In this model, each arm is controlled by its own CPG, which coordinate with the CPG of the other arm. The CPG circuits are thought to be their own sets of spinal neurons, and not simply using existing interneuron networks that are activated in pattern generating manner. The CPG circuits can be stimulated by supraspinal descending commands or from proprioceptive feedback. In most cases, however, the sensory feedback would enhance or reinforce the CPG activity and not initiate it on its own (Adapted from Zehr, E., Carroll, T. J., Chua, R., Collins, D. F., Frigon, A., Haridas, C., et al. (2004). Possible contributions of CPG activity to the control of rhythmic human arm movement. *Canadian Journal of Physiology and Pharmacology*, 82(8–9), 556–568. © 2008 Canadian Science Publishing or its licensors. Reproduced with permission.)

Concepts in Action

Body-Weight Supported Training

Body-weight supported (BWS) training is treadmill walking by a partially paralyzed or injured individual supported by a harness system. Presumably, this type of training forces the walking pattern CPG into action and causes the spinal cord or lower brain stem to learn (Van de Crommert et al., 1998). Results are preliminary, but a small number of studies (e.g., Barbeau & Visintin, 2003, see review by MacKay-Lyons, 2002) have shown BWS training to be more effective than traditional physical therapy in getting stroke and hemiparetic patients to walk, or walk better (faster, more symmetrical). Other investigators have shown BWS training to have effectiveness for children with neurological disorders such as cerebral palsy and Down's syndrome (Damiano & DeJong, 2009). A current focus of some research is to use electrical stimulation to activate the spinal pattern generators. Minassian et al. (2007) did an elegant study in which they implanted electrodes in the spinal cord to provide a tonic stimulation to the lumbar region. With stimulation the patients began a stepping pattern in the legs. The researchers also gave lumbar cord stimulation during BWS training and found much greater leg muscle activation with the stimulation than without.

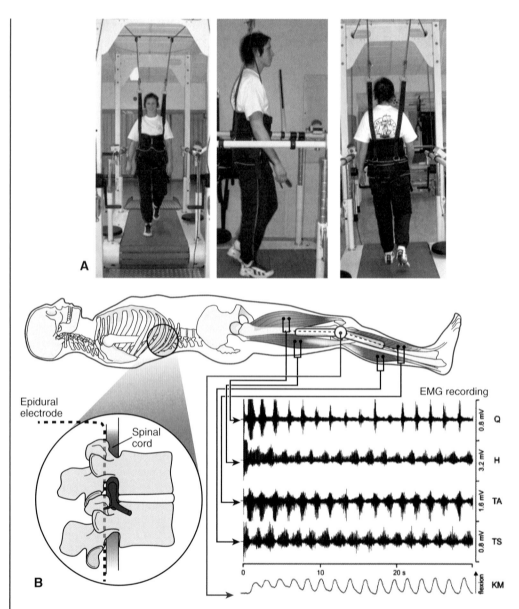

A. BWS training to take advantage of CPGs for walking. It is necessary for the patients to be supported by a harness system. This type of training requires some motor commands and sensory feedback, hence it is done with partially paralyzed, or hemiparetic, patients. (Reprinted from Aaslund, M., Helbostad, J., & Moe-Nilssen, R. (2011). Familiarization to BWS treadmill training for patients post-stroke. *Gait & Posture, 34*(4), 467–472, 2011, with permission from Elsevier.) **B.** Rhythmical stepping motions are produced from electrically stimulating the spinal cord with epidural electrodes above the lumbar spinal cord. The electrodes stimulate at a constant rate of 25 Hz. Surface EMG and goniometers record muscle activity and leg stepping movements. The EMG traces of the quadriceps (Q), hamstrings (H), tibialis anterior (TA) and triceps surae (TS) muscles show an alternating pattern of activation consistent with walking motion as shown in the goniometer trace (KM). These data provide strong evidence for the presence of walking CPGs in the spinal cord in humans. (Reprinted from Minassian, K. K., Persy, I. I., Rattay, F. F., Pinter, M. M., Kern, H. H., & Dimitrijevic, M. R. (2007). Human lumbar cord circuitries can be activated by extrinsic tonic input to generate locomotor-like activity. *Human Movement Science, 26*(2), 275–295, with permission from Elsevier.)

in turn modifies the signals and routes them out to the next lower levels. Sensory feedback greatly modifies the command signals at each level. These motor commands may be in the form of setting stretch reflex thresholds (*equilibrium point hypothesis*) or activating series of synergistic muscle actions (*uncontrolled manifold hypothesis*). According to Latash (2010), sensory feedback modifies motor commands to create desired levels of muscle stiffness that are set to achieve minimal muscle action necessary to achieve the movement goals. Raibert and Hodgins (1993) described the actions of the CNS as offering "suggestions" to the musculoskeletal systems that are governed by mechanical laws and constrained by the goals of the task and the physical laws of the environment. These models have been called **hierarchical** (top–down) by some, but they better represent a codependent or **heterarchical** command structure between CNS and PNS. This heterarchical structure relies heavily on sensory feedback or the manipulation of muscle spindle gain. Thus these models are considered here as feedback-based models.

More recent models have emerged in part based on discoveries of synergistic muscle and limb actions. **Synergies** are ensembles or groupings of muscles and limbs that work together as a functional unit, and by their actions also constrain one another (Latash, 2007). Synergies involve inherent neural pathways, muscle and limb biomechanical properties, and learned behaviors. Because a group of muscles and limbs act as a single unit, the degrees of freedom are reduced and the nervous system command structure is simplified (Neilson & Neilson, 2010). According to Latash (2010), the nervous system may or may not choose to use synergies, may learn new synergies, and modify existing ones. By themselves, synergies are neither open loop nor closed loop but simply represent an organizational structure of the nervous system. But like CPGs, synergies may be closely linked to hardwired spinal circuitry and sensory feedback loops that represent a high degree of spinal and peripheral nervous system (PNS) control (Ting et al., 1998).

Arm action during hammer striking provides a well-researched example of synergies in action. In broad terms, hammer head is ultimately controlled by the wrist and hand, which is controlled by the elbow, which is controlled by the shoulder. Actions at a joint complex are closely tied to the other joint complexes in terms of neural, physiological, and mechanical coupling, and also in terms of purpose. Relatively gross and variable actions of the proximal joint and limb segments (e.g., shoulder) become refined at the distal joints (e.g., wrist), but at the same time, the simultaneous muscle and joint actions occurring in each component of the synergy impose limits or restrictions on the other components. In the example of the hammer strike, the shoulder is limited in what it can do (e.g., speed and range of motion) because the final motions of the wrist and hand to hone the final trajectory are dependent on the shoulder actions.

Synergies are often found in pairs of agonist and antagonist muscles that work in alternating fashion. The action of an agonist muscle is often determined by the action or capability of its antagonist, and vice versa. Experiments with rapid and targeted limb movements have shown that the ability to go fast is limited by the ability to stop. In other words, the timing and activation levels of the agonist muscle to accelerate the limb are constrained or tied to the ability of the antagonist muscle to stop the limb at the target (Ives et al., 1999). These muscles work in tandem, suggesting that synergies enable a movement goal to be initiated and executed with a relatively simple motor command that sets the action in motion. This action is carried out and refined by the peripheral neuromuscular and sensory systems working as a cohesive synergistic team.

Another well-researched example of motor synergies is **coordinative structures**. Coordinative structure is another term for synergy as applied to the coupling between opposite limbs during bilateral movements. Kelso and his colleagues (1979) noted that arm and hand movements in one limb are predisposed to move with the same relative timing either in the same direction (in-phase) or exactly the opposite direction (antiphase) of the opposing limb. For instance, a rhythmical flexion–extension movement of the right arm is easily matched by a rhythmical flexion–extension or extension–flexion movement of the left arm with the same timing. Attempts to break out of the coordinated structure, such as swinging the left arm faster than the right arm, or have the left arm abduct and adduct, causes the limbs to assimilate each other back into a similar timing and muscle activation pattern.

Experiments with bicycle ergometer pedaling with one leg (unilateral) or both legs (bilateral) have revealed further mechanisms of coordinative structures. In an elegant experiment by Ting et al. (1998), the neural control of a single leg during unilateral pedaling was showed to be uncoordinated and less efficient than during bilateral pedaling. These authors noted that each leg must rely on sensory information from the other leg to set coordination patterns and that the limb reciprocal activation pattern (one leg flexes, the other extends) is strongly coupled, providing evidence that this coordinated structure may be part of some CPG system.

■ Thinking It Through 5.1 Uncoordinated Structures

A simple experiment can help you grasp the workings of coordinated structures. Sit comfortably in a chair with both feet on the ground. Extend your right knee and plantar flex your right ankle to point your right leg straight out ahead of you. Using your whole leg, draw clockwise circles in the air. While continuing to draw circles with your right leg, point your right finger and arm straight out ahead of you halfway between completely horizontal and vertical. Maintain the clockwise circles with your leg. Now, draw a six ("6") in mid air with your right arm. What happens to your leg? Try this experiment by varying which leg and arm you use and whether your leg is circling clockwise or counter clockwise. Can you explain these results based on coordinative structures?

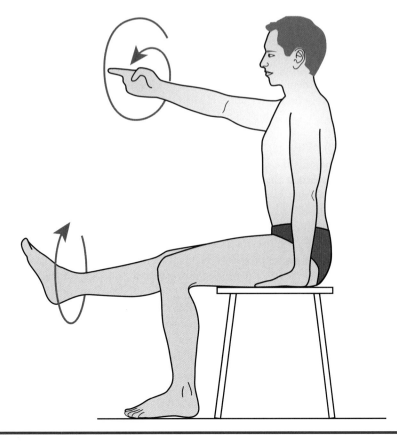

Despite the considerable evidence for synergies, pattern generators, feedback control, and the role that peripheral neuromechanical systems play in movement execution, the current closed loop and codependent models cannot easily account for behavioral nuances that influence movement execution (Houk, 2010; Scott, 2004). Brain imaging studies of healthy and brain-injured humans and primates, including recordings of individual neurons, show widely distributed and highly complex actions of the brain that may vary as much with behavioral intention as they do with actual movement outcomes (Scott, 2004). These findings raise many questions regarding the generalizability of movement models that downplay the role of the brain.

OPEN-LOOP AND HIERARCHICAL MODELS

In contrast to hardwired neural circuit models that need only low-level neural control, traditional hierarchical models are based on strict top–down control. In other words, higher brain centers send comprehensive commands to lower brain centers, lower brain centers send those commands to the spinal cord, and the spinal cord sends signals to the muscles. Movements arising based on these comprehensive sets of commands are said to be *centrally preprogrammed*. Like a puppeteer controlling a marionette, hierarchical models suggest that the body cannot do any purposeful and coordinated movement without precise manipulation from a highly and continually involved controller. Hierarchical systems presume that open-loop systems dominate over closed-loop systems. Feedback information from sensory systems comes back into the brain centers but is largely used to prepare or modify the next movement. The initiation of movement is purely open loop because there has been no preceding movement to provide feedback.

The Schema Theory

The most notable and long-standing open-loop model reinforcing central preprogramming is Schmidt's schema theory. The schema theory posits the existence of **generalized motor programs (GMPs)** and memory **schemata** stored in brain higher centers. The GMP is defined as a general representation of various motor actions or a class of actions. The schemata are separate memory components in which movements are recognized and recalled, essentially the decision-making and learning processes for the GMP (Shea & Wulf, 2005). When the brain wants to make a movement, it selects the most relevant motor program, which contains the necessary information to execute the movement. Stored in the GMP and schemata are **invariant characteristics** and **parameters**. Invariant characteristics are those features of the class of actions that do not change, and includes relative force, relative timing (rhythm) of the skill components, and sequencing of the components. Parameters are features that change within the class of actions, and include overall force, overall duration, and the specific muscles used. The schema theory does not discount the idea of CPGs, synergies, or other hardwired mechanisms but simply incorporates them as part of motor programs. Neither does the schema theory disregard the role of closed-loop feedback that may modify a perturbed movement and provide information for adapting the GMP for later movements.

Over 30 years of experimentation to document GMPs has provided explanations for a number of movement questions, such as bilateral transfer of motor skills across the limbs. For example, individuals can sign their name in recognizable script with their nondominant hand and even their feet, suggesting that the essential features of writing are stored in the brain and then applied under different contexts. Similarly, strength training in only one arm may produce strength gains in the unexercised arm (Hortobagyi et al., 1997), and imagined strength training exercises in one limb have been shown to increase strength in the opposite limb (Yue & Cole, 1992). One explanation for this phenomenon is that the motor program used to produce movement in one limb is simply used for the other limb. During training (real or imagined), the trained limb gets stronger, in part, due to changes in the motor commands that were part of the motor program. This new and improved motor program can then be applied to the untrained limb.

Among the most compelling data for preprogrammed movements come from an experiment by Wadman et al. (1979), who examined rapid and targeted elbow extension movements. These researchers collected EMG data from the agonist triceps b. muscle and antagonist biceps b. muscle and found a normal pattern of agonist activity to accelerate the limb, antagonist activity to stop the limb at the target, and then another burst of agonist activity to help clamp the limb at the target. This three-burst pattern of EMG activity, called the triphasic pattern, has a characteristic timing of agonist to antagonist muscle firing. In one of their experimental manipulations, the authors unexpectedly blocked the arm from moving, but the triphasic pattern still emerged (see Fig. 5.5), providing strong evidence that feedback from a moving limb is unnecessary to generate precise coordination patterns.

Other evidence for strict top down control is the presence of postural muscle activation that occurs prior to the muscle activation of self-initiated movements for the purpose of stabilizing the body. This phenomenon is explored in much more detail in Unit 3, but for now, consider that the brain may activate leg and trunk muscles prior to an individual moving his or her arm. This leg and trunk muscle activation comes without the person being consciously aware of it and can change based on the

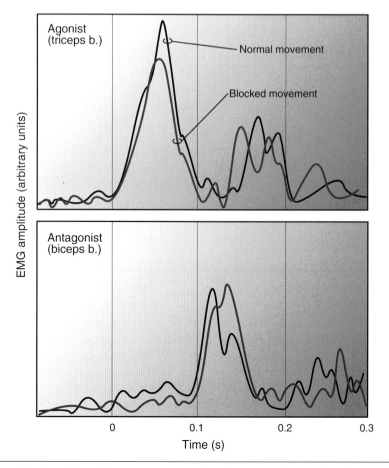

Figure 5.5 • The idea of central preprogramming of motor commands is reinforced by data shown here, adapted from Wadman et al. (1979). In their experiment, rapid elbow extension movements to a target were done normally (*dark lines*) and then under conditions in which the movement was unexpectedly blocked from starting (*light lines*). In both cases, a characteristic triphasic pattern of reciprocal agonist–antagonist–agonist muscle activity progressed. The appearance of an antagonist burst even after the movement was blocked suggests that it was preprogrammed prior to the movement. See text for more details.

anticipation of environmental and sensory information, not actual information. These findings demonstrate convincingly that the brain can set forth preprogrammed motor commands in the absence of relevant feedback and that somewhere the brain must store some form of motor skill-related commands.

■ Thinking It Through 5.2 Evidence for the GMP?

Motor program theory suggests that the basic plan for handwriting is stored in memory and can be applied to any relevant muscle group. To test this theory, sign your name with your dominant hand using a careful pace, and then with your nondominant hand. Compare the signatures for similarities in form and style. Next, sign your name on a wall-hung whiteboard (or chalk/chalkboard) by only using shoulder motions. To do this, hold the marker in your hand like a sword and rigidly hold your arm straight out with an extended elbow. Keep your wrist and elbow rigid and only move at the shoulder. Also try signing your name by holding your shoulder rigid and moving the marker by moving up and down with your legs. How do the signatures compare? What features of the motor program would make the signatures similar across each of the different movements?

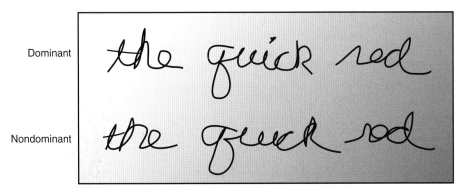

One piece of evidence for hierarchical control systems is the evidence for motor programs. Motor programs would predict that handwriting between left and right hands would have similar characteristics due to shared motor programs. This handwriting sample with the dominant right hand **(top)** and nondominant left hand **(bottom)** show marked similarity in form and shape and reinforces the idea of a stored representation of motor actions.

Internal Models

Though the idea of a GMP is attractive and the term "motor program" continues to have widespread use in scientific and nonscientific circles, it has some shortcomings as a movement model. The main criticisms of GMPs and the schema theory are the implausibility of the brain being able to store GMPs and schemas for so many different movements, questions over how entirely novel movements are created, and the need for a highly intelligent executive controller to make never-ending rapid fire decisions (Mathiowetz & Haugen, 1994; Turvey & Fonseca, 2009). Further, researchers have shown that the concept of a movement's invariant characteristics may not be so invariant (for review, see Schmidt, 2003). These cracks in the schema theory have prompted even its originator to suggest that it requires modification and it is time for a new model to emerge that provides better explanatory and predictive power (Schmidt, 2003).

Hierarchical models have more recently focused on what are termed internal models (Kawato, 1999; Wolpert & Ghahramani, 2000) (Fig. 5.6). In an internal model, the brain sends a movement plan to both the target body part and internally to itself through efference copy. Efference copy includes the movement plan and a prediction of what the sensory outcome will be. According to Wolpert and Ghahramani (2000), the task itself determines the nature of the motor action, but the actual planning and initiation of the motor commands is based much on prediction of outcomes. When feedback of

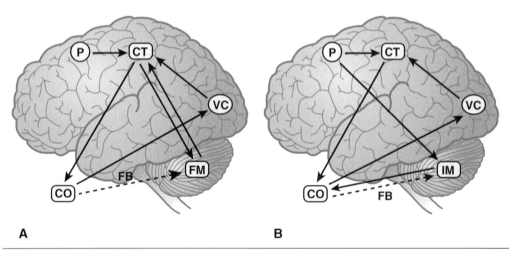

Figure 5.6 • Internal models are proposed to describe how the CNS devises a plan of movement action. **A.** A forward internal model plan is devised by a planner (P) somewhere in the premotor cortex, association cortex, or other areas. This plan is sent to a controller (CT) in the motor cortex, which sends the commands to the controlled object (CO), which could be the spinal interneurons, lower brain center, or motor units/muscles. The commands are also sent via efference copy to the forward model (FM) comparator in the cerebellum, where it is compared to sensory feedback (*dashed line*) and this difference relayed back to the controller. Visual information in the visual cortex (VC) is also relayed to the controller. The efference copy in the forward model contains a prediction of sensory feedback, which is then compared to the information from actual feedback, and a new plan is revised based on errors. **B.** In the inverse internal model the plan—not the specific motor commands—is also sent to storage in the cerebellum, and the inverse model (IM) compares outcome feedback to the original plan. The inverse model structures then send their own commands to complement the commands sent by the motor cortex to refine the movement. The inverse model largely differs from the forward model by the use of feedback in devising plans of action. (Adapted by permission from Macmillan Publishers Ltd., Ito, M. (2008). Control of mental activities by internal models in the cerebellum. *Nature Reviews Neuroscience*, 9(4), 304–313.)

the movement process and outcome arrives back in the brain, it is compared to what was predicted. Differences between the actual movement feedback and the predicted feedback are used not only to refine subsequent motor commands but also to filter out sensory information. Selecting the best motor commands, therefore, is based on the brain understanding the relationship between the original motor commands and the actual output, and in doing so, altering the commands to meet the task and environmental constraints (Kawato, 1999).

Because the CNS is often predicting outcomes in the face of changing environmental contexts, internal models are inherently dealing with uncertainty, variability, and error. This prediction and even the amount of error may aid the CNS in regulating the amount of incoming sensory information, may help it process information faster, and eventually may enhance the learning process (Wolpert & Ghahramani, 2000)

SIMILARITIES AND CONSENSUS POINTS AMONG MODELS

These models all suffer from a reductionist viewpoint and fall short of describing the vast array of complex movement enabled by our bodies. Nonetheless, three consensus points have emerged that span models old and new, and open loop and closed loop. The first point is that it appears that the nervous system is more concerned with movement outcomes or *endpoint effect* than specific muscle action. Regardless of the nature of the nervous system command structure, ultimately the goal is to produce a final movement outcome that minimally varies, can withstand disturbances, and in some cases, can self-correct itself back to the movement goal (Kawato, 1999; Latash et al., 2010). This endpoint effect may be the spatial location of a foot placement, the force of a hand grip, or the velocity of a golf club head; and a pathway may be selected based on minimal muscle activation, efficiency, or some other parameter (Latash, 2010). The second point is that the nervous system must take into account the chronic and current psychological, biological, and biomechanical properties of the body, the movement goals, and the environmental context (Kawato, 1999). Put differently, what is happening in the external environment and the internal bodily environment directly and indirectly influences movement outcome and movement planning. The entire motor process, from planning, initiating, and executing, is not isolated from internal and external feedback arriving at all levels of the CNS. The third point is the presence of hard-wired, pre-formed, and synergistic movements that form building blocks for more complex movements.

This leads us to our final model, the systems model. This model has unique features and also incorporates many other ideas presented above. Perhaps most important, this model is most closely aligned with the best motor learning strategies presented in Unit 2.

THE SYSTEMS MODEL AND APPROACH

The systems model (Fig. 5.7) describes the formation and execution of movement from a different perspective than the models above. Rather than describing the specific functions of individual components within the nervous and muscular systems, it approaches the production of skilled and purposeful

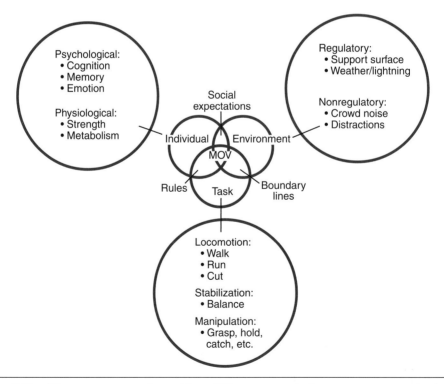

Figure 5.7 • The systems approach provides a different way to look at movement organization. The emphasis is on factors that influence movement production and outcome, and less on the specific physiological, psychological, and biomechanical properties that contribute to motor skill production. By examining the interaction of these individual factors with task and environmental demands, better frameworks for practice and training can be developed.

movements as a natural outcome of the person interacting with the environment. Specifically, given a task goal the characteristics and capabilities of the individual interact with the characteristics and features of the environment, and from these interactions a movement solution emerges. Thus the task requirements and the environmental context cannot be separated from how movement is planned and what movement eventually emerges. Because an individual's physiological and psychological capabilities strongly engage with the task and the environment, no single characteristic is considered most important. Open- and closed-loop systems are both at work, and for these reasons, the systems model is considered heterarchical and not hierarchical in forming a command structure. The systems model has proved fruitful as the basis for designing effective interventions in rehabilitation (Hoch & McKeon, 2010; Mathiowetz & Haugen, 1994), child development (Corbetta & Vereijken, 1999), wellness (Ives & Keller, 2008), and training of athletes (Buekers, 2002; Handford et al., 1997).

The systems model is based on a compilation of different theories and models, namely, the dynamic systems theory, ecological approaches, and action theory (Mathiowetz & Haugen, 1994). Shumway-Cook and Woollacott (2001) termed their description of this model as the systems approach. The use of the word approach indicates that this model underlies an entire framework for not only understanding movement but also practical solutions for improving movement behavior. These authors suggest that the fundamental concept of this theory is that movement "emerges from an interaction between the individual, the task, and the environment in which the task is being carried out. Thus, movement is not solely the result of muscle-specific motor programs or stereotyped reflexes, but results from a dynamic interplay between perceptual, cognitive, and action systems" (p. 22). Put differently, the requirements of the motor skill task itself and the features of the environment in which the task is carried out directly influence how movement is planned, initiated, and executed, and how sensory information is acquired and used. In this systems approach sensory information is important, but how this information is perceived is vital to the planning and overall movement process. It is important for the practitioner to know these factors and their interactions, for they can be manipulated and exploited for better motor learning and performance.

Identifying Dynamic Systems and Constraints

The individual (or person), the task, and the environment are systems that interact and each of these systems contain multiple subsystems that also interact. The dynamic interplay among these systems identifies them as **dynamic systems**, a term specifically describing systems that are dependent upon one another and change in relationship to one another. What these systems are and why they are important is best understood by examining how they influence movement. Systems are assemblies or groups of components that together have certain features or characteristics that are task specific. Synergies as described earlier are part of human systems, as are cardiopulmonary, endocrine, neuromuscular, and psychological systems.

The features and characteristics of systems impose **constraints** to movement (Newell, 1986). A constraint is a barrier or restriction that must be used, avoided, or overcome for effective movement to take place. Constraints may dictate precisely how a movement must be done, or what movement must be done. In some cases, a constraint may be exploited to offer an advantage or an enabling situation depending on the task. For instance, a pitching rubber constrains how a pitcher may throw the ball, but also provides an advantage to the pitcher by providing solid footing from which to push off. *Task constraints* and *environmental constraints* are considered external and individual systems produce *internal constraints*.

Task constraints often dictate the nature or type of movement. A task like diving, for example, requires rotational body mechanics and large joint ranges of motion. Conversely, diving is not a prolonged activity and thus does not require high aerobic fitness. Other tasks may require hand–eye coordination and object manipulation, fast running, jumping, or single-leg balance. A task's cognitive demands, rules, scoring objectives, and coach instructions provide other task-related constraints. For instance, football linemen and soccer players are both constrained in how they can use their hands, and basketball players and team handball players are limited by the number of steps they can take while holding the ball.

The environment provides constraints that can be considered *regulatory* versus *nonregulatory*, and physical versus sociocultural. Regulatory conditions are those that directly impact the production and execution of motor skills, such as weather, support surface traction, lighting, other people, objects, and boundary lines. Nonregulatory conditions are those that often influence movement but theoretically should not. The most notable nonregulatory conditions are crowd noise distractions and playing road games. Most of the regulatory conditions also fall in the category of the physical environment, that is, the actual physical surroundings. In contrast to the physical environment is the sociocultural environment. Sociocultural factors, including customs, education, economic status, culture, and gender role expectations, often influence one's movement choices or motivation.

An individual's physiological and psychological subsystems create their own sets of internal constraints. For example, muscle strength, maximal motor unit firing rate, reaction time, and metabolic reserves are just a few of the physiological properties that constrain motor performance. Intelligence, experience, values, and emotional state are just a few psychological constraints. One example of dynamic systems at work is these systems interacting continually to maintain homeostasis such as core body temperature. A change or disruption in one system may have a small or large influence on one or all other systems, and moment to moment adjustments in blood flow, hormone release, metabolism, and autonomic nervous system control are necessary. No single system always dominates over the others, revealing that the systems approach is not fully hierarchical but has heterarchical controllers. Effective motor skill performance emerges from the individual in response to the dynamic interplay of individual internal constraints with external task and environmental constraints.

Behavior of Biological Dynamic Systems

A key feature in dynamic systems is that each system, working as an individual unit and interacting with other systems, has **self-organizing properties**. Given a set of circumstances, the system tries to maintain a stable and patterned mode of operation that is relatively resistant to change. These stable points are called **attractor states**.

For instance, one's preferred walking pace is stable, comfortable, and metabolically efficient. This preferred pace is consistent with the natural pendular motion of the legs, suggesting that the nervous system has matched itself to the natural inertial and viscoelastic properties of the limb segments (Holt et al., 1991). Slight perturbations during walking, like stumbling or ducking under a low branch, may only produce a momentary disruption. Gait cycles are quickly attracted (or self-corrected) into normal and stable gait patterns. A slower walking speed occurs during uphill walking not because the nervous system commands it, but because it emerges as a functional outcome of physiological systems self-organizing in the presence of physical laws and environmental constraints. The dynamic walking tinkertoy illustrated in Chapter 3 is an example of a mechanical system that self-organizes itself into a walking pattern when given a little nudge to walk downhill. Additional examples of self-organization are observations that reaching and grasping movements are automatically coupled with stages of breathing, possibly to take advantage of intrathoracic pressure that may aid in postural stability (Mateika & Gordon, 2000).

Though we see each system works to maintain stability, there is a degree of unavoidable and necessary variability that accompanies dynamic biological systems (Davids et al., 2005). Variability is seen even under highly stable circumstances like treadmill walking, when there is variation in step speed, direction, and length from step to step (Danion et al., 2003). This variation enables a degree of flexibility to accomodate changing conditions, and thus actually helps to maintain stability. During moderate changes in uphill and downhill grades, for instance, the walking systems can readily adapt with changes in step speed and length.

Given a large-enough disruption or change, however, a biologic system may not have enough flexibility to adapt and may become entirely unstable. Under these circumstances, the system may self-destruct or be forced to transition into a new stable state. The **transition phase** from walking to running demonstrates that high speeds or high internal workloads destabilize the stable walking pattern and forces a transition to the new attractor state of running. Speed (or workload) is a **control parameter**, which is a factor that when disrupted or changed causes a wholesale change throughout the entire system. The rest of the system components that follow suit are called **order parameters**. Order parameters are those parts of the system that essentially define or describe the movement. Thus in the case of transitioning from walking to running, order parameters are muscle coordination and gait repatterning (e.g., running has a flight phase), and vertical center of mass movement. The locomotion system has enough built-in variability to be stable at various walking speeds, but given a strong enough perturbation, it self-organizes from walking to a new stable state of running. Dynamic systems can make these sudden changes from one stable state to another or can do so progressively over time (Corbetta & Vereijken, 1999).

■ Thinking It Through 5.3 Transitions and Stable States in Walking and Running

Walking and running provide well-researched examples of dynamic systems. In this mini experiment you will examine the transition of one attractor state to another. Begin walking at a very slow pace of 1 mph on a treadmill and walk at this pace for about 30 seconds. Have a partner control the pace of the treadmill and block the readouts so you cannot see your speed. Your partner should observe the actions of your arms and legs while increasing the speed by about 0.5 mph every 10 seconds (or 0.1 mph every 2 seconds if possible). Have your partner record the speed at which you transition from a walk to a run, and then continue to increase the speed by another 2 mph. Continue to run at this speed for about 15 seconds, and then have your partner slow the treadmill at 0.5 mph every 10 seconds. Note at what speed you transitioned from a run to a walk. After cooling down and stopping the treadmill, switch positions with your partner.

From the very slow walk to the fast walk is a transition phase and another transition phase from walk to run. Can you identify them and what occurs during each transition? Compare the walk to run transition speed to the run to walk transition speed. Are they different? If so, why? Do you think these results would differ based on fitness or training status? For insight into these questions read Diedrich and Warren (1995), Raynor et al. (2002), and Beaupied et al. (2003).

It is often necessary to purposefully cause destabilization in order to promote new and better system functioning. Most physical training aims to progressively cause destabilization, such as mechanical and fatigue stress brought on by strength training over periods of weeks and months. This stress breaks down tissues, which in turn causes repair processes to work to create new and stronger tissues. Destabilization, however, does not always have such positive outcomes. Changing one variable, even for the "better" may have a minimal impact on overall performance. Improving strength, for example, may have no affect on sport performance. Sometimes, other systems must adapt in a negative manner in order to stabilize the system. Injuries themselves are a common form of destabilization that results in adaptations that are not always positive. Shoulder weakness, for instance, may lead to adaptive actions at the elbow and wrist that may predispose one to further injury. Fatigue is an order parameter that must be monitored closely to ensure that it contributes to positive and not negative transitions. Acute fatigue during an event may result in coordination and behavioral changes that contribute to poor performance and even injury. On the other hand, fatigue during training is used to stimulate adaptations in tissues and metabolism. Too much training fatigue may lead to chronic maladaptations and overtraining syndrome.

Affordances and Perception–Action Coupling

Constraint-based information from the environment continually merges with internal sensory information and task-based constraints. Perceptual systems interpret the nature of these constraints and determine ways to take them into account for movement planning and execution. This process is known as searching for **affordances** and closely ties together what is perceived by an individual and what action subsequently takes place. The idea of affordances is based on Gibson's ecological psychology research on how individuals learn and adapt within environments (Gibson, 1966). According to Gibson, environmental constraints may be used, misused, or ignored. As individuals learn to account for environmental and task constraints, within the bounds of their internal constraints, the nature of what kinds of actions are afforded begin to emerge. For example, if the lights go out and darkness falls upon a busy supermarket, sighted people slow down or stop and reach out with their hands to feel for obstacles, whereas blind persons may not change their behavior at all.

Affordances directly link what is perceived and what action may take place. The coupling between perception and a subsequent motor action, that is, perception-action coupling, is closely associated with sensorimotor processes. Perception–action coupling is both an innate and learned behavior that links a motor action with environmental and task-related sensory inflow. Perception–action coupling makes the need for precise motor programs unnecessary because the information regarding movement planning and action is largely contained in the environment and revealed when the person interacts with the environment (Buekers, 2002).

Within the systems model perception–action coupling is the key to the emergence of purposeful and effective motor skills. The environment acts upon the person through the person's sensory system, but this information only interacts once it is processed and perceived by the CNS. The huge amount of information arriving via somatosensation, vision, and hearing is interpreted as what movements are possible and effective given the functional task goals and constraints, and the physiological, psychological, and physical constraints that are inherently imbedded in the person–environment system (Davids et al., 2005). Like the general motor program, this amount of information processing would seem as if it would overwhelm the CNS. The nervous system, however, has a remarkable ability to filter irrelevant information and find the perceptual information most relevant to the situation.

The search for affordances and the process of filtering sensory information so that it can be coupled with actions is not well understood, especially for highly complex movements and environments. For some "simple" actions, such as catching or hitting a ball, a number of perception–action coupling mechanisms have been identified. Optic flow, for instance, provides single-source information on moving objects and time to contact that is inextricably linked to motor actions.

In short, the systems model does not discount the idea of brain-based high-level executive controllers but considers these controllers to be just one part of the overall mechanism from which effective and purposeful motor skills emerge. Exactly what type of motor commands arise from the brain and race down the spinal cord, and the nature of the information contained within those commands, are unknown. Current models, namely the systems model, suggest that these commands are based on information perceived from the environment and are focused toward meeting task goals enabled based on the environmental and personal circumstances.

Applying the Systems Approach

From a practitioner's standpoint, the systems model and approach provides a framework from which to address movement-related problems. In particular, it makes available ways to answer questions, such as, "Why is this motor skill performed poorly?" and "How can the training be changed to maximize improvement?" The practitioner can look to environmental and task-related factors and how they interact with the individual's own constraints and abilities, leading to individual-specific assessments and interventions. Moreover, understanding the importance of the environment enables the practitioner to bring those situation-specific constraints into the practice and training environment. Consider the apparently simple case of a field-goal kicker whose kicking form and performance is outstanding during practice but not in games. At first glance, it may seem that game-related anxiety may be the culprit (and it may), but there are other factors worth investigating. The full crowd in an enclosed stadium creates ambient or focal visual information that is different than practice, and the crowd noise may produce similar differences. The pressure of the game situation may cause the snapper and ball holder to behave differently, throwing off the kicker's timing or confidence. The systems

SIDE**NOTE**	**PERCEPTION–ACTION COUPLING**

Perception–action coupling implies that flow of information coming into the brain is somehow processed and automatically linked up with an appropriate movement to meet the task goals within the environmental context. This idea seems hard to grasp, but experimental evidence shows this indeed happens. Consider an experiment by Mohler et al. (2007) in which they had subjects walk on a large treadmill surrounded by a virtual reality environment of walking down a hallway. Subjects were instructed to pay attention to doors opening and closing in the virtual hallway in order to keep their attention off walking and on the external environment. The treadmill was free running and thus the subjects were free to adjust their walking speed at will. The experimenters could adjust the virtual visual environment to make progressing down the hall consistent with tread-mill speed, or could make the virtual environment move faster or slower than the actual treadmill speed. When the virtual environment was sped up or slowed down the subject's walking speed increased or decreased, respectively. Moreover, the transitions from walk to run and run to walk were also changed by the virtual environment. These authors concluded that the optic flow and perception of self-motion are coupled with locomotor actions, perhaps even with CPGs. Similar results from an experiment by Varraine et al. (2002) in which optic flow was manipulated during treadmill walking led these authors to conclude that changing one sensory input leads to modifica-tion in the integration of other sensory inputs and thus the coupling between perception and action depends on the environmental constraints.

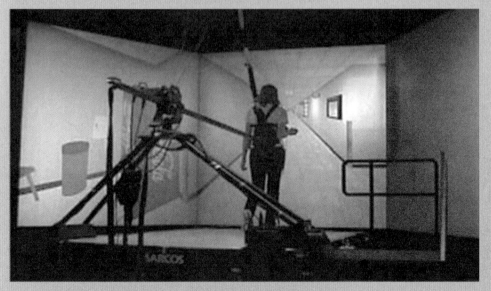

Virtual reality experiments with treadmill walking illustrate perception–action coupling. In this experiment, the subject is walking on a treadmill surrounded by a virtual reality projection of walking down a hallway. The "speed" of the virtual world can be matched or mismatched to the speed of the treadmill. (From Mohler, B., Thompson, W., Creem-Regehr, S., Pick, H., & Warren, W. (2007). Visual flow influences gait transition speed and preferred walking speed. *Experimental Brain Research, 181*(2), 221–228, with permission from Springer.)

approach enables the practitioner to take a holistic approach to movement performance, and then address those components of the system likely to have the most beneficial effect to the entire system.

SUMMARY

Models have been created to explain how movements are put together in an organized and logical fashion. Closed-loop style models posit that many fundamental movement patterns and behaviors, such as walking, are simply automated hardwired circuits controlled at low levels of the nervous system that require minimal thinking or decision making. Hierarchical or open-loop models are just the opposite and posit that higher brain centers control movement through a definitive command structure. Various aspects of movements are stored in memory as motor programs and can be modified to different circumstances. Evidence for both open- and closed-loop systems can be found, but neither model type provides workable solutions for many complex movement behaviors.

The systems model approaches the control of movement in a different way. The systems model posits that purposeful movement arises from an interaction of environmental factors, task-related factors, and individual-specific factors. Underlying the systems model is the existence of dynamic systems that when working alone or with other systems, self-organize into stable patterns of behavior. Self-organization arises to fit within the constraints of environmental and individual systems and is bound by functional task goals. Environmental systems interact with an individual through perception, and perceptual systems seek to find affordances in the constraints imposed by the environment. Perception is then coupled with motor actions and thus purposeful motor skills emerge from the individual in the context of the environmental circumstances, individual capabilities, and task goals.

STUDY QUESTIONS

1. Explain the degrees of freedom problem and the way that each movement model deals with this problem.
2. Define motor redundancy. Explain if redundancy is a good thing or a bad thing for the body to have.
3. What are the advantages of having a model to describe movement?
4. What are the real differences between feedback and feedforward based models?
5. Describe reflex models and CPGs. Explain the shortcomings of these models in describing an all-encompassing view of motor skill planning, initiating, and executing.
6. Define GMP and describe its features. Discuss some of the research support for this model and its ultimate shortcomings.
7. Explain in detail the concept of a synergy and provide examples.
8. What are the three consensus points among open-loop and closed-loop theories?
9. How does the systems model and approach differ from the other models?
10. Define the systems model and explain the fundamental concepts in detail.
11. Define constraints and identify individual, environmental, and task constraints.
12. Explain the nature of dynamic systems, including self-organization, and provide examples.
13. Define affordance and perception–action coupling and explain the relationship between them.
14. How can a coach or instructor use the concept of the systems theory to improve performance?
15. A volleyball player lifts weights to increase leg strength in order to improve vertical jump and thus, her play on the volleyball court at the net (blocks, hits). Using the systems model, explain the potential inadequacy of this approach. Mention the role of the individual, the task, and the environment. Use the terms constraints, affordances, perception–action coupling, and self-organization.

References

Barbeau, H., & Visintin, M. (2003). Optimal outcomes obtained with body-weight support combined with treadmill training in stroke subjects. *Archives of Physical Medicine and Rehabilitation*, *84*(10), 1458–1465.

Beaupied, H. H., Multon, F. F., & Delamarche, P. P. (2003). Does training have consequences for the walk-run transition speed? *Human Movement Science*, *22*(1), 1–12.

Buekers, M. J. (2002). Coaches and teachers at the crossroads of emerging patterns and direct perception. In S. P. Shohov (Ed.) *Advances in psychology research* (Vol. 9, pp. 75–90). Hauppauge, NY: Nova Science Publishers.

Corbetta, D. D., & Vereijken, B. B. (1999). Understanding development and learning of motor coordination in sport: The contribution of dynamic systems theory. *International Journal of Sport Psychology*, *30*(4), 507–530.

Damiano, D., & DeJong, S. (2009). A systematic review of the effectiveness of treadmill training and body weight support in pediatric rehabilitation. *Journal of Neurologic Physical Therapy*, *33*(1), 27–44.

Danion, F., Varraine, E., Bonnard, M., & Pailhous, J. (2003). Stride variability in human gait: The effect of stride frequency and stride length. *Gait & Posture*, *18*, 69–77.

Davids, K., Renshaw, I., & Glazier, P. (2005). Movement models from sports reveal fundamental insights into coordination processes. *Exercise and Sport Sciences Reviews*, *33*(1), 36–42.

Diedrich, F. J., & Warren, W. H. (1995). Why change gaits? Dynamics of the walk-run transition. *Journal of Experimental Psychology: Human Perception and Performance*, *21*(1), 183–202.

Dimitrijevic, M., Gerasimenko, Y., & Pinter, M. (1998). Evidence for a spinal central pattern generator in humans. *Annals of the New York Academy of Sciences*, *860*, 360–376.

Gabbett, T. J., & Domrow, N. (2007). Relationships between training load, injury, and fitness in sub-elite collision sport athletes. *Journal of Sports Sciences*, *25*(13), 1507–1519.

Gibson, J. J. (1966). *The senses considered as perceptual systems*. Boston, MA: Houghton Mifflin.

Handford, C. C., Davids, K. K., Bennett, S. S., & Button, C. C. (1997). Skill acquisition in sport: Some applications of an evolving practice ecology. *Journal of Sports Sciences*, *15*(6), 621–640.

Hoch, M. C., & McKeon, P. O. (2010). Integrating contemporary models of motor control and health in chronic ankle instability. *Athletic Training & Sports Health Care*, *2*(2), 82–88.

Holt, K. G., Hamill, J. J., & Andres, R. O. (1991). Predicting the minimal energy costs of human walking. *Medicine and Science in Sports and Exercise*, *23*(4), 491–498.

Hortobagyi, T. T., Lambert, N. J., & Hill, J. P. (1997). Greater cross education following training with muscle lengthening than shortening. *Medicine and Science in Sports and Exercise*, *29*(1), 107–112.

Houk, J. C. (2010). In search of common ground. *Motor Control*, *14*(3), e9–e14.

Hughes, G. M., & Wiersma, C. A. G. (1960). The co-ordination of swimmeret movements in the crayfish, *Procambarus clarkii*. *Journal of Experimental Biology*, *37*, 657–670.

Ives, J. C., Abraham, L., & Kroll, W. (1999). Neuromuscular control mechanisms and strategy in arm movements of attempted supranormal speed. *Research Quarterly for Exercise and Sport*, *70*(4), 335–348.

Ives, J. C., & Keller, B. A. (2008). Functional training for health. In: J. K. Silver & C. Morin (Eds.) *Understanding fitness. How exercise fuels health and fights disease*. (pp. 71–90). Westport, CT: Praeger Publishers.

Kawato, M. (1999). Internal models for motor control and trajectory planning. *Current Opinion in Neurobiology*, *9*(6), 718–727.

Kelso, J., Southard, D., & Goodman, D. (1979). On the coordination of two-handed movements. *Journal of Experimental Psychology. Human Perception and Performance*, *5*(2), 229–238.

Latash, M. L. (2007). No, we don't need internal models. *Motor Control*, *11*(Suppl), S10–S11.

Latash, M. (2010). Motor synergies and the equilibrium-point hypothesis. *Motor Control*, *14*(3), 294–322.

Latash, M., Levin, M., Scholz, J., & Schöner, G. (2010). Motor control theories and their applications. *Medicina*, *46*(6), 382–392.

MacKay-Lyons, M. (2002). Central pattern generation of locomotion: A review of the evidence. *Physical Therapy*, *82*(1), 69–83.

Marder, E., & Bucher, D. (2001). Central pattern generators and the control of rhythmic movements. *Current Biology*, *11*(23), R986–R996.

Mateika, J., & Gordon, A. (2000). Adaptive and dynamic control of respiratory and motor systems during object manipulation. *Brain Research*, *864*(2), 327–337.

Mathiowetz, V., & Haugen, J. (1994). Motor behavior research: Implications for therapeutic approaches to central nervous system dysfunction. *American Journal of Occupational Therapy*, 48(8), 733–745.

Minassian, K. K., Persy, I. I., Rattay, F. F., Pinter, M. M., Kern, H. H., & Dimitrijevic, M. R. (2007). Human lumbar cord circuitries can be activated by extrinsic tonic input to generate locomotor-like activity. *Human Movement Science*, 26(2), 275–295.

Misiaszek, J. F. (2006). Neural control of walking balance: IF falling THEN react ELSE continue. *Exercise and Sport Sciences Reviews*, 34(3), 128–134.

Mohler, B., Thompson, W., Creem-Regehr, S., Pick, H., & Warren, W. (2007). Visual flow influences gait transition speed and preferred walking speed. *Experimental Brain Research*, 181(2), 221–228.

Mulloney, B., & Smarandache, C. (2010). Fifty years of CPGs: Two neuroethological papers that shaped the course of neuroscience. *Frontiers in Behavioral Neuroscience*, 4, 45, doi: 10.3389/fnbeh.2010.00045.

Myer, G., Ford, K., & Hewett, T. (2011). New method to identify athletes at high risk of ACL injury using clinic-based measurements and freeware computer analysis. *British Journal of Sports Medicine*, 45(4), 238–244.

Neilson, P., & Neilson, M. (2010). On theory of motor synergies. *Human Movement Science*, 29(5), 655–683.

Newell, K. M. (1986). Constraints on the development of coordination. In M. G. Wade & H. T. A. Whiting (Eds.) *Motor development in children: Aspects of coordination and control* (pp. 341–360). Dordrecht: Nijhoff.

Noyes, F. R., & Barber Westin, S. D. (2012). Anterior cruciate ligament injury prevention training in female athletes: A systematic review of injury reduction and results of athletic performance tests. *Sports Health: A Multidisciplinary Approach*, 4(1), 36–46.

Raibert, M. H., & Hodgins, J. K. (1993). Legged robots. In R. Beer, R. Ritzman, & T. McKenna (Eds.) *Biological neural networks in invertebrate neuroethology and robotics* (pp. 319–354). Boston, MA: Academic Press.

Raynor, A., Yi, C., Abernethy, B., & Jong, Q. (2002). Are transitions in human gait determined by mechanical, kinetic or energetic factors? *Human Movement Science*, 21(5–6), 785–805.

Schmidt, R. A. (2003). Motor schema theory after 27 years: Reflections and implications for a new theory. *Research Quarterly for Exercise and Sport*, 74(4), 366–375.

Scott, S. H. (2004). Optimal feedback control and the neural basis of volitional motor control. *Nature Reviews Neuroscience*, 5(7), 532–544.

Shea, C., & Wulf, G. (2005). Schema theory: A critical appraisal and reevaluation. *Journal of Motor Behavior*, 37(2), 85–101.

Shumway-Cook, A., & Woollacott, M. (2001). *Motor control: Theory and applications* (2nd ed.). Baltimore, MD: Lippincott Williams & Wilkins.

Ting, L., Raasch, C., Brown, D., Kautz, S., & Zajac, F. (1998). Sensorimotor state of the contralateral leg affects ipsilateral muscle coordination of pedaling. *Journal of Neurophysiology*, 80(3), 1341–1351.

Turvey, M., & Fonseca, S. (2009). Nature of motor control: Perspectives and issues. *Advances in Experimental Medicine and Biology*, 629, 93–123.

Van de Crommert, H. W., Mulder, T. T., & Duysens, J. J. (1998). Neural control of locomotion: Sensory control of the central pattern generator and its relation to treadmill training. *Gait & Posture*, 7(3), 251–263.

Varraine, E., Bonnard, M., & Pailhous, J. (2002). Interaction between different sensory cues in the control of human gait. *Experimental Brain Research*, 142(3), 374–384.

Wadman, W. J., Denier van der Gon, J. J., Geuze, R. H., & Mol, C. R. (1979). Control of fast goal directed arm movements. *Journal of Human Movement Studies*, 5, 3–17.

Wilson, D. M. (1961). The central nervous control of flight in a locust. *Journal of Experimental Biology*, 38, 471–490.

Wolpert, D., & Ghahramani, Z. (2000). Computational principles of movement neuroscience. *Nature Neuroscience*, 3 (Suppl), 1212–1217.

Yue, G., & Cole, K. (1992). Strength increases from the motor program: Comparison of training with maximal voluntary and imagined muscle contractions. *Journal of Neurophysiology*, 67(5), 1114–1123.

Zehr, E. P. (2005). Neural control of rhythmic human movement: The common core hypothesis. *Exercise and Sport Sciences Reviews*, 33, 54–60.

Zehr, E., Carroll, T. J., Chua, R., Collins, D. F., Frigon, A., Haridas, C., et al. (2004). Possible contributions of CPG activity to the control of rhythmic human arm movement. *Canadian Journal of Physiology and Pharmacology*, 82(8/9), 556–568.

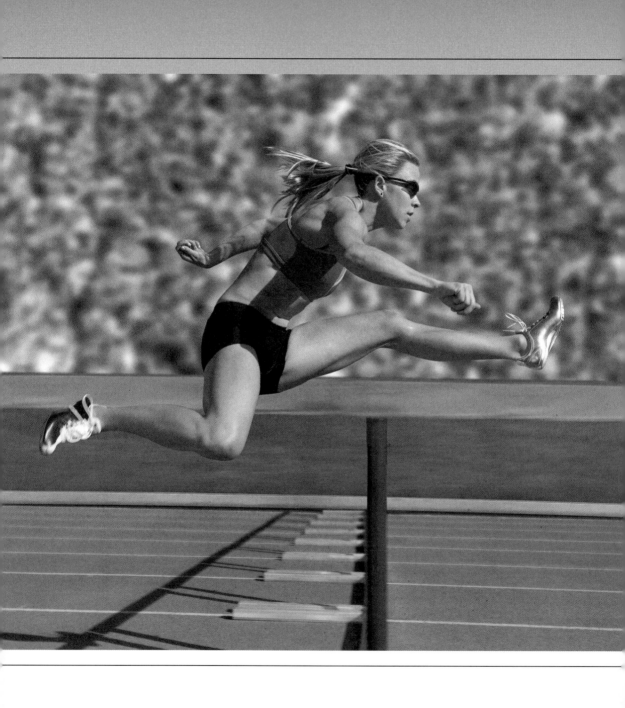

II

Motor Learning

Motor learning is the study of how the brain plans, learns, and executes movements and those factors that influence these processes. Essential to understanding these actions are the measurement and classification of motor skills. In this unit, we also look at important information processing factors, especially attention, memory, and decision making, and finally look at practice and instruction methods.

6 | Understanding Motor Skill and Motor Abilities

PURPOSE, IMPORTANCE, AND OBJECTIVES OF THIS CHAPTER

The purpose of this chapter is to describe the nature of motor skills and abilities, how they are classified, how they are measured, and how they relate to one another. By understanding these concepts, the practitioner and researcher have a framework for recognizing and understanding strong and poor motor skill performance and, therefore, the tools to address motor skill improvement.

After reading this chapter, you should be able to:

1. Explain how motor skills and abilities are identified and classified and the purpose of classifying skills and abilities in these ways.
2. Explain how a person's abilities contribute to motor skill learning and performance.
3. Explain how to go about measuring motor skills and abilities in reliable and valid ways.
4. Explain why measurement of motor skills is vital to the learning process.
5. Explain how response outcome and response production performance measures differ and why it is important to assess one versus the other.
6. Explain the significance of reaction time as a performance measure and what the different components of fractionated reaction time reveal.
7. Explain the different types of error measurements and when and why each type of measure should be used.
8. Explain the difficulty in using abilities as predictors of performance.

As presented back in Chapter 1, motor skills are defined as voluntary and purposeful actions requiring body and limb movements to achieve a goal, and abilities were defined as attributes that provide the capability to produce motor skills. The differences between motor abilities and motor skills are not always clear and can be subtle. The lack of distinction comes into play when abilities seem to be skills, such as muscle strength in weightlifters. In this case, muscle strength (ability) appears synonymous with weight lifting performance (skill). However, muscle strength is a physiological ability that along with other physiological and psychological attributes, and technical skills, contributes to weightlifting performance.

Concepts in Action

Ability versus Skill

Herb Washington was a world record–holding sprinter in the early 1970s before he was signed by the Oakland Athletics major league baseball club to be a designated pinch runner. Despite having unmatched running speed ability, he managed to successfully steal a base only 63% of the time. To put this in perspective, 67% is considered the "break-even" point, and Carlos Beltran holds the highest percentage at 88%. Herb Washington's statistics demonstrate that even in a skill like base stealing that seems to be near synonymous with an ability, they are not one and the same.

To understand what constitutes strong motor skill performance and the process to acquire such performance, it is imperative to understand the fundamental qualities of motor skills. Understanding begins by identifying, classifying, and then measuring motor skills, which then enables the identification of those abilities that may contribute to skilled performance. This chapter begins with concepts underlying motor skill performance and ends with discussion of abilities.

IDENTIFYING AND CLASSIFYING MOTOR SKILLS

Identifying and classifying motor skills are necessary because movements vary so greatly. Sometimes these actions are not easily observable, for instance, the actions of the pelvic girdle to stabilize the trunk during sitting. Some movements require adaptation to a changing environment. Other movements are done with external objects like sticks. Some movements are rapid and violent. Some are slow, sustained, and precise. And though the definition of motor skills requires actions to be purposeful and voluntary, some actions are so highly automatic and learned that it seems that we need not think about them. Classification enables similarities and basic characteristics among diverse movements to be teased out, which helps in teaching motor skills, monitoring progression through rehabilitation, and prescribing training and exercise regimens. Furthermore, these characteristics may further help identify some of the underlying abilities contributing to execution of the motor skill.

Over the years there have been numerous classification schemes developed to meet the needs of researchers and practitioners (see Burton and Miller, 1998, for a review), but we present here what we believe is the simplest and most applicable classification scheme useful for exercise scientists. This scheme uses characteristics of movements based on (a) the precision of movement, (b) the stability of the environment, and to a lesser extent (c) movement continuity.

Classifying Motor Skills Based on Movement Precision

Classification based on movement precision generally refers to **gross motor skills** versus **fine motor skills**. Gross motor skills use large muscle groups and generally have little precision and often use whole-body movements and multiple limb segments. Many gross skills, including walking, running, jumping, kicking, and basic throwing actions, are further considered to be fundamental motor skills. Fundamental motor skills are those that are typically learned early in development and are foundational to other motor skills. Fine motor skills use small muscles and are precise, such as writing and sewing. Fine motor skills are almost by definition perceptual motor skills.

Some skills are hard to classify as strictly gross or fine, that is, a continuum exists between fine and gross motor skills. Ballet dancing provides a notable example of gross motor actions (jumps, kicks, spins) done with extreme precision and timing, making it unseemly to classify them as gross motor skills. Yet because the underlying movements are fundamental, such as running, jumping, and leaping, most ballet movements would indeed be placed in the gross motor skill category. Other movements

Concepts in Action

Reflexes or Automatic Skills?

Some motor skills happen so fast and are so automatic they seem like reflexes. Consider, for example, a hard hit line drive hit right back at a pitcher (a "comebacker") who makes what seems to be an instantaneous and instinctual catch of the ball. Players in such situations are often commented on as having lightning fast reflexes, but in fact, this is a motor skill and not a reflex. The fundamental patterns of the motor skill may look like a reflex, but through practice and experience the player has learned to react in a directed and coordinated manner and in fact may be suppressing some reflexes. Even though these dangerous situations may be uncommon, players should still practice for them. One technique for baseball pitchers is to have the pitcher face away from the coach who is hitting the "fungoes" from just 55 feet away, and as the coach is preparing to hit the ball, the pitcher is signaled to turn around as fast as possible. This spin disorients players and forces them to quickly and simultaneously ready themselves while looking for an oncoming ball. Clearly this type of practice is for experienced players only, but even younger players can engage in practice designed to develop reaction movements.

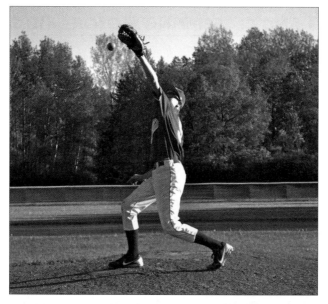

Photo credit Whitman R. Ives.

include both fine and gross skills. Some throwing actions require gross movement of the legs, trunk, and arm followed by a fine motor action of the wrist and hand to control the projectile. Dart throwing would be on the fine motor skills side of the continuum whereas javelin throwing would be on the gross motor skill side.

The importance of gross versus fine classification is best seen in the development and learning of motor skills. Developing children and new learners most often acquire gross motor skills first and then fine skills, and may lose gross and fine skills in differential amounts following injury or disease (Kuhtz-Buschbeck et al., 2003). In addition, fine skills and gross skills may require different practice or training regimens because of the inherent differences between them, such as the level of metabolic effort required of gross skills and the attention demands of fine skills. Piek et al. (2006) even showed that social, academic, and emotional factors were influenced differently by a child's performance on gross versus fine motor skills. There are certainly some exceptions to these gross versus fine differences; nevertheless, it is important to understand that it is generally suggested to develop the gross motor skill components of movement first followed by the fine motor component.

Classifying Motor Skills Based on Environmental Stability

Motor skills are performed in many different settings or environments. The number of settings seems innumerable, but researchers have found that classifying motor skills based on the stability of the sur-rounding environment reveals essential components of the skill. Classification based on environmental stability refers to **closed skills** versus **open skills**. Closed skills are performed in an environment that is stable and predictable. The environment, or objects in the environment, waits to be acted upon by the individual. Examples include bowling, stationary target shooting, and golf. Closed skills are **self-paced**, meaning that the individual chooses their own pace of action.

Open skills are done in a changing and unpredictable environment. The performer acts according to what is happening in the environment. Batting a ball, dribbling a ball through defenders, automo-bile driving, and running a football are examples of open skills. Open skills are generally **externally paced**, meaning that the environment influences the timing and initiation of the motor skill. Thus, open versus closed skills relate to what dictates *what* the performer does; self-paced versus externally paced relates to what dictates *when* the performer acts.

As with fine and gross skills, a continuum exists between open and closed skills. Running on a track is a closed skill, yet running through congested city streets has a large amount of environ-mental instability and may be classified as more of an open skill. Trail running may be classified as midway between open and closed depending on the terrain. Some activities can be open or closed depending on how the individual approaches the task. In the case of activities like parkour or free running (urban acrobatic running), the environment need not physically move or change, but the movement of the performer himself creates unpredictability. For instance, as the free runner jumps over an obstacle or dashes around a corner, an unknown environment appears that may dictate the specific action and pace of action: an open skill. On the other hand, if the course is set in advance, the runner can encounter each obstacle with a preplanned and self-paced action in a closed skill fashion. A common example of open versus closed skills being dependent on environmental- and task-dependent situations is musical instrument playing. In its basic form, playing most instru-ments is a closed skill. Emphasis is on the technical manipulation of the instrument in an ordered and consistent fashion. High-level musicians, however, may play in response to an audience and accompanying musicians. Tempo, loudness, and other musical qualities become tuned into the environment.

The distinctions of open versus closed and externally versus internally paced are important ones. Most motor skills are commonly learned first in a closed environment even if they are naturally open skills. In fact, much of what should comprise "functional training" is the taking of skills and abilities developed in a closed environment and adapting them to the open environment. While this progres-sion is often necessary, it is more challenging than it sounds, because the development of motor skill proficiency in the closed environment is different from the development of proficiency in the open environment. For closed skills, emphasis is placed on consistency of performance, often with precise mastery of technique. In contrast, high-level performance in open skills is marked by adaptability and flexibility of techniques and decision-making skills that are necessary to accommodate changing situations.

Open and closed skills also differ in how regulatory conditions determine motor skill planning and execution (Gentile, 2000). In Chapter 5, we saw how regulatory conditions are those environmental factors that directly or indirectly influence which motor skill is selected and how it is performed. In closed skills, the regulatory conditions are relatively stable, for example, the slickness of a bowling lane is stable and accounted for by the bowler by altering wrist action to change the speed or spin of the ball. Regulatory conditions in an open environment may be relatively stable, such as a smooth turf playing surface, or entirely unstable, such as moving defenders.

SIDE**NOTE**	**ADAPTING FROM CLOSED SKILL TO OPEN SKILL**

Sometimes closed skills need to be rapidly followed by open skills, for example, a pitcher after pitching the ball (mostly closed) needs to ready herself for fielding (open). Practicing the transition from closed to open is necessary to maximize performance, but sometimes a closed skill becomes an open skill without warning. These moments are ripe for injuries as the individual is unprepared for subsequent actions. This squat lift in the photo below is one such example. Due to uneven lifting (and no collars!), the right side weight plate has begun to slide off the bar without notice by the lifter. As soon as this weight falls off the bar, this closed environment becomes open as the lifter must now react to an unstable environment. The need to change attention from a preplanned action in a stable environment to a chaotic situation will make it difficult for this lifter to make appropriate adjustments.

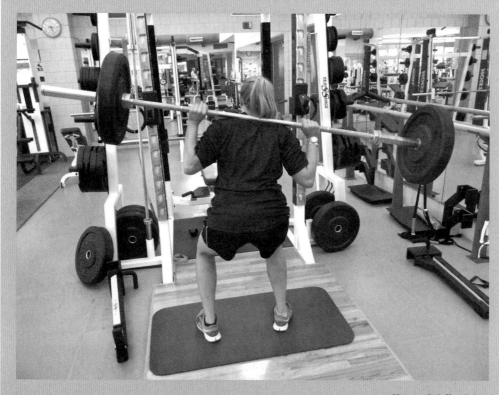

Photo credit Jeffrey C. Ives.

■ Thinking It Through 6.1 Closed versus Open Vertical Jump Actions

Shown in the photos below are two maximal vertical jumps by collegiate volleyball players. The one on the left is done in the lab, the one on the right as part of a spike in a volleyball game. Describe the open and closed skill nature of each and contrast the regulatory conditions that influence jump performance. Next, read the review by Ziv and Lidor (2010) and their conclusions regarding the weak association between laboratory measures of vertical jump height and volleyball. Comment on these findings with respect to open and closed skills.

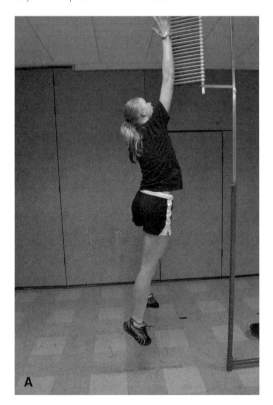
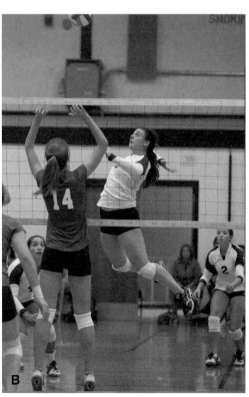

A. Photo credit Jeffrey C. Ives. **B.** Photo credit Tim McKinney.

Classifying Motor Skills Based on Movement Continuity

Another way to categorize movements is based on defining the movement beginning and endpoint. **Discrete skills** have a clear beginning and endpoint, such as a finger snap or punch. Discrete skills can be complex and use the whole body, as seen in a throwing motion. **Serial skills** (or **sequential**) are a series of discrete movements or motor skills done in order to produce a larger or compound motor skill. Some serial skills repeat that same type of motor action, such as playing the piano or typing, while others string together completely different actions. In the latter example are layups in basketball (comprising dribbling, jumping, and shooting) and a gymnastics or dance routine that may have jumps, spins, glides, and more. The operation of many types of industrial equipment provides good examples of serial skills. For instance, running a piece of fabric though a sewing machine requires pressing a foot switch combined with arm motions to push the fabric through the sewing apparatus. **Continuous skills** are repetitive skills such as swimming and running that have arbitrary beginning and endpoints. The endpoints are determined by the performer and the skill itself. Sometimes the distinction between a discrete skill, a serial skill, and a continuous skill is small. For example, shifting gears in a car—requiring depressing the clutch, shifting the gear shift lever, and then releasing clutch—is generally considered a sequential skill. On the other hand, the simultaneous act of braking and depressing the clutch during a normal slowing action in a manual shift vehicle would be considered a discrete skill. Musical instrument playing may sometimes be considered any of the three categories. The emphatic strike on the drum's cymbals may be considered discrete, the repetitive striking of the base drum with the foot pedal may be continuous, and the combination of arm and foot strikes may be considered serial.

Classifying movements based on continuity is used in both research and applied situations. For the practitioner, understanding the continuity and components of a movement helps with breaking down movement sequences for instructional purposes. From an instructional standpoint, it is valuable to determine if a motor skill can or even should be broken down into smaller or discrete segments. It is often difficult, for example, to logically break down a discrete movement into a smaller component, whereas it is relatively easy to do so for serial movements.

A Two-Dimensional Taxonomy of Motor Skill Classification

Gentile (2000) devised a classification scheme combining movement precision and environmental stability. Movement continuity is not considered within this model but can be used in conjunction with the model as necessary. In Gentile's model, environmental context refers to closed skilled (stationary) and open skilled (in motion) motor skills. Gentile's original classification scheme included trial to trial variability, which refers to whether the environmental context changes from one time or trial to another. Trial to trial variability is exemplified in pitching, in which each pitch presents a different situation with new goals. The model presented in Table 6.1 has been simplified by excluding trial to trial variability. Movement precision (action function) in this model has been broken down into those movements that require a stable body (e.g., sitting, standing) versus a mobile body (e.g., gross motor skills like running, swimming, jumping), and object manipulation versus no manipulation (generally fine motor skills with the hands but also includes kicking, heading balls). Shumway-Cook and Woollacott (2007) refined the original model by adding a "quasi-mobile" action function. Originally, body transport referred only to locomotion type activities, but the quasi-mobile distinction includes any movement in which there is a significant linear or angular displacement in the center of mass, such as rising from a chair, falling, and whole-body rotation.

In the taxonomy presented in Table 6.1, tasks generally become more complex as they move from closed to open skill, as more body action is added, and as object manipulation is added. Do not mistake this as meaning that tasks without these factors are easy. For instance, playing most musical instruments are done without body motion in a closed environment (but see previous discussion), yet it takes years of practice to become proficient. Nevertheless, the use of this scheme is useful in many circumstances, including determination of factors that increase the complexity and difficulty of motor skill performance. Classifying the complexities of a movement aids in teaching and rehabilitation, primarily as a guide to progress from simple to complex. For example, orthopedic rehabilitation programs often progress from the simplest components, like standing balance, to the more complex components, like running while simultaneously manipulating an external object. Determining the complexities of movement further aids in understanding what psychological and physiological abilities contribute to the motor skill performance.

Applying the Classification Taxonomy

In a broad sense, the classification of a motor skill using the two-dimensional taxonomy helps to understand the skill's components, complexities, and regulatory influences. This information can be used to break the skill down into simpler components to facilitate learning and provide direction for continued skill development. Consider, for example, basketball dribbling. The first step is to determine its classification and then, from that point, identify ways to simplify and instruct. Chapter 9 provides an in-depth look at instruction, so we will not elaborate further at this time. Table 6.2 outlines the steps to this process and provides examples. Note that identifying key regulatory conditions is an important part of understanding the open and closed environment.

Classifying a motor skill is also the first step to understanding the abilities that provide the foundation for successful performance. From the example in Table 6.2, dribbling is seen to be a complex skill

TABLE 6.1	A Modified Version of Gentile's Taxonomy of Motor Skills with Examples

	Action Function					
	Stable Body		Quasi-Mobile Body		Mobile Body	
Environmental Context	No Object Manipulation	With Object Manipulation	No Object Manipulation	With Object Manipulation	No Object Manipulation	With Object Manipulation
Closed skill: stationary	Sitting, static hamstring stretches	Industrial sewing, free throw shooting, guitar playing	Rising from a chair, sitting up on a bed, jumping jacks	Squat exercises with weight bar, golf	Running on a treadmill, swimming, diving	Bowling, pole vaulting
Open skill: in motion	Riding a roller coaster, balance platform	Assembly line work, video games, driving	Dance, dance revolution, round-house karate kick	Batting, wrestling throw	Running outdoors among traffic	Most team sport play, tennis

Note: Tasks Generally Get More Difficult or Complex Moving from the Upper Left Corner to the Lower Right Corner.

TABLE 6.2	Guidelines for Using Gentile's Taxonomy to Classify and Then Simplify Motor Skills

Identifying the Motor Skill Taxonomy of Basketball Dribbling		
Classification Dimension	**Classification Decision**	**Simplification Ideas**
1. Is the environment open or closed? Why? What are the key regulatory conditions?	Open. Primarily because players (offensive and defensive) are moving about Location of other players, ball characteristics, speed of player's movements, presence of a defender, boundary lines, and floor characteristics	Make the skill closed by practicing without other players Remove or ignore difficult conditions, such as defenders and boundary lines
2. Action: body transport	Generally yes. Player runs/walks up and down court. May include sideways and backward movements	Remove the need to run or walk by dribbling in place or while slow walking
3. Action: object manipulation	Yes, handling the ball	Simplify ball characteristics, such as making the ball larger and with a better grip

requiring, among other things, agility, hand–object coordination, and the ability to "read" the court to determine patterns of play. Successful coaches are able to evaluate players to determine which areas of a player's performance are in need of most practice or training and create practice conditions to work on those weaknesses.

■ Thinking It Through 6.2 Steps in Classifying and Simplifying

1. Using the taxonomy of motor skills shown in Table 6.1 and the classification guidelines in Table 6.2, classify the movements below. In order to understand the movement well enough to classify it, you must observe the movement or experience it for yourself. If you are unable to personally observe or experience the movements, either watch a video (e.g., YouTube) or mentally image the act as best you can and proceed from there.

   a. Walking down a flight of spiral stairs in the Statue of Liberty
   b. Exercising on a cross-country ski simulator
   c. Playing hopscotch
   d. Performing open heart surgery
   e. Driving a manual shift automobile
   f. Rock climbing

   Based on the classifications, order the tasks from easiest to most difficult. Also identify the movement continuity classification (discrete, serial, continuous) of these skills. Does your perception of difficulty match up with the classification scheme? Why or why not?

   Next, using the guidelines presented in Table 6.2, simplify for instructional or rehabilitation purposes one of the activities listed above.

MEASURING MOTOR SKILL PERFORMANCE

Determining the type of motor skill and its constituent components is important, as is measuring the quality of performance. Measuring movement quality enables an assessment of progression of improvement during training and rehabilitation, identifies areas of weaknesses and strengths, and provides information for feedback. Knowing the quality of performance allows persons to be compared to standard metrics or to others. The measurement of motor skills necessarily includes the measurement of motor abilities. In fact, measuring abilities may give insight to how an individual performs a skill. For example, after determining a volleyball player's hitting skill, it would be useful to measure contributing abilities like agility and vertical jump height.

Procedures for Measuring Motor Skills and Abilities

Evaluating motor skills and abilities is the topic of many textbooks in physical education, physical rehabilitation, and sport performance training (e.g., Burton & Miller, 1998; Gore, 2000). Here we highlight the two essential steps necessary to provide useful information. The first is determining the appropriate and valid **performance measure** (or **criterion measure**), and the second is to test the performance measure with accuracy and reliability. Both sound simple, but both steps are in fact difficult and when done incorrectly lead to assessments that may be incorrect and misleading.

Establishing the appropriate performance measure in terms of validity is filled with potential problems. In general, validity refers to the measurement actually measuring what you want to know, or being a true reflection of the performance item in question. Consider a collegiate cross-country running coach evaluating high school runners. The coach wants to recruit the best athlete to help her team win. What is the coach going to evaluate? The obvious choice would be to look at the athletes' running times, but how could she compare an athlete running at sea level versus an athlete living in the mountains? She could base her evaluation on winning percentage, but competition so varies from school to school that the star at one school might not even make the team at another. She could evaluate abilities, like maximal oxygen consumption (VO_2max), but how much does this really contribute to success? Perhaps she could get hold of psychological profiles of hardiness and confidence, but again, are there clear associations among these and running success? Thus, the question of what is the most important thing to measure to determine the athlete's future success is not an easy one.

Determining the relevant and valid motor skills and abilities requires experience and trial and error. A great deal of scientific literature exists on assessing the skills and abilities of athletes, laypersons, and persons with injuries or disease, though it is difficult to find consensus on what should be measured for a given situation. Rehabilitation situations provide good examples that the important criterion measures are not always obvious. For example, it may be more helpful in evaluating progression of cardiopulmonary rehabilitation to know depression scores rather than oxygen consumption, because depression scores directly relate to the patient's quality of life. Likewise, an injured athlete's hamstring to quadriceps strength ratio and figure-8 running speed may be less important indicators of return to play than a subjective measure of movement smoothness.

■ Thinking It Through 6.3 Performance Measurements

Select one of the disease or injury conditions below and conduct a scientific literature search on how functional performance is measured on patients with the condition. Comment on whether these performance measures are valid or reliable.

a. Cardiac or cardiopulmonary conditions
b. Idiopathic low back pain
c. Chronic fatigue syndrome
d. Hip replacement

After the performance measure is chosen, testing must take place. Unless the testing is accurate, reliable, and repeatable, it is a waste of time. It is out of the scope of this book to discuss testing methodology, but it is important for practitioners to know that if testing procedures are poor, then there is little point in testing at all. Reliability of a performance measure refers to the ability to get similar results over repeated testing and is based on the performer, the tester, and the testing procedures. Because of biological variation and psychological factors such as motivation, the human performer tends to be plagued by inherent variation. Being able to test people and account for this variation to get reliable results is a necessary skill for all exercise scientists.

There are no specific rules for choosing the right performance measure, but there are some guidelines. In keeping with the essential elements of testing, the measure must be reliable in terms of administering the test and the subject's performance on the test. Deviations in performance measures should thus reflect real changes in performance and not inconsistencies in how the test was administered. The measure must be valid, that is, performance on the criterion measure must reflect performance of the motor skill. Validity may be the most problematic and most overlooked aspect in testing human motor performance, in part because of entrenched measurement systems. Even at the highest level of sport, for example, the highly touted National Football League (NFL) scouting combine, prediction tests are questionable in terms of identifying future star players (Kuzmits & Adams, 2008). In particular, some of the NFL combine tests, such as the 40-m dash and the NFL 225–bench press test, are questionable in terms of how important they are. Consider, for instance, that New England Patriot quarterback Tom Brady recorded the slowest 40-m dash of any quarterback up to that time. Apparently this did not slow him down from being one of the most successful quarterbacks of all time and certainly a future Hall of Famer. The National Hockey League (NHL) has a similar combine, which continues to use a cycle ergometer test for VO_2max even though it is poorly associated with the outcome of on-ice VO_2max tests (Durocher et al., 2010). In sum, it is essential that the measurement reflects accurately what the practitioner wants to know, which may be the outcome of performance or how the performance outcome was accomplished. These differences are described below.

Categories of Performance Measures

In choosing a performance measure, the practitioner or researcher must determine what kind of information is important. Performance measures can be loosely grouped into two categories regarding the nature of the information provided: response outcome and response production measures. **Response (or performance) outcome** measures evaluate the result of a particular skilled action. These measures reveal what happened, not how it happened. Specific response outcome measures generally include measures of speed (e.g., velocity), time (e.g., 0.25 seconds), accuracy, and direction. **Response (or performance) production** measures, on the other hand, reveal how a response was produced. Note that these categories are not mutually exclusive. Sometimes a response production measure can be used for response outcome measures and vice versa.

Response production measures are those that pertain to how, or even why, a movement was done. Kinematic measurements of displacement, velocity, and acceleration and kinetic measures of force and torque describe characteristics of movement without necessarily revealing the outcome of the movement. These biomechanical measures can be made with sophisticated goniometric and videographic technology but are often done in a more subjective or qualitative manner by observation (Knudson & Morrison, 2002). For instance, a coach may identify a poor ball toss as a reason why a tennis serve hit the net. Electromyography (EMG) and mechanomyography (MMG) are other sophisticated tools to provide response production information. EMG and MMG may give information on muscle timing, strength of contraction, and muscle function that underlie motor skill performance. Either can be used to examine muscle dysfunction and have other clinical uses in rehabilitation such as biofeedback.

Concepts in Action

Using EMG to Evaluate Exercise Performance

The use of EMG as a response production measure can reveal much about how the movement is being carried out. In the illustration below, the top trace is movement of the elbow through flexion and extension during two rapid push-up exercises. The middle trace is EMG activity from the triceps b. muscle, and the bottom trace is EMG activity from the biceps b. muscle. The triceps b. EMG reveals a rapid onset of muscle activity at the bottom of the push-up to stop the body's downward movement and propel it upward. Biceps b. activity comes on a bit later during the extension, probably as part of horizontal shoulder flexion, perhaps as cocontraction to stabilize shoulder and elbow. The triceps are moderately active during descent of the body (elbow flexion), probably as a way to control downward speed. These data reveal that movement form and quality are dependent on a coordinative action of both flexor and extensor muscles.

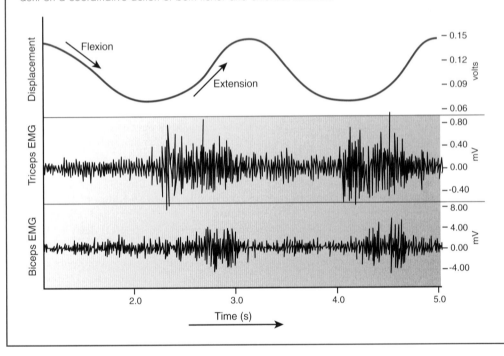

Measuring Information Processing

The aforementioned response outcome and production measures assess physiological performance. Measures to assess the cognitive aspects of movement are often more complex and less user-friendly. The most common measurement of cognitive performance is the response outcome measure **reaction time (RT)**. RT is the measure of the time from a stimulus to the onset of a response. It does not include movement and is thus used to measure the information processing time involved in a task. **Information processing** is the essential job of our brain—to take in information and interpret it, store it, and manipulate it (see Chapter 8). RT is not the only way to measure information processing but in most instances is the most practically useful way to measure the cognitive components that accompany motor skill performance.

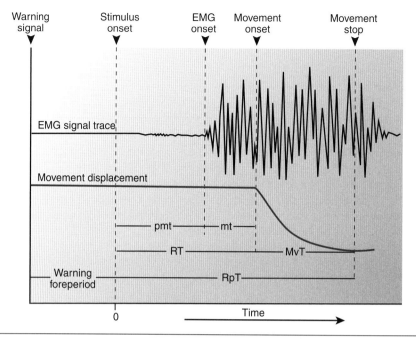

Figure 6.1 • The components of fractionated response time and RT are illustrated in this schematic. The stimulus may be any sensory signal, including light, sound, and touch. A warning signal gives advance notice, but is not the stimulus. Total RT is made up of premotor time (pmt) and motor time (mt). RpT is made up of RT and movement time (MvT).

RT can be fractionated into premotor time and motor time. Figure 6.1 illustrates that **premotor time** is the time from the stimulus to the onset of muscle electrical activity and reflects the pure information processing component. **Motor time** (also called **electromechanical delay** or **EMD**) is the time from the onset of muscle electrical activity to the initiation of the motor response and reflects peripheral neuromuscular delays. These delays include neural transmission times and time for excitation–contraction coupling in the muscle. RT itself is one component of total response time (RpT). RpT is the time from a stimulus to the completion of the response and thus includes RT and movement time (MvT). **Movement time** (MvT) is defined as the time from the onset of movement to movement completion. When RT is paired with a movement response, it is specifically called motor RT.

RT paradigms can range from *simple RT* with just one stimulus paired with one response to very complex, in which there are multiple stimuli and multiple responses. Complex RT tasks are further categorized as *choice RT* or *discrimination RT*. Choice RT paradigms have two or more stimuli, with each stimulus coupled to a specific response. Discrimination RT paradigms have multiple stimuli, but only one stimulus is relevant and only one response is coupled to that stimulus. According to *Hick's Law* (Hick, 1952), RT slows logarithmically as the number of stimulus and response choices increases. The fastest RTs with a motor response are about 150 to 200 ms and occur in simple RT situations of one stimulus and one response. Complex RT paradigms are the most difficult and result in the slowest RTs, as individuals must assess the nature of the stimuli and an appropriate response. Complex RT tasks done in the lab may slow RT by 50% to 100% over a simple RT task, and very complex RT tasks may take seconds rather than milliseconds.

Complex RT paradigms serve to challenge information processing and may include stimuli that are unpredictable, situations in which the stimulus is not compatible with the response (e.g., a right arrow stimulus prompts a movement to the left), and when the stimulus or the response are very complex by themselves. Note, however, that the demands of the movement response may or may not impact information processing speed. Automobile driving illustrates all of these concepts. Consider the case of driving down the road and a dog unexpectedly runs out from between two parked cars, running from right to left toward the middle of the road. The dog itself is the visual stimuli. Had the dog been seen in advance on the sidewalk (a warning), preliminary steps would have been taken to plan a potential response and reduce uncertainty (e.g., prepare to step on the brake). The dog's direction, speed, and body actions provide information to the driver regarding potential responses. If the dog sprints with no hesitation, the stimulus is relatively simple, but if it hesitates or changes direction, the driver is forced to process a more complex situation. Responses are to stop (compatible response), swerve to the left or right (either is compatible or incompatible depending on prior experience), do nothing (incompatible based on prior experience), or simultaneously brake and swerve (complex). Each response has a consequence, and each response is situation dependent. Most drivers would slam on the brakes (not complex, compatible), but that may be a poor choice in heavy traffic or high-speed situations. In both situations, rapid braking may end up in a loss of control or being rear-ended by the cars following. Swerving left into oncoming traffic or swerving right into parked cars are even worse choices. The best choice may be to do nothing, which for most drivers is highly incompatible with the stimulus.

In the laboratory, simple and complex RT paradigms are easily set up and manipulated with various stimuli and various responses. Visual, auditory, and tactile stimuli are the ones most investigated in the laboratory, but stimuli from all of sensory receptors give rise to movement reactions. This includes taste, smell, and all the signals from our visceroreceptors and somatoreceptors monitoring body processes. In the laboratory, responses are most often simple discrete movements like key presses, but developments in technology are enabling measurement of whole-body actions to complex stimuli. Experimental paradigms may include warning signals that precede a stimulus. A warning is not the stimulus itself, but may provide some information to enable the individual to anticipate that a stimulus is coming and even what that stimulus may be.

Reaction tasks have provided a wealth of information on information processing concepts, but unfortunately performance on simple RT tasks do not seem to translate well outside the laboratory to real-world skills. For example, Vanttinen et al. (2010) found no difference in simple laboratory visual RT scores between elite U16 and U19 youth soccer players. Over the past several decades, a number of researchers have examined if basic laboratory measures of RT were valid in identifying or discriminating higher level athletes, but no consensus has been found (see Emre & Kocak, 2010, for a brief review). Mouelhi Guizani et al. (2006) concluded that using RT tests to discriminate and identify athletes need to be made much more similar to the actual information processing demands of the sport or activity. Recently, Australian researchers have begun developing reactive agility tests designed to test for open skill choice RT (Farrow et al., 2005). These tests, as diagrammed in Figure 6.2, hold promise in being more appropriate in assessing sport-specific RT abilities.

Some RT tests, even relatively simple tests, have been made to assess task-dependent information processing in areas outside of sport. The older adult driver RT test from the American Association of Retired Persons (AARP) is a simple paper and pencil test used to assess elderly drivers for driving-specific information processing (Fig. 6.3). As part of a larger test battery, this test has been shown to help predict the risk for driving accidents in older drivers (Stutts et al., 1998).

In recent years, two techniques have become popular in assessing information processing in the motor skill environment: visual gaze tracking and visual occlusion. Gaze tracking uses specialized equipment to follow the pupil of the eye, which enables researchers to identify visual search strategies and attention control strategies. Occlusion techniques are methods used to limit visual information to the subjects to assess their ability to predict forthcoming actions. One way to occlude visual information is to have the subject watch a motor skill performance on video that is stopped at certain points during the action (temporal occlusion) or certain aspects of the movement are hidden from view

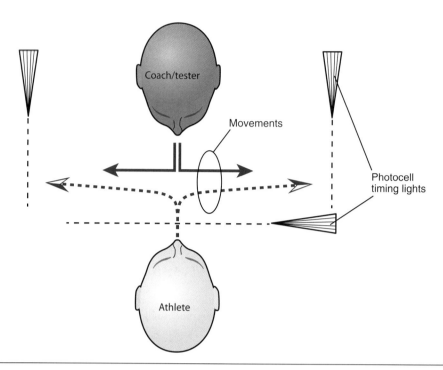

Figure 6.2 • A reactive agility testing paradigm based on Farrow et al. (2005). This test measures RpT in an agility test without fractionating RT from movement time. In the test, the athlete and tester face each other from about 5 yards apart. The athlete initiates a movement directly toward the tester, which triggers the onset of timing by the photocell timing light. As soon as the athlete begins movement, the tester takes a step toward the oncoming athlete and makes a cut to the right or left. The athlete must respond to the cut and follow the tester to the left or right and through the photocell timing light to stop the clock. The RpT is a combination of agility speed and ability to react to the tester's movement stimulus.

(spatial occlusion) (see accompanying "SideNote"). When the video is stopped, the subject is instructed to predict what action of the performer comes next, such as the direction of a volleyball or tennis serve. Responses by the subject may include simple verbalization, key strokes, or whole-body actions. Another occlusion technique uses special glasses that can turn opaque almost instantaneously. This allows researchers to stop the visual information coming to the subject during real-life action. These techniques have revealed that expert performers predict or anticipate actions faster and more accurately than novices, even with less information available to them.

Measuring Error

Among the most common performance measures are measurements of error. Error measurements are used to determine accuracy of response outcomes as well as response production measures, both of which can include spatial (in space) or temporal (in time) errors. Several different types of error measures, used with both temporal and spatial accuracy, can be used to gain an understanding of what caused the error and how to instruct performers to better their performance. Each error score provides one bit of information and thus must be interpreted carefully to gather important information. Often a single error score is compiled after several trials that summarizes the trials.

Constant error (CE) is simply the average error over a given number of trials. The score is based on both the magnitude and direction of error and thus provides not only a measure of how much error but a bias or tendency in the performance. Absolute error (AE) is the average over a given number of trials

Test steps

1. Find the number 1 in the upper left corner of the photo. Start the timer for 10 seconds.
2. As quickly as possible, touch the other numbers in numerical order (2, 3, 4, 5, 6, etc.).
3. Stop after 10 seconds. The last number you touch is your score.

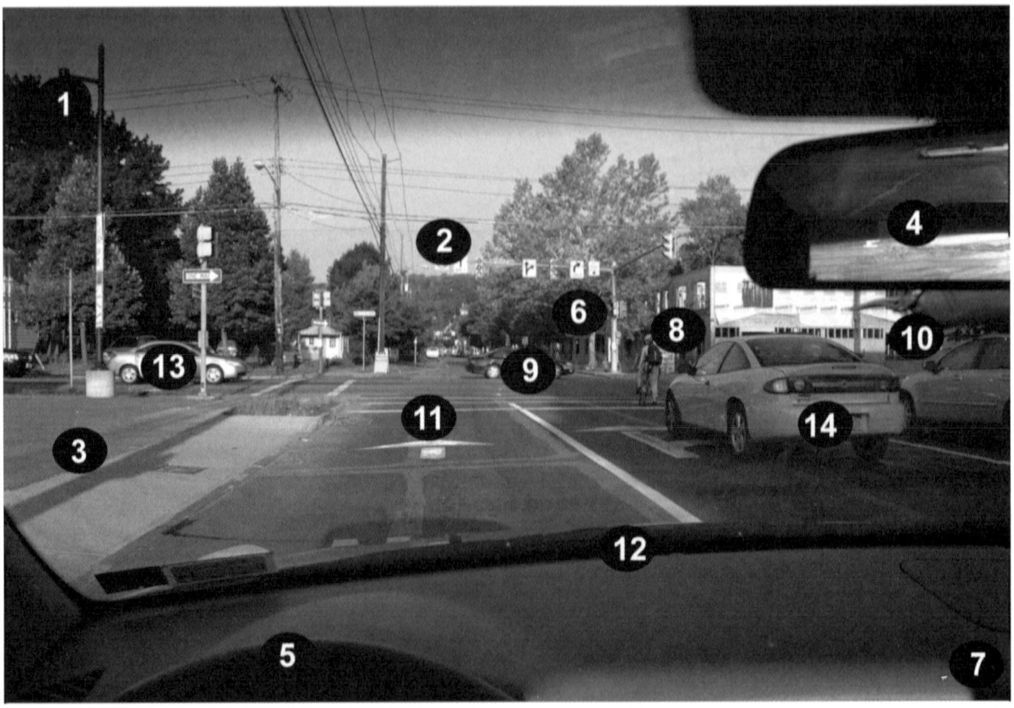

Scoring	Age	<18	18-29	30-39	40-49	50-59	40-49	70+
	Above average	14	14	14	13-14	13-14	13-14	10-14
	Average	12-13	11-13	11-13	10-12	9-12	8-11	6-9
	Below average	1-11	1-10	1-10	1-9	1-9	1-7	1-5

Score: Find your score in one of the columns under your age

Figure 6.3 • A RT test for older adult drivers from the AARP. The test simply has the drivers tap each number in numerical sequence and marks the highest number reached in 10 seconds as the score. Perhaps not an RT test in a direct sense, it does require the driver to search the photo for stimuli (numbers) and react to the stimuli. The task requires visual search as well as the ability to pick up incidental information (location of numbers) as the search process continues. (Test adapted from American Association of Retired Persons. (1992). *Older driver skill assessment and resource guide: Creating mobility choices*. Washington, DC: American Association of Retired Persons; *http://emedicine.medscape.com/article/318521-overview*.)

of the error absolute values. Thus, no plus or minus or direction of the scores is provided, just the error magnitude. **Variable error** (VE) is the standard deviation of the group of error scores. It is a measure of the consistency of the responses and not the amount of error. Figure 6.4 gives examples of the types of errors and basic interpretations of what they could indicate.

Videos are shown on a computer screen with various amounts of temporal (A) or spatial (B) information. (A) The video is stopped at different points during the serve: from early (T1) to late (T4). In each instance, the experimental subject is instructed to respond as fast as they can verbally or with keystrokes regarding where they think the served ball is going to land. Accuracy of the response and RT are measured.
(B) The video actor has been erased to varying amounts, limiting the amount of information. With more information in panel 1, the subjects react faster and more accurately than in panels 4 or 5. Compared to novices, sport-skilled subjects react faster and with more accuracy to images with less information.

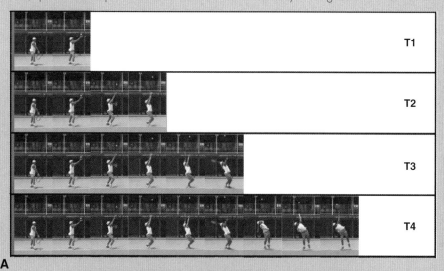

A

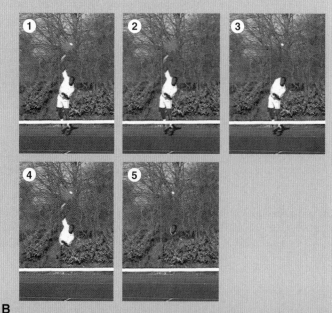

B

A. From Farrow, D., & Abernethy, B. (2002). Can anticipatory skills be learned through implicit video-based perceptual training?. *Journal of Sports Sciences*, *20*(6), 471–485, Reprinted by the publisher Taylor & Francis Ltd; *http://www.tandf.co.uk/journals*, with permission. B. From Jackson, R., & Morgan, P. (2007). Advance visual information, awareness, and anticipation skill. *Journal of Motor Behavior*, *39*(5), 341–351. Reprinted by the publisher Taylor & Francis Ltd; *http://www.tandf.co.uk/journals*, with permission.

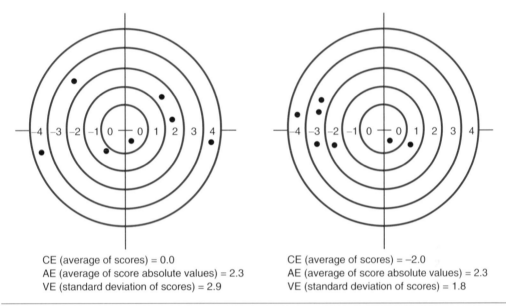

CE (average of scores) = 0.0
AE (average of score absolute values) = 2.3
VE (standard deviation of scores) = 2.9

CE (average of scores) = –2.0
AE (average of score absolute values) = 2.3
VE (standard deviation of scores) = 1.8

Figure 6.4 • Two examples of error scores using rifle targets as examples. Negative scores represent shots to the left, positive scores are shots to the right. On the left, the CE is zero, indicting no left/right bias. The far from center shots result in an AE of 2.3 and a wide scatter results in a large VE. The scores on the right target have the same AE, but because the scores are more clustered, there is a smaller VE. The scores are biased to the left of the target, leaving a negative CE. Interpretation of these error scores between left and right may be vastly different. The left side may indicate an inability of the shooter to hold a steady hand, whereas on the right the systematic error may indicate a problem in the rifle or scope. The simplicity of the scoring does not account for high and low shots, which could be additional sources of error.

As we will see in the next few chapters, the majority of instruction given to learners to improve their performance is based on error information, or more specifically, the deviation from a standard or idealized performance score. Errors in performance, even if using high-speed video, are generally assessed using qualitative or subjective observations by coaches or instructors. These methods can be very successful (Knudson & Morrison, 2002). Quantification of production errors, that is, a precise numerical analysis of error, is typically made from video assessment and software-enabling quantified measurements. As illustrated in Figure 6.5, movements can be broken down using proper video software and measurements taken. Response outcome error measurements tend to be more easily quantified, as in the case of target shooting and precisely measuring the distance from the target. Whether the error measurement is qualitative or quantitative, it is important to understand that VE, AE, and CE provides different types information regarding performance and thus must be interpreted in the context of identifying the most important or meaningful performance errors.

The use of video—both high speed and standard—to provide instruction feedback for athletes and persons undergoing physical rehabilitation, is now considered normal. Consider the javelin thrower in Figure 6.5. Close inspection of the athlete's body biomechanics, javelin trajectory, or performance outcome (javelin distance) may reveal a number of different errors ranging from a poor release point to overstriding. The coach and athlete must determine if these errors are consistent (low or high VE), if they are biased in one direction or another (CE), or if they are large or small in magnitude (AE). Inconsistent performance may be caused by one thing, biased performance another, and large errors still another. Instructors may decide to address just one aspect of performance error or may decide to identify a root cause leading to multiple error types. Clearly no single type of error always reveals the most about performance, but instructors and learners must be able to evaluate all different types of error.

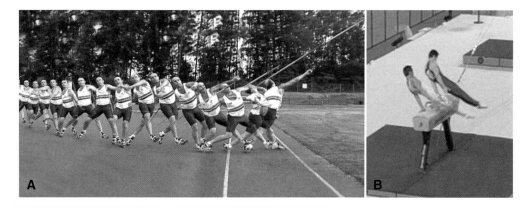

Figure 6.5 • Performance errors can be assessed by using digital videography. **A**. A strobe image of a javelin thrower enables the athlete and coach to break down and evaluate each component of the approach and throw. Errors can be evaluated by comparing to previous performances, and even overlaying a previous performance onto the video. Sometimes the measurement of error is subjective, with the coach and athlete making comparisons to mental images they may have. **B**. Another way to evaluate performance is by comparison of one person to another. In this overlayed strobe image, two different gymnasts are compared on the pommel horse performance. (Photos courtesy of Dartfish Software, Switzerland.)

ABILITIES AND INDIVIDUAL DIFFERENCES

If there is one thing that is revealed by testing of motor skills, it is that people are all different. A vast array of qualities, alone or in combination, provide each person with unique abilities. These abilities give rise to different skill sets and proficiencies, which enable people to solve problems and overcome challenges in vastly different ways. Two football running backs, for example, may be equally successful (yards gained per carry), but one gains yards by avoiding tacklers while the other runs through tacklers. The first running back may rely on abilities like agility, perceptual decision making, and visual search. In contrast, the second running back may make use of leg power, body mass, and an aggressive personality.

Both runners in this example use motor abilities that contribute to their football running skill. There are many such abilities, some of which are easily identifiable, some of which are difficult to

SIDE**NOTE**	**VIDEO, THE INTERNET, AND PERFORMANCE EVALUATION**

Using the Internet to view videos of professional athletes has turned many individuals into self-proclaimed professional performance evaluators. Athletes with hallmark traits, such as Andy Roddick's worlds' fastest tennis serve, have come under intense qualitative and quantitative analyses by individuals with all levels (or lack thereof) of expertise. But even among experts, the evaluation of performance may differ. For instance, the USA Today newspaper quoted former Roddick coaches who claimed that Roddick's success was due to leg and body power (http://www.usatoday.com/sports/tennis/andy-roddick-serve.htm). In contrast, motor control experts noted the importance of trunk, arm, and wrist rotation as reported in Popular Mechanics magazine (http://www.popularmechanics.com/outdoors/sports/physics/4221210). The take-home point is that performance evaluations are often complex, particularly with complex motor skills, and relying on single sources of information may not be wise.

identify, and some of which are yet to be uncovered by researchers. This is just one of the problems in trying to identify the essential abilities that underlie successful motor skill performance, or for identifying athletic potential in individuals. In this section, we will first look at the nature of abilities and how to identify them and then the problems with using abilities to predict future motor skill success.

CLASSIFYING ABILITIES

Unlike motor skill classification, abilities fall into three broad categories: (1) physical proficiency, (2) psychological, and (3) psychomotor (Table 6.3). Physical proficiency abilities are those that are based largely on physiological and anatomical characteristics. These abilities include those that are highly modifiable through training, such as muscle strength, muscle mass, flexibility, maximal oxygen uptake, and metabolic properties. These abilities also include those that are static or have limited potential to change, such as muscle fiber type, height, lung size, and many others. Keep in mind that these static abilities are largely genetic, but that does not mean that all genetic abilities are unmodifiable. Genetic abilities (and perhaps some genetic skills) that contribute to specific motor performance are defined here as **talent**.

Psychomotor abilities are physical proficiency abilities that require a great deal of cognitive processing. Generally, this includes hand–eye coordination and precision capabilities, RT, and decision making for motor actions. Catching and interceptive actions are examples of psychomotor abilities. Psychological abilities are numerous, but their contributions to successful motor performance are much less clear compared to physical proficiency abilities. General psychological abilities that have been identified as important in many sport situations include motivation, desire and enthusiasm, concentration, self-efficacy and confidence, task-related information processing, and hardiness (Humara, 2000; Morgan et al., 1988; Sheard & Golby, 2010). Other cognitive abilities with an uncertain relationship to motor performance, or that may vary depending on the motor task, include general intelligence, emotional coping, aggression, personality, and hope (e.g., Gould et al., 2002; for a review, see Gould & Maynard, 2009).

Physical proficiency abilities are often simple to identify either through direct observation or testing. Indeed, physical proficiency and physiological measures form the majority of testing across the range from athletic performance to medical testing in clinical populations. Strength, speed, power, and metabolism form the bulk of athlete testing, and measures like heart rate, blood pressure, and blood tests are just a few of the basic measures taken in nearly every medical evaluation. Though some psychomotor abilities, like RT, are easy to measure in the laboratory, the validity of these measures to

TABLE 6.3	Categories of Abilities with Examples		
	Categories of Abilities		
	Physical Proficiency	**Psychomotor**	**Psychological**
Description	Physiological, anatomical, biomechanical characteristics	Movements and motor skill components requiring considerable perceptual and cognitive processing	Behavioral and psychological characteristics
Examples	Lung capacity, fiber type, muscle strength, tissue strength, immunity	Motor RT, limb coordination, movement precision, dexterity	Emotional control, cognition, hardiness, attention, optimism

contribute to real-life and sporting environments is often uncertain. Psychological abilities, generally measured by pen and paper tests, are plagued by validity and reliability issues (Adams & Kuzmits, 2008), which is one reason why only a few psychological abilities have been decidedly identified as important.

GENETIC AND LEARNED ABILITIES

Compared to physical proficiency abilities, the genetic predisposition and trainability of the psychological and psychomotor abilities has been little investigated (Bouchard & Malina, 1983; Rankinen et al., 2006). Moreover, the psychological factors that give rise to psychological abilities, for instance, identifying psychological traits that enable one to gain more sport-related information processing, are largely unknown. Despite the cloud of ambiguity that surrounds the identification and measurement of psychological abilities, there is a growing recognition that psychomotor and psychological abilities are the key to performance at the highest levels. For example, even a simple agility test with a RT component (perceptual motor open skill) is a much better discriminator of higher level athletes than a simple closed skill agility test without the RT component (Sheppard et al., 2006).

Among all the abilities one can list, vision is critical to performance of a vast array of motor skills, particularly open skills involving the need to monitor the external environment. Vision plays a considerable role in feedback but more than any other sensory system plays a role in movement preparation, that is, feedforward (see Chapter 4). In particular, information gathered during visual searching enables the performer to anticipate and preselect and preset limb and body movements relative to the environment.

Vision, like other sensory systems, involves both a physiological detection component and a "software" perception component. It was thought that perfect vision (20/20 on the Snellen's eye chart) was a prerequisite for any hand–eye coordination sport and that athletes in these sports had better visual hardware (both foveal and peripheral vision). This, however, is not likely the case. There is not a lot of evidence that experts in a chosen field have better vision (e.g., acuity, foveal and peripheral vision) nor is there compelling evidence that better visual acuity can be improved with visual training. Certainly, there are reports of athletes with better than average vision, such as the 20/10 vision of Hall of Fame baseball player Ted Williams. Williams, however, dismissed this as being the important factor in seeing the ball, but rather, he maintained that it was his intense discipline and visual concentration that was important.

Visual sensation is genetically linked, but is visual perception also genetic? Is it possible to improve both sensation and perception of vision? It is well known that experts have better visual search and that visual search is modifiable through training. Exactly how much one's visual perception can improve, though, is unknown.

COMBINING ABILITIES FOR SKILLED MOTOR PERFORMANCE

Successful motor skill performance, whether driving, knitting, or playing linebacker, nearly always requires multiple abilities. The contribution of some abilities to performance seems obvious, like vertical jump height to basketball playing. Yet the importance of a particular ability to performance varies considerably among individuals. Basketball Hall of Famer Larry Bird had only average jumping ability by National Basketball Association (NBA) standards yet along with Michael Jordan (outstanding vertical leap) were the stars of their day. Bird used other abilities—court sense, knowledge, shooting touch, and body control—to succeed on the court.

There are a few athletes that seem able to do it all; so-called natural athletes that step out onto any field or court and excel. The performance of multiple sport stars, like Jim Thorpe and Babe Didrikson Zaharias from days past, or Deion Sanders and Jackie Joyner-Kersee more recently, seems to imply the existence of a singular global motor ability that contributes to ultimate motor skill performance. In other words, is there some motor ability that is required for success in any sport, or in any given sport, is there some ability that all the successful athletes have? The answer to the question appears to be a resounding "no." Research extending back to the 1950s has been unequivocal in documenting that success—even high-level success—in one sport or motor skill does not in any way guarantee success in any other sport or motor skill. In like manner, it does not appear that there is a general motor educability, that is, the ability to learn different motor skills with the same proficiency or efficiency.

The all-around athlete, sometimes called the natural athlete, is best explained by an athlete having many abilities or a few extremely good abilities that are relevant to many skills. For example, power, speed, and visual search are abilities that are important to many sports, and some athletes manage to exploit these abilities and transfer them to other sports. This does not mean that any athlete with these skills can easily apply them across the board nor does it imply that there is a general motor educability.

ABILITIES AND TALENT IDENTIFICATION

It makes sense that if one's motor abilities can be determined, then practice and training can be more deliberate in enhancing strengths and overcoming weaknesses. Moreover, it seems reasonable that prediction of motor skill proficiency would be possible if one's underlying motor abilities were identified. Both of these suggestions have merit, and both are widely practiced. However, there are a number of issues that make teaching and prediction based on motor abilities difficult.

Challenges in Determining Abilities for Talent Identification

The practice of predicting future performance based on current abilities is widespread, and is often referred to as **talent identification**. Remember, talent is defined as genetic abilities, though in this context, "talent" is more broadly used as a combination of skills and abilities contributing to overall success in a particular sport or activity. For example, personality tests, like the Myers-Briggs Inventory, are used in business to assess the qualifications and potential for success for managers and executives. The NFL participates in the "scouting combine," a 4-day series of physical and mental proficiency tests to rate the potential for college players to succeed in the NFL.

The first challenge in talent identification is the measurement of one's abilities. As we saw earlier, some abilities are difficult to measure or even categorize. The second issue concerns the matching of one's abilities with performance in a particular motor skill. There have been numerous studies that have identified certain features of athletes participating in certain sports. The best hitters in volleyball, for example, tend to be tall and have good vertical leaps. There are many players, though, that are tall with good vertical leaps that are not good hitters. Abernethy et al. (1995) noted that muscle strength is able to discriminate players in many sports, but only to the extent of identifying high-level from low-level athletes. Within a performance level (e.g., NFL), strength does not appear to discriminate one athlete from another. These examples illustrate the difficulty in identifying the essential abilities necessary for good performance and that individuals bring their own ability mixture to motor skill performance.

The Effectiveness of Talent Identification Programs

Perhaps the most striking example of talent identification is the selection of children by the Chinese to enter their Olympic training programs. In China, talent selection officers travel from elementary school to elementary school and measure flexibility, RT, body and bone anthropometrics, and other abilities. Children with outstanding abilities are sent to sport training schools specific to their abilities, like gymnastics school for children with high flexibility or weight lifting school for children with specific leg to torso to arm length ratios. While the Chinese authorities may marvel at this model of efficiency, there is little evidence that such a selection process has merit. Vaeyens et al. (2009) have looked at state-sponsored Olympic talent identification programs and concluded that they remain questionable and, further, noted that the extended institutional sport-specific training for adolescents is not necessarily associated with elite sport achievement. Even the validities of the highly touted NFL scouting combine (Kuzmits & Adams, 2008) and NHL combine (Vescovi et al., 2006a,b) are in question. All these cases, particularly the testing of children and adolescents, fail to adhere to the two key principles of testing: (1) identifying the essential abilities of the target skill and (2) the validity and reliability of the tests used.

■ Thinking It Through 6.4 Professional Scouting Combines

The ability to predict performance in professional athletes is the purpose of scouting combines. These combines involve a multiday series of physiological, motor skill, and psychological testing. The NHL draftee in the photo below is performing the NHL combine medicine ball throw. Despite being at the highest level of sport, these combines are controversial in their prediction success. For instance, Vescovi et al. (2006a,b) cast doubt on the usefulness of the NHL combine, whereas Tarter et al. (2009) supported its use. Read through the articles below and come to your own conclusions regarding the usefulness of the NHL scouting combine.

Tarter, B., Kirisci, L., Tarter, R., Weatherbee, S., Jamnik, V., McGuire, E., & Gledhill, N. (2009). Use of aggregate fitness indicators to predict transition into the National Hockey League. *Journal of Strength and Conditioning Research, 23*(6), 1828–1832.

Burr, J., Jamnik, R., Baker, J., Macpherson, A., Gledhill, N., & McGuire, E. (2008). Relationship of physical fitness test results and hockey playing potential in elite-level ice hockey players. *Journal of Strength and Conditioning, 22*(5), 1535–1543.

Vescovi, J., Murray, T., Fiala, K., & VanHeest, J. (2006). Off-ice performance and draft status of elite ice hockey players. *International Journal of Sports Physiology and Performance, 1*(3), 207–221.

Vescovi, J. D., Murray, T. M., & VanHeest, J. L. (2006). Positional performance profiling of elite ice hockey players. *International Journal of Sports Physiology & Performance, 1*(2), 84–94.

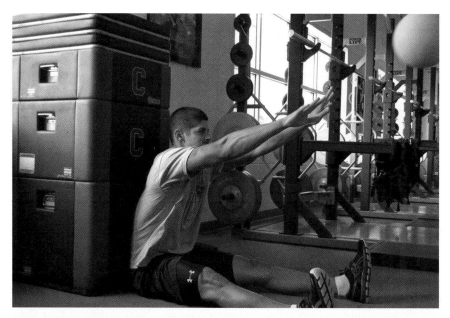

(Jeffrey C. Ives photo)

Part of the challenge in using abilities to predict later success is similar to the difficulty in predicting later success based on initial achievements in children and novice learners. Generally speaking, initial success (good or bad) does not solidly predict future performance, because the abilities for success at an early stage are often different from those at a later stage. As performers go through learning stages, they must acquire or make use of new abilities. For example, strength is a strong predictor of high school wrestling success but not so at high levels such as Olympic level wrestlers. Though predicting growth and height is reliable, maturity and adaptability to practice and training are not. For example, there is no way to assess a child's capability for strength development.

At this time, the evidence points to one factor or ability that may contribute to success in a number of sports or activities. This factor is **relative age**, and it simply means that the older or more mature children within an age group will be more likely to succeed at each age progression (Cobley et al., 2009; Musch & Grondin, 2001). Though maturational level may not play a role in some sport-specific skills (Malina et al., 2005), it is thought in general that older children are bigger and more biologically advanced than their counterparts, which are clear advantages at an early age. These advantages contribute to more success, and because of this success more time and effort are provided to these children. Moreover, this early success is a strong motivator for these children to continue to participate and work hard for more success. Mujika et al. (2009) described this bias toward older children and the resources provided them as a loss of a lot of potential talent in the younger age group children.

Proper Uses of Talent Identification

Identifying the essential abilities behind any motor skill is difficult, particularly as the motor skill becomes more complex. As described previously, individuals may achieve high levels of success even with abilities that do not seem characteristic of the sport or activity. On the other hand, it is possible to identify abilities that contribute to **domain selection**. Domain selection is the identification of a particular field or area in which particular abilities may be more important. For example, short individuals may be drawn toward activities in which a slight stature is a definite advantage, such as gymnastics or some equestrian events. Individuals with a large percentage of fast twitch muscle fibers may avoid aerobic type activities. Domain selection, whether done "forcibly" by the government or by one's own volition, may have a large genetic component and may serve to eliminate activities rather than select specific activities.

Despite the problems and pitfalls of measuring abilities, there are reasons to measure them beyond domain selection. Measuring abilities provides a metric upon which the effectiveness of practice, training, and rehabilitation may be evaluated. Knowing the abilities that seem to characterize the athletes in certain sports provides some direction for individuals regarding training and practice. For example, physiological characteristics of Australian high-level female netball players include a 1.98 seconds 10-m sprint, a 2.47 seconds agility score (the 505 agility test), a 15.5 cm sit-and-reach flexibility score, and a 53.4 cm vertical jump (Gore, 2000). These scores do not define what it means to be an expert player, but they do provide a general description of abilities that may be more or less important (e.g., the 53.4 cm jump is large compared to other athletes, the sit-and-reach is similar). Measurement of these abilities then provides goals and focus areas for training.

SUMMARY

Motor skills can be classified according to characteristics of the motor actions, including overt body movement and manipulation of objects, and the open versus closed environment in which the skill is performed. Classification schemes enable a better understanding of how motor skills are performed and are critical in setting up learning, training, and rehabilitation programs.

Measuring the quality of performance is a challenge because of measurement difficulties and validity and reliability issues. Nevertheless, is it important to measure performance as a way to gauge progression of improvement and to infer if learning is taking place. Two general types of performance measures—outcome and production measures—offer a different way of assessing performance level and interpreting learning. Response outcome measures reveal what happened, and production measures give insight to how the movement was performed. It takes trial and error and experience for instructors to recognize the important performance measures to assess. RT, as a measure of information processing, is an underutilized performance measure in sport and exercise settings, but conversely, the typical laboratory-based measures of RT are not seen to hold much validity in actual sport and life settings. The increasing use of eye tracking equipment is enabling researchers and practitioners to better understand decision-making and other information processing abilities of performers.

Error measurements are the most common performance measures as they reveal a deviation from an ideal or a desired level of performance. Errors may reveal the magnitude of deviation (AE), tendencies or bias in performance (CE), or the consistency in performance (VE). No single form of error measurement is better than another as each reveals different insights into motor skill performance. Measurement of errors from video analyses are in common use and offer simple and effective ways to evaluate errors.

Individuals have a wide array of motor abilities that alone or in combination provide the basis for successful motor skill performance. These abilities include those that are physical proficiency, psychomotor, and psychological. Though some abilities have been clearly identified as major components of success in specific motor skills, determining the essential abilities for most all motor skills has proved difficult. What is clear is that individuals can succeed at particular motor skills with different combinations of abilities. This does not imply that any motor skill activity can be accomplished with a high level of success with just any combination of abilities. Some abilities help discriminate potential activities through domain selection, either by providing a clear advantage or disadvantage. Aside from domain selection (though it too is questionable), attempting to predict a child or novice performer's potential for motor skill success based on the evaluation of abilities is filled with problems. There are simply too many factors involved with motor skill success to take stock in measuring just a few motor abilities, even in those cases where the ability testing is reliable and valid.

Ability testing does have its uses, however. It is well understood that for many sports and motor skills there is a base or minimal level of abilities, such as strength, speed, body size, visual acuity, and so forth, that empirically and theoretically contribute to performance. These measures provide minimal goals for individuals to strive for during practice and training. Measurement of abilities also helps identify overt weaknesses and strengths and provides measurements upon which progression may be monitored during training or rehabilitation.

STUDY QUESTIONS

1. Externally paced skills tend to also be open or closed skills?
2. Describe the important differences between open skills and closed skills, and gross skills versus fine skills. What are the practical implications of classifying motor skills in these ways?
3. Using Gentile's modified taxonomy, what movement characteristics tend to make motor skills more difficult?
4. What are the difficulties in determining a valid performance measure for both motor skills and abilities?
5. What are the general ways to measure errors? What information does each of these error measurements reveal?
6. On average, typical simple and choice reaction times for young adults would be about how fast? Identify some situations in which these small changes (e.g., slowing) of reaction times would be of great importance and some situations where it would matter little.
7. What are the differences between response time and reaction time?

8. Define and describe the differences between response production measures and response outcome measures. Give examples when one type of measure would be preferable to the other.

9. Why is reaction time somewhat unique among performance measurements used in exercise science and kinesiology?

10. Define and describe the relationships and differences among skill, ability, and talent.

11. What are the ways abilities are categorized? Among these categories, which are most measured in motor skill performance?

12. What is visual search and how can it be measured?

13. What is talent identification and what are effective uses of talent identification?

14. What factors make it difficult to predict future performance based on initial performance?

15. The visual–perceptual skills of superior athletes differ from that of lesser athletes in what way(s)?

16. List and describe the factors that influence the speed of reaction time.

References

Abernethy, P., Wilson, G., & Logan, P. (1995). Strength and power assessment. Issues, controversies and challenges. *Sports Medicine, 19*(6), 401–417.

Adams, A. J., & Kuzmits, F. E. (2008). Testing the relationship between a cognitive ability test and player success: The National Football League case. *Athletic Insight, 10*(1), 5.

Bouchard, C., & Malina, R. (1983). Genetics of physiological fitness and motor performance. *Exercise and Sport Sciences Reviews, 11*, 306–339.

Burr, J., Jamnik, R., Baker, J., Macpherson, A., Gledhill, N., & McGuire, E. (2008). Relationship of physical fitness test results and hockey playing potential in elite-level ice hockey players. *Journal of Strength and Conditioning, 22*(5), 1535–1543.

Burton, A. W., & Miller, D. E. (1998). *Movement skill assessment*. Champaign, IL: Human Kinetics.

Cobley, S., Baker, J., Wattie, N., & McKenna, J. (2009). Annual age-grouping and athlete development. *Sports Medicine, 39*(3), 235–256.

Durocher, J., Guisfredi, A., Leetun, D., & Carter, J. (2010). Comparison of on-ice and off-ice graded exercise testing in collegiate hockey players. *Applied Physiology, Nutrition, and Metabolism, 35*(1), 35–39.

Emre, A. K., & Kocak, S. (2010). Coincidence-anticipation timing and reaction time in youth tennis and table tennis players. *Perceptual and Motor Skills, 110*, 879–887.

Farrow, D. D., Young, W. W., & Bruce, L. L. (2005). The development of a test of reactive agility for netball: A new methodology. *Journal of Science and Medicine in Sport, 8*(1), 52–60.

Gentile, A. M. (2000). Skill acquisition: Action, movement, and neuromotor processes. In J. H. Car & R. B. Shepherd (Eds.) *Movement science: Foundations for physical therapy* (2nd ed., pp. 111–187). Rockville, MD: Aspen.

Gore, C. J. (Ed.) (2000). *Physiological tests for elite athletes. The Australian Sports Commission*. Champaign, IL: Human Kinetics.

Gould, D. D., Dieffenbach, K. K., & Moffatt, A. A. (2002). Psychological characteristics and their development in Olympic champions. *Journal of Applied Sport Psychology, 14*(3), 172–204.

Gould, D., & Maynard, I. (2009). Psychological preparation for the Olympic Games. *Journal of Sports Sciences, 27*(13), 1393–1408.

Hick, W. E. (1952). On the rate of gain of information. *Quarterly Journal of Experimental Psychology, 4*, 11–26.

Humara, M. M. (2000). Personnel selection in athletic programs. *Athletic Insight, 2*(2), http://www.athleticinsight.com.ezproxy.ithaca.edu:2048/Vol2Iss2/Personnel.htm

Ivančević, T., Jovanović, B., &Ddash;ukić, M., Marković, S., & &Ddash;ukić, N. (2008). Biomechanical analysis of shots and ball motion in tennis and the analogy with handball throws. *Facta Universitatis: Series Physical Education & Sport, 6*(1), 51–66.

Knudson, D., & Morrison, C. (2002). *Qualitative analysis of human movement* (2nd ed.). Champaign, IL: Human Kinetics.

Kuhtz-Buschbeck, J. P., Hoppe, B., Gölge, M., Dreesmann, M., Damm-Stünitz, U., & Ritz, A. (2003). Sensorimotor recovery in children after traumatic brain injury: Analyses of gait, gross motor, and fine motor skills. *Developmental Medicine and Child Neurology, 45*, 821–828.

Kuzmits, F. E., & Adams, A. J. (2008). The NFL combine: Does it predict performance in the National Football League? *Journal of Strength and Conditioning Research, 22*(6), 1721–1727.

Malina, R., Cumming, S., Kontos, A., Eisenmann, J., Ribeiro, B., & Aroso, J. (2005). Maturity-associated variation in sport-specific skills of youth soccer players aged 13–15 years. *Journal of Sports Sciences, 23*(5), 515–522.

Morgan, W. P., O'Connor, P. J., Ellickson, K. A., & Bradley, P. W. (1988). Personality structure, mood states, and performance in elite male distance runners. *International Journal of Sport Psychology, 19*(4), 247–263.

Mouelhi Guizani, S., Tenenbaum, G., Bouzaouach, I., Ben Kheder, A., Feki, Y., & Bouaziz, M. (2006). Information-processing under incremental levels of physical loads: Comparing racquet to combat sports. *Journal of Sports Medicine and Physical Fitness, 46*, 335–343.

Mujika, I., Vaeyens, R., Matthys, S. J., Santisteban, J., Goiriena, J., & Philippaerts, R. (2009). The relative age effect in a professional football club setting. *Journal of Sports Sciences, 27*(11), 1153–1158.

Musch, J. J., & Grondin, S. S. (2001). Unequal competition as an impediment to personal development: A review of the relative age effect in sport. *Developmental Review, 21*(2), 147–167.

Piek, J. P., Baynam, G. B., & Barrett, N. C. (2006). The relationship between fine and gross motor ability, self-perceptions and self-worth in children and adolescents. *Human Movement Science, 25*, 65–75.

Rankinen, T., Bray, M., Hagberg, J., Pérusse, L., Roth, S., Wolfarth, B., et al. (2006). The human gene map for performance and health-related fitness phenotypes: The 2005 update. *Medicine and Science in Sports and Exercise, 38*(11), 1863–1888.

Sheard, M., & Golby, J. (2010). Personality hardiness differentiates elite-level sport performers. *International Journal of Sport and Exercise Psychology, 8*(2), 160–169.

Sheppard, J., Young, W., Doyle, T., Sheppard, T., & Newton, R. (2006). An evaluation of a new test of reactive agility and its relationship to sprint speed and change of direction speed. *Journal of Science and Medicine In Sport, 9*(4), 342–349.

Shumway-Cook A., & Woollacott, M. H. (2007). *Motor control. Translating research into clinical practice*. Philadelphia, PA: Lippincott Williams & Wilkins.

Stutts, J. C., Stewart, J. R., & Martell, C. (1998). Cognitive test performance and crash risk in an older driver population. *Accident Analysis and Prevention, 30*, 337–346.

Tarter, B., Kirisci, L., Tarter, R., Weatherbee, S., Jamnik, V., McGuire, E., & Gledhill, N. (2009). Use of aggregate fitness indicators to predict transition into the National Hockey League. *Journal of Strength and Conditioning Research, 23*(6), 1828–1832.

Vaeyens, R., Gullich, A., Warr, C. R., & Philippaerts, R. (2009). Talent identification and promotion programmes of Olympic athletes. *Journal of Sports Sciences, 27*(13), 1367–1380.

Vanttinen, T., Blomqvist, M., Luhtanen, P., & Hakkinen, K. (2010). Effects of age and soccer expertise on general tests of perceptual and motor performance among adolescent soccer players. *Perceptual and Motor Skills, 110*, 675–692.

Vescovi, J., Murray, T., Fiala, K., & VanHeest, J. (2006a). Off-ice performance and draft status of elite ice hockey players. *International Journal of Sports Physiology and Performance, 1*(3), 207–221.

Vescovi, J. D., Murray, T. M., & VanHeest, J. L. (2006b). Positional performance profiling of elite ice hockey players. *International Journal of Sports Physiology and Performance, 1*(2), 84–94.

Ziv, G. G., & Lidor, R. R. (2010). Vertical jump in female and male volleyball players: A review of observational and experimental studies. *Scandinavian Journal of Medicine and Science in Sports, 20*(4), 556–567.

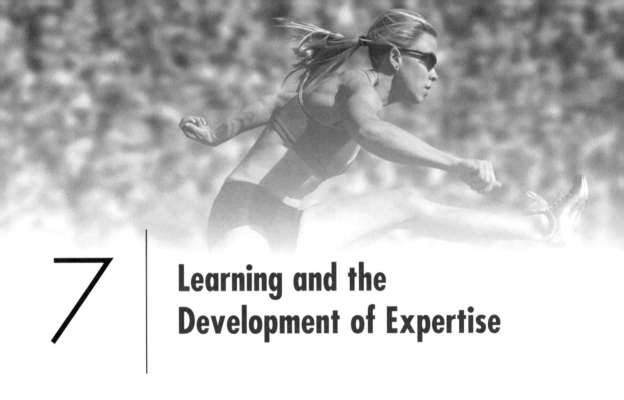

7 | Learning and the Development of Expertise

PURPOSE, IMPORTANCE, AND OBJECTIVES OF THIS CHAPTER

The purpose of this chapter is to describe motor learning and the basic principles and characteristics that define the progression of learning motor skills, and the characteristics that distinguish high-level performers. These principles help the practitioner identify if learning is taking place and provides the rudimentary framework for creating the best learning environment.

After reading this chapter, you should be able to:

1. Define and explain the definition of motor learning and the factors indicating if learning has taken place.
2. Define and explain the definition of transfer of learning, why it occurs, and how to maximize it.
3. Explain how and why performance plateaus occur.
4. Explain the use of transfer and retention tests to assess performance and learning.
5. Explain the 3-stage and 2-stage models of learning and how to identify the characteristics of performance that correspond to the learning stages.
6. Explain the characteristics that distinguish the highest-level performers apart from less accomplished performers.
7. Explain how to use the learning stage models to provide general directions and strategies for planning training and practice sessions.

How do we know that learning has occurred? The answer to this question seems obvious; that is, someone with improved performance apparently has learned to perform better. Such an improvement seems to imply that learning has taken place, but in fact, we do not directly observe learning; we only observe behavior and thus must determine if the motor behavior reflects learning.

DEFINING AND DETERMINING LEARNING

Performance is the observable and measurable outcome of executing a motor skill. In contrast, **learning** is defined as a relatively permanent change in one's capability to perform a skill as a result of practice or experience. The definition of learning implies that the potential, or capability, is improved, not necessarily the actual performance. There are a number of factors that may inhibit performance despite learning taking place. Motivation, anxiety, and fatigue are just a few of the things that can cause performance to fall even as learning continues. The definition of learning also states that learning is a result of practice or experience, which means that improved performance due to growth or maturation or luck does not reflect learning.

Theoretically we cannot directly assess learning because it is an internal phenomenon that is not directly observable. Instead, performance is measured, and learning is inferred from performance measurements. Performance scores usually give good indication of what has been learned, but not always. In order to infer learning, several performance characteristics are assessed. The first is *persistent improvement* over time. This means that better performance stays better, even after periods of no practice or training. Better learning is reflected in performance improvements that are more resistant to forgetting over longer and longer time periods. The second is *better consistency*. Performance should become less variable from trial to trial and day to day and so forth. Consistency is perhaps best evaluated by looking at response production measures, including biomechanical and EMG variables. The third characteristic is *stability of performance*. Stability is related to consistency, but refers to performance remaining stable in the face of disruption, either internal or external. Internal disruptions may be physiological, such as fatigue or injury, or psychological, such as mental fatigue or poor mood states like stress. Common external disruptions are poor weather and lighting, and even a different venue for performance. Of course, many of these factors will cause performance decrements, but highly learned motor skills are less affected by these factors than skills that are not learned as well. The last factor is *adaptability*, which refers to the ability of the learned motor skill to be applied in different contexts. Skills that are better learned are better able to adapt or change in order to be incorporated into different contexts, environments, and situations. For example, an individual with a well-learned tennis serve is better able to adapt to straight and spin serves and change the serve to fit the slickness characteristics of the court (e.g., grass vs. concrete). Moreover, the same player may be able to use the overhead striking motion for a volleyball serve or spike.

Assessing and Inferring Learning

To determine if learning has taken place, performance must be assessed for improvement, consistency, stability, or adaptability after periods of practice. In research and school-based settings, testing is done in the form of evaluating *performance curves* with *retention tests* and *transfer tests*. A performance curve, as shown in Figure 7.1, simply illustrates the change in performance over time. After a period of practice in which performance has typically improved, retention tests—one or more—are given after a period of no practice to determine if performance is still elevated. Assessing performance directly after periods of practice, when the skill is still fresh, does not provide a good indicator of persistence. Repeated retention tests provide evidence of consistency. If performance level or consistency drops to baseline levels, it is assumed that learning has not taken hold. Figure 7.1 illustrates this concept.

Transfer tests assess motor skill performance in a context different from that in which the motor skill was practiced (see later for more on transfer of motor skill learning). Transfer tests assess the stability or adaptability of the learned skill. The most common type of transfer test is testing the motor skill in an open or complex environment versus the closed or very structured environment of practice. Another form of transfer test is testing the motor skill with different types of performance feedback or no feedback at all regarding performance. Consider learning the tennis backhand, first off of a ball machine that provides a very structured, albeit open, environment. The learner may consistently perform the stroke beautifully. A transfer test could have the learner faced with hitting strokes on the run, of

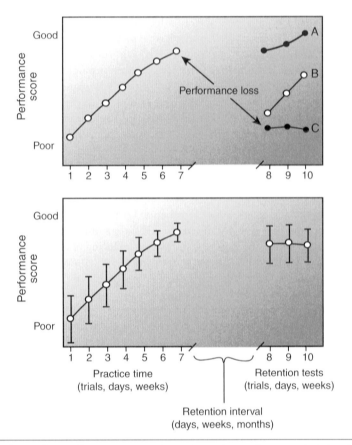

Figure 7.1 • The **top figure** illustrates a typical practice and retention test schedule with three possible outcomes (A,B,C). The schedule involves extensive practice over trials, days, or weeks and is dependent on the particular motor skill and the level of previous knowledge of the learner. Retention tests, normally more than one, follow after a period of no practice (retention interval). The degree of performance loss over the retention interval is dependent on the length of the retention interval and the amount of original learning. In scenario (A) there is no drop in performance, and even a rise in performance over the retention tests. The amount of original learning was persistent, at least within the retention interval. In (B), there is a large drop in performance over the interval followed by a rapid reacquisition of performance during the retention tests. The amount of reacquisition may be due to the testing itself that may serve as practice, the length of time between retention tests, and the amount of original learning. Interpreting these results can be difficult. In (C), there is a large drop in performance that does not recover, indicating poor learning of the motor skill. The **bottom figure** illustrates performance scores with variability. Each score is the average of a block of trials and is shown with the standard deviation error bars (variable error). Over practice the performance improves and consistency improves (smaller error bars). Retention tests show that performance is still elevated, but performance consistency has dropped considerably. Interpreting these results can be challenging as they may reflect incomplete learning or that the learner is trying new approaches.

different paces, and varying between forehand and backhand. Regardless if the test is a retention test or a transfer test, it is imperative that the test be conducted with minimal instructor feedback or instructions (this may prod the learner's memory), and follow guidelines for valid and reliable testing.

Apart from research and school settings, retention and transfer tests are seldom administered in a formal manner. Individual skill sport instructors, such as tennis and golf coaches, may observe their students at the start of a practice session to see if they retain anything from the previous lesson, but assessment is normally cursory and subjective. In a like manner, a team sport coach may have their team run a play at the start of the practice to evaluate what they retained and to serve as a starting point for the next phase of practice. In most cases, however, a team runs through a series of drills or plays in a simple or closed environment, and then progresses to more a complex or open environment. This progression is essentially a built-in transfer test, because if the performance is poor during the complex skills, it is assumed the players failed to learn during the simple practice.

All too often, though, these informal transfer and retention tests are not done or not done in a manner to truly indicate if learning has taken place. A case in point is the practice of rundowns ("pickles") in youth baseball. In a rundown, the base runner is caught off base, and the fielders throw the ball back and forth to get in position to tag the runner out. During practice, the fielders can become highly skilled at this maneuver, often taking just one or two throws to catch the runner. Seeing a high level of competence by the fielders, coaches often assume the tactic has been learned, only to see it break down during an actual game situation. The reason for this failure is that the highly structured environment of practice did not allow for the situational factors during the game, such as additional base runners, the number of outs, the score, stress, and more. During practice, the players have time to mentally rehearse and prepare for the drill, but in the game, the rundown situation appears suddenly, forcing the players into action with little preparation. What had been "learned" in practice is abandoned or forgotten because it does not fit the actual game situation. To assess that learning has taken place, it is recommended that coaches routinely insert transfer tests into their practice schedules, and do it without warning insofar as possible. For example, during routine infield and outfield practice at cut-off throws, the coach may direct a player to get on base and purposefully get into a rundown. The fielders are forced to change their mindset and adapt to the new situation. Poor performance in this transfer test indicates the learning has not taken hold.

Performance Plateaus and the Learning Process

Improvement in performance over time rarely follows a steady path. Sometimes performance curves reveal a rapid progression; sometimes, it levels out. In Figure 7.2, the performance curve shows areas of little or no improvement. These areas are called **plateaus**. For both the learner and instructor, plateaus are challenging. Not only is the lack of improvement discouraging, but trying to determine the cause of the stagnation can be frustrating. Learners and instructors should understand that even if performance improvement has stopped, that learning may still be continuing. It is thus essential to determine why the plateau occurred and if it reflects both learning and performance or simply performance.

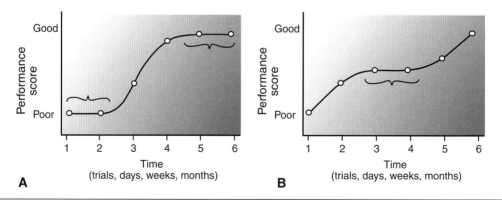

Figure 7.2 • Performance plateaus (*areas in brackets*) showing that performance may level out at any point in the learning process. (**A**) A plateau during the initial phase of practice for beginners may indicate a change in instructional approach is necessary. A plateau occurring after extended practice may indicate learner fatigue. (**B**) A plateau after a lot of initial learning may indicate the need to learn a new skill set.

Plateaus may be caused by numerous factors that can be categorized as *learner-based factors, instructor-based factors*, and *task-based factors*. Among the learner-based factors are psychological factors such as a lack of motivation or poor attentional focus and physiological and psychophysiological factors such as injury, fatigue, or overtraining. Factors such as these may be considered **performance variables** in that they may affect performance but not necessarily learning. Sometimes these influences, attentional focus and motivation in particular, may at times also cause learning itself to stagnate. These are then called **learning variables** because they affect both learning and performance. Other learning variables include quality of instruction and time spent in practice.

Instructor-based factors are largely a result of poor instructional strategies. For instance, if the instructor chooses the wrong performance measure, it could seem as if performance has plateaued. Measuring a task that is so easy that the person maximizes the score quickly and leaves little room for improvement is the **ceiling effect**. Likewise, the **floor effect** occurs if the task being measured is so difficult that improvement is difficult to achieve, resulting in a plateau in performance. Sometimes an area of skill improvement is missed because the wrong performance measure was evaluated. In Chapter 6, we saw the difficulty in choosing the correct performance measure, and selecting the wrong measure could indicate that performance has stagnated. In addition, a learner may hit a plateau when instruction is not appropriate or specific to meet the needs of the learner. Consider, for instance, a youth hockey coach providing instruction on stick handling skills when the players' skating abilities are not sufficient to enable proper balance and stability for upper body stick handling movements. Player–coach communication difficulties may contribute to discouragement and poor motivation, resulting in poor performance and learning. When the plateau is a result of poor measurements or inappropriate teaching strategies, it is the responsibility of the instructor and learner to recognize these shortcomings and change the practice environment and their own strategies.

■ Thinking It Through 7.1 Overcoming Slumps

Slumps are short-term (hopefully!) performance plateaus. Slumps may include physiological abilities, such a lack of improvement on the bench press exercise or motor skills, such as baseball batting. Craig Counsell, a major league baseball player for the Milwaukee Brewers, tied a modern-day batting slump record by going 45 at-bats without a hit during the 2011 season. Using these examples of weight lifting and batting, identify what you believe may be potential causes of slumps and possible solutions for getting out of the slump.

Task-based factors leading to plateaus are among the most common and frustrating for learners. Task-based plateaus are caused by the need for the learner to learn new skills, tactics, or strategies in order to rise to the next level of performance. As performance improves and tasks are mastered, it is necessary to begin learning entirely new skill components or acquire new abilities. Learners must often discard familiar ways of doing things, break old habits, and adopt new techniques. Not only can this be difficult to do, but performance may suffer, and frustration is common. Learning the proper soccer-style kick from the immature toe-kick (Fig. 7.3) inevitably leads to poor kicking performance and even physical discomfort. Novice snow skiers can master the snowplow turn quite readily and can use the snowplow technique to conquer all but the steepest slopes. Yet, higher-level skiing requires development of the parallel turn technique, which predictably results in falling and demotion to the beginner slopes. This type of plateau is not restricted to children and novices and, in our experience, is a main contributor to intermediate level performers not progressing. For instance, overreliance on muscle strength and size rather than technique for football linemen and unwillingness to learn nondominant ball handling and shooting skills in basketball players are just two examples. Instructors and learners must work together to progress through these plateaus.

In the discussion and examples provided above, plateaus appear to be somewhat of an artifact; that is, they are circumstantial and not a real indicator that learning has stopped or that performance has

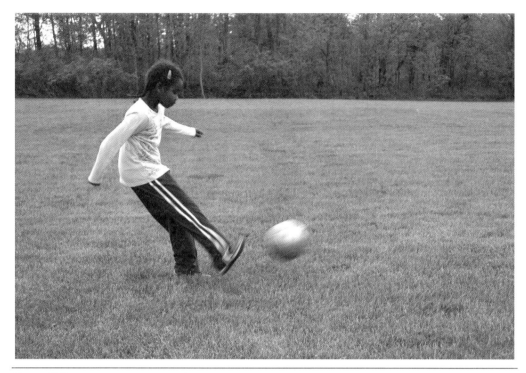

Figure 7.3 • Toe-kicking a soccer ball is intuitively easy and produces successful results for this child. Why would she want to change to a mature soccer-style kick that requires a lot of work to learn? (Photo courtesy Whitman R. Ives.)

peaked. Further, it seems that if the cause of the plateau could be determined, modifications could be made to the practice and learning environment to get back on the right track. Conversely, is it possible that plateaus are a result of real biological limitations, that is, that they do reflect a maximal level of performance capable by an individual? If this is the case, then it may be useful to know these limitations such that time and effort are not wasted in futility. Certainly there are limitations in human performance, but we believe the evidence shows that the human capability for improvement, regardless of genetic makeup, is so vast that attempting to identify genetic limitations as a training constraint is not useful at this time. Rather, it appears more prudent to identify those modifiable factors that contribute to performance stagnation and engage in practice and training designed to overcome the plateau.

■ Thinking It Through 7.2 Performance Curves and Plateaus

1. Access the webpage "CognitiveFun.net." Open the link to "Tests" and then "Attention Tests." Perform the visual RT tests in accordance with the directions. Perform a block of 10 to 12 trials, writing down your average RT over the trial block (the computer will calculate this in the results link). Reset the trials to begin again, and do another block of 10 to 12 trials and recording the average block score. Continue this until you have completed at least six trial blocks. Graph out your scores over blocks, and note if you reached a plateau in performance. If so, why?
2. Repeat the experiment above but this time with the visual Go/No Go reaction time tests and with the "Fast Counting" test. Did plateaus occur in these tests? If they did, did they occur at the same time? Compare your results here to the first experiment, and explain any difference in plateaus based on the concepts discussed in the text.

Concepts in Action

Overcoming Plateaus through Training Changes

Concepts involving the development of motor skill expertise and plateaus pertain as much to sports that are more dependent on fitness requirements and less dependent on precise motor skills, such as distance running. Jones' (2006) longitudinal (1992–2003) examination of the world's best female marathon runner provides a picture on the development of expertise from age 18 to age 29, at which time she set the world marathon record. Over this time, her maximal oxygen consumption (VO_2 max) remained relatively stable and essentially plateaued. However, her running economy (run faster at the same VO_2) improved markedly and was suggested to be central to her success. The exact mechanisms behind improved running economy were thought to come from a broad array of changes, including improved blood lactate handling, a more lean body composition, reduced recruitment of fast twitch muscle fibers, increased muscle strength and stiffness, and changes in cardiac output. Changes in these mechanisms were likely a result of two distinct changes in training. First, she increased her weekly running mileage by fivefold, and second, she engaged in rigorous strength and power training. The summary of her story is that development took place in many different systems in very small increments using many different training methods. Even though it looked like a plateau had been reached (VO_2 max), other more subtle changes enabled her to continue improving.

TRANSFER OF LEARNING

One of the identifying features of learning is that learning enables transfer to take place. This phenomenon, called **transfer of learning**, is defined as previous learning and experiences influencing the learning of subsequent motor skills. Transfer enables individuals to take what is learned in one situation and apply it in another situation, which facilitates the learning of new skills and enables diversification of their movement repertoire. It is one of the most powerful phenomena in the learning process, and underlies many of the learning and instructional techniques described in this and subsequent chapters. Transfer may be in the form of **positive transfer** that facilitates the learning of the secondary motor skill, **negative transfer** that impedes learning of the secondary skill, or neutral transfer that has no net effect.

How Transfer Occurs

Transfer occurs more when there is similarity, or **identical elements**, among the skill components or context under which the skills are performed. For example, an overhand throw has elements similar to an overhand serve in volleyball and tennis. More transfer also occurs when there is **similarity of information processing** requirements or previous experiences. This type of transfer is often seen in applying team tactics and strategies from one sport to another sport, such as the basis for a zone defense used in many team sports. Another common example is that experienced athletes know the type of feints and moves that throw a defender off balance, which can work in multiple sport settings.

There is more transfer when there are both identical elements and similarity in information processing, but this transfer is not always welcome. Transferring learning from one skill or context to another usually leads to positive secondary performance, at least initially. In some cases, however, this transfer is negative and impedes the learning of the secondary skill because the individual finds it difficult to break away from the initial learning. Hockey and baseball players, for example, may have negative transfer when playing golf. At first, these players may have positive transfer of basic hand–eye coordination and rotational body mechanics, but after time, the automatic hockey and baseball swings fail to enable progression in the golf swing, which requires a more calculated and precise action. The swing patterns of hockey and baseball have thus become a difficult-to-break bad habit for golf. Learning in these cases may become difficult and confusing for the learner, though negative transfer should always be thought of as a temporary phenomenon. If the learned skill takes advantage of intrinsic synergies or pattern generators, negative transfer may be more pronounced or more difficult to overcome if those synergies need to be changed.

More positive transfer occurs when the conditions of information processing and identical elements are more similar between the previously learned skill and the new skill. Often this occurs when learning a progression of skill components from simple to complex. Gentile's taxonomy of motor skills (Chapter 6, Table 6.1) provides a basis to examine transfer of skills from simple to complex. Tasks that are seen as more simple involve either gross movements or fine movements, but not both together. In addition, movements in a closed environment may be simpler than those in an open environment. By developing and refining basic or simple movement patterns, the learner has a platform upon which to advance by transferring those patterns to more complex situations. Consider novices learning to shoot a basketball (Fig. 7.4). At first, new learners typically shoot a two-handed set shot. The basics of timing and rhythm of the fundamental shoulder, elbow, and wrist actions are learned. In addition, effective projectile motion for the basketball is beginning to be understood (e.g., high and soft arc). These characteristics are then transferred to the single-handed set shot, which may necessarily include more whole-body transfer of force from the legs to the arms. Next may come shooting with the ball over the head and then a true jump shot. The single arm shooting coordination has already been learned, but is now diversified to apply during jumping. These qualities may then be further diversified to off balance and in-motion shots and different shots (e.g., hooks shots, scoop shots). During this time, the learner may also be practicing these shots with a defender, putting them at the most complex point on Gentile's taxonomy of motor skills, open skills being done with body motion and object manipulation. Because of transfer, each progression builds upon what has already been learned. Put differently, the learner has early on focused on specific motor skills and then diversified those skills into different contexts or motions using the transfer of learning phenomenon.

This basketball shooting example paradoxically also provides examples of negative transfer. In our experience, the progression from a two-handed shot to a one-handed shot can be difficult because the action of the nonshooting hand must now be different. The off-hand is now involved in ball stabilization and not projectile motion, and learners have a difficulty uncoupling the off-hand from doing the shooting action. The progression to shooting from over the head versus from the chest also poses negative transfer problems for some learners. Some learners may still continue to initiate the shot from chest level, finding it difficult to change their motion and rhythm to begin that shot above the head. In addition, some learners revert back to the two-handed shot when attempting to shoot over their head (Fig. 7.4). This shooting position is comfortable for them, particularly considering the need to control the ball and provide enough force to shoot from longer distances.

Perhaps the most common form of negative transfer is learning a new response to an old stimulus. Our examples of reaction time and driving from Chapter 6 provide evidence of negative transfer, particularly in response to rapid braking to obstacles in the road. Most drivers automatically hit the brake when something runs into the road, but often times, doing nothing is a safer and better response. Learning to do nothing can be learned, but it takes considerable practice. Another example is baseball players learning to get out of the way of a pitched ball coming at them. Inexperienced players universally duck or jump out of the way, but this is poor technique. Experienced players rotate their trunks to move their bodies out of the way. Perhaps most important is that the trunk rotation keeps the body in a hitting position for a longer period of time in order to adjust to a curve ball. Unlearning the duck and jump action in response to a speeding baseball coming at one's head is indeed a difficult task.

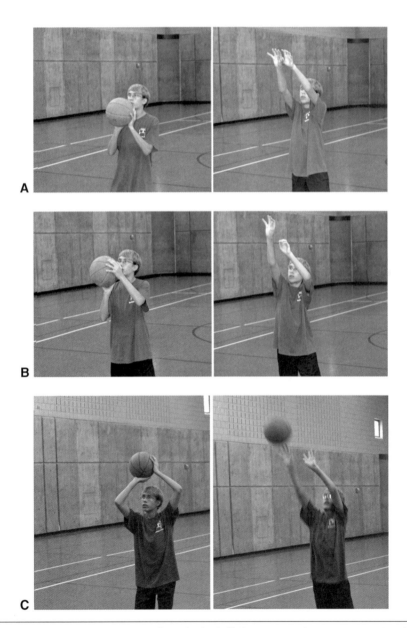

Figure 7.4 • Positive and negative transfer in basketball shooting. In photo sequence **(A)**, the player is shooting a two-handed set shot and follows through with a two arm extension. In **(B)**, the player is shooting a one-handed set shot, using the nondominant hand to stabilize the ball rather than propel it. In the follow-through, the extension is similar as is the projectile motion and general sequence of trunk to arm action. These similarities facilitate transfer. In photo **(C)**, the player is attempting the advanced over-the-head shot. Though the initial form of the shot look okay, a look at the follow-through shows that he reverted back to using both hands to propel the ball. His initial learning of the single-handed chest shot was not sufficient to overcome the complexity and challenge of the overhead shot, causing him to revert back to his original learning. See text for more details. (Photo courtesy Jeffrey C. Ives.)

Bilateral Transfer

Our exploration brain plasticity in Chapter 2 and generalized motor programs in Chapter 5 provide a backdrop for additional concepts in transfer. In Chapter 2, we learned of cross-transfer of strength from one arm to the contralateral arm following unilateral strength training, and in Chapter 5, we saw that handwriting with one hand could be applied, or transferred, to the other hand. These specific cases of transfer from one limb to the other are called **bilateral transfer**, or in the specific case of the wrist and hand, **bimanual transfer**. Bilateral transfer is defined as the learning of a motor skill in one limb applied to the contralateral limb, and is essential in the development of many motor skills. The use of surgical equipment, instrument playing, and even the firing of weapons with either hands makes use of bilateral transfer. In our basketball shooting example above, bilateral transfer would facilitate the transfer of shooting performance from one hand to the other, such as in the case of doing layups first with the dominant hand and then with the nondominant hand. Figure 7.5 illustrates the concept of bilateral transfer during layup practice, but it also illustrates that the intrinsic coupling of limbs may facilitate negative transfer as well, making some learning more difficult at the start.

The amount and nature of bilateral transfer may be related to the learner's age, handedness, and the nature of the motor task, particularly with respect to motor skills requiring force versus accuracy or changes in movement frequency (Fagard & Corroyer, 2003; Stöckel & Weigelt, 2012; Vangheluwe et al., 2006). Stöckel and Weigelt (2012) found more bilateral transfer in accurate throwing tasks when the learners practiced first with the nondominant hand, but more transfer in forceful throwing tasks when the learners practiced first with the dominant hand. These authors ascribed the differences to

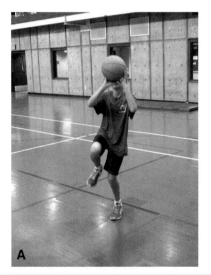 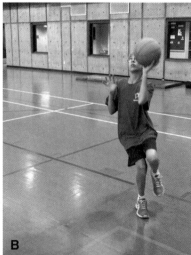

Figure 7.5 • Bilateral transfer and negative transfer. Though bilateral transfer is a real phenomenon that aids in motor skill learning, it should not be considered an easy process. In this sequence, the basketball player is learning to shoot a layup with his nondominant (left) hand. This action requires that he also jumps off his opposite (right) foot. **A.** The player attempts to shoot with his left hand but has difficulty because he "forgot" to jump off the right foot. Instead, he jumps off his left foot, and thus, his natural inclination is to shoot with the right hand even though he wants to shoot with his left hand. As a result of negative transfer exacerbated by leg–arm synergies, he ends up shooting with both hands. **B.** The player is now jumping off his correct leg, but is so right arm dominate that the only way he can eliminate its effects is to remove it from the ball altogether. As a result, the player shoots the ball without any right arm stabilization. Once he learns to jump off this right leg and get his right arm out of the way, his actual left arm shooting motion is relatively smooth and effective due to bilateral transfer. See text for more details. (Photo courtesy Jeffrey C. Ives.)

SIDE**NOTE**	**TRANSFER OR NO TRANSFER IN REHABILITATION?**

Bilateral transfer, including cross-transfer of strength, has been hailed as a great benefit for rehabilitation. Ausenda and Carnovali (2011), for instance, found improvement in fine motor skill performance in the partially paralyzed arm of patients following practice designed to facilitate bilateral transfer. These patients, all suffering hemiparesis from stroke, extensively practiced a fine motor skill with their nonaffected arm for 3 days. After practice, the patients had a 22% improvement in performance in their affected arm, demonstrating bilateral transfer. Bilateral transfer, however, has limits. Individuals with injured or paralyzed limbs may highly overcompensate with the healthy limb, but the skills and abilities developed in the intact limb may not transfer to the affected side. It was speculated by Dr. Edward Taub at the University of Alabama that persons with paralysis on one side of their body, as a result of brain injury, would give up using their affected arm because of difficulty. This would cause "unlearning" to take place, regardless of how much was being learned in the intact limb. To counter this, he forced his patients into using the affected arm by covering the intact arm with a large mitt, sling, or cast, to effectively disable it (Taub & Morris, 2001). Called constraint-induced movement therapy (CIMT), patients were forced into use their affected arms during therapy and during normal activities of daily living, often 6 to −10 hours a day every day over 2 to 3 weeks. The results have been very promising, showing improved function in a variety of patients and conditions (Gauthier et al., 2009). Brain imaging has shown that cortical brain regions are reorganized following CIMT, including enhanced activation of brain area contralateral to the damaged area of the brain (Stark et al., 2012; Sutcliffe et al., 2009). These areas are likely different from what would be gained from bilateral transfer learning.

differences in brain lateralization. Other authors have found that transfer of movement frequency patterns may actually be strongly negative, suggesting that movement patterns in synergistic limbs are coupled and sometimes transfer may try and interfere with these patterns (Vangheluwe et al., 2006).

Using and Maximizing Transfer

Without transfer, it would be impossible to progress from simple to complex motor skill learning. In addition, transfer enables those skills learned in practice settings to be applied in real situations. Practice settings are often closed, and transfer provides the basis to apply the skills learned in the closed setting to the open real-world setting. Because of transfer, we can gain a better understanding of the theoretical process of learning and how to go about sequencing the learning of a complex skill. For example, fundamentals motor actions are learned before complex movement patterns, which is especially important for dangerous skills such as platform diving and some gymnastics routines.

Maximizing the amount of transfer is firmly rooted in the similarity between the conditions of the original learning and the secondary task, that is, the more similar the conditions, the more transfer. Proteau et al. (1992) termed this concept the *specificity of learning* (or *specificity of practice*) hypothesis. In particular, these authors suggested that the greater the similarity in sensory and environmental information, the better the transfer because the motor commands are sensitive to afferent information. These authors based their conclusions on studies in which movement tasks were learned with or without vision (Mackrous & Proteau, 2007; Proteau et al., 1992), for example, when vision was added, to a transfer test the performance suffered even though vision theoretically should have helped performance. These authors also noted that the amount of transfer is dependent on the amount of initial learning and variability in the practice environment (Soucy & Proteau, 2001).

■ Thinking It Through 7.3 Virtual Reality Simulation and Transfer

Computer simulations of real-life tasks, such as flying and driving, are common video games. Microsoft's "Flight Simulator" was one of the first home-based computer simulators accessible to a wide audience, and is currently used professionally to train pilots. With your understanding of transfer of learning, describe the amount and nature of transfer from computer flight simulator to learning actual flight.

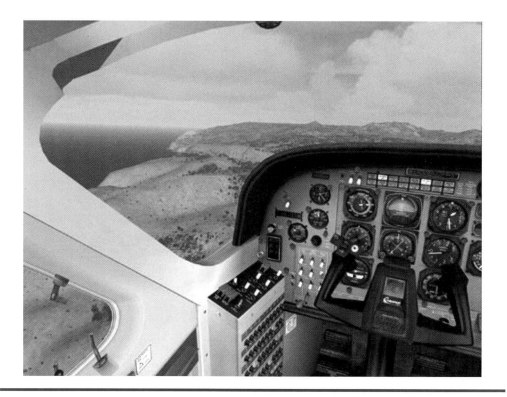

STAGES OF MOTOR SKILL LEARNING

The previous sections on plateaus and transfer of learning from simple to complex imply that learning occurs in stages over time. Indeed, as learning progresses, there are various times or stages in which different aspects of the motor skill, whether cognitive or physical, become more or less important in the learning process. Sometimes previously learned skills need to be abandoned. Sometimes new abilities must be gained to provide the foundation from which new skills can be learned. At each stage, the teaching and learning strategies may also need to change. Two learning stage theories, **Fitts and Posner's 3-stage model** (Fitts & Posner, 1967) and **Gentile's 2-stage model** (Gentile, 2000), provide frameworks of what changes learners go through as they progress from one stage to another. The Fitts and Posner model emphasizes a description of motor skill performance from stage to stage, whereas the Gentile model focuses on the learning process and instruction occurring during the stages. Together these models help to identify where the learner is at, and what to expect for further improvement. Both models assume that learning starts cognitively and ends with automatic movements. Table 7.1 puts these two models side by side so that their overlap may be better seen.

TABLE 7.1	Learning Stage Theories Compared between Fitts and Posner's 3-Stage Model and Gentile's 2-Stage Model

Learning Stage Theories			
Fitts and Posner's Learning Stage Theory		**Gentile's Learning Stage Theory**	
Learning Stages	**Stage Characteristics**	**Stage Characteristics**	**Stages**
Cognitive stage	Learning rules, strategies, and technique concepts, basic movement patterns, many gross errors, unable to detect or correct body errors, poor efficiency	Learning rules, strategy, and technique concepts; basic movement patterns; understanding the relationship between a motor action and its outcome; emphasis placed on figuring out the best movements	Idea of movement
Associative stage	Able to detect and correct some errors, associate body actions with movement outcomes, less variation in performance	Emphasis placed on refining skills to a high degree of automaticity and then adapting skills to other contexts and situations	Fixation and diversification
Autonomic stage	Able to detect and correct errors, even during movement; execute task with limited attention; consistent performance with efficiency; few errors		

Defining the Learning Stages

Stage 1 of the Fitts and Posner model is the verbal–cognitive stage, or simply the *cognitive stage*, implying that most of the learning is not reflected in motor skill performance changes. Instead, during this stage, learning is dominated by cognitive factors such as understanding rules, getting a feel for the concepts for movement, learning tactics, and even learning how to learn. Gentile termed this stage the *idea of movement stage* as the learner begins to grasp the fundamental ideas of movement and determines what must be done to move effectively. To do so, the learner determines proper stimuli and establishes movement patterns. In determining the proper stimuli, the learner identifies stimuli or cues that are relevant to the movement, like ball speed, and nonrelevant stimuli or distractions that must be ignored. There is improvement and learning in actual motor skill performance, but the improvement in task knowledge likely exceeds motor performance. Performance in stage 1 is characterized by many errors, large errors, and high variability. Learners are not aware of how to correct the errors. The learner is also beginning to establish movement patterns, which may include footwork and limb coordination.

Stage 2 of the Fitts and Posner model is the *associative stage*. Fundamentals are learned, and fewer and smaller errors are made. At this stage, learners begin to associate a motor action with an outcome, providing them with a basis to detect and correct errors. Concentration is on skill refinement as learners begin to modify their actions to determine what works and what does not. Thus, learners can alter their own practice and reduce performance variability.

Stage 3 of the Fitts and Posner model is the *autonomous stage*. It only comes with much practice, after which the skill becomes automatic. The learner is able to perform the skill without "thinking" about it or paying close attention to the movement itself. Errors can be detected and corrected by the individual, often while the task is ongoing. The most important feature of the autonomous stage is that attentional resources are freed to be placed on things other than the movement. Gentile combined the Fitts and Posner stage 3 with stage 2, calling this a single stage of *fixation and diversification*. The learner fixates on specific movements developed early, refining them to make them more effective, more consistent, more efficient, and automatic. For learning to continue, the movements are then adapted to different situations, or adjustments are made to fit specific needs. This means that a larger number of motor patterns must be developed. Gentile termed this adaptation to be diversification, effectively expanding the learner's movement repertoire.

The three stages of Fitts and Posner are sometimes labeled as beginner, intermediate, and expert, but these labels are misleading. There is a great range of skill levels that can fall within each stage. Automaticity, for instance, does not make one an expert. Bicycle riding is automatic for many people, but few people would be considered expert cyclists. Conversely, an expert gymnast may struggle in learning a new routine, temporarily rendering them as beginner or intermediate performer. Figure 7.6 provides an example of characteristics and features of overarm throwing during the learning from the novice stage to what are considered "mature throwers" (Haywood, 1993). It is hard, perhaps, to understand the cognitive actions of throwing a ball, but this stage is marked by getting a feel for the ball and ongoing revelations about how to use the trunk and legs rather than just the arm. Initial leg action is often ipsilateral, that is, the leg used to step and the arm used to throw are on the same side of the body. Learning to step in a contralateral matter takes a concentrated and intentional action. By the time the learner reaches the autonomic stage, they demonstrate a mature throwing action, but this by no means indicates they are ready for the big leagues!

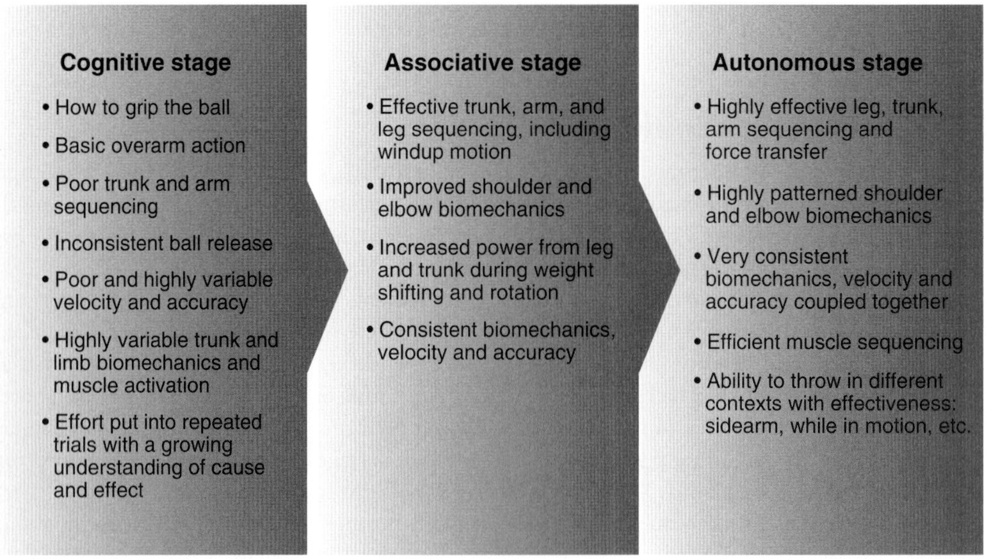

Cognitive stage	Associative stage	Autonomous stage
• How to grip the ball	• Effective trunk, arm, and leg sequencing, including windup motion	• Highly effective leg, trunk, arm sequencing and force transfer
• Basic overarm action	• Improved shoulder and elbow biomechanics	• Highly patterned shoulder and elbow biomechanics
• Poor trunk and arm sequencing	• Increased power from leg and trunk during weight shifting and rotation	• Very consistent biomechanics, velocity and accuracy coupled together
• Inconsistent ball release	• Consistent biomechanics, velocity and accuracy	• Efficient muscle sequencing
• Poor and highly variable velocity and accuracy		• Ability to throw in different contexts with effectiveness: sidearm, while in motion, etc.
• Highly variable trunk and limb biomechanics and muscle activation		
• Effort put into repeated trials with a growing understanding of cause and effect		

Figure 7.6 • Example of learning stages for overarm throwing. The development of overarm throwing, including children and adults, follows a predictable pattern from the cognitive stage to the autonomic stage. From novice to mature throwers, the largest changes are in the use of the legs and trunk to create high velocities at the hand, the development of consistent throwing actions that are stable across many different contexts, and the ability to adapt the throw when needed.

CHARACTERISTICS OF LEARNING STAGES AND NOVICE–EXPERT DIFFERENCES

Identifying the stage a learner is at is not an easy task. Simply inferring automaticity, identifying errors in performance, and observing error correction are insufficient in placing an individual in a certain stage of learning. This difficulty arises, in part, because the learner may be at different stages for different components of a complex motor skill. A gymnast, for example, may have outstanding jumping ability and the technical skill to rotate the required number of times in a vault, but she may not have the skill to adapt the rotations in case a slight error is made in the jump take-off, leading to inconsistent performances. There are other characteristics to look for that help identify a learner's progression and overall level of skill proficiency besides the magnitude of error and error detection and correction. It may seem that identifying strong proficiency versus poor proficiency is obvious; after all, the better performers win more often. In addition, the best athletes are often thought to be bigger, faster, and stronger, and these are the reasons for their success. Winning is certainly a characteristic of high-level performers, but physiological abilities do not easily distinguish the high-level performers (Abernethy et al., 1995).

There are a number of changes that accompany the progression through the learning stages of motor skills, and even more, develop into specific characteristics and traits that distinguish high-level performers from lower level performers. By understanding these changes, instructors and learners can develop the steps necessary to progress to high-level motor skill performance. The general characteristics that distinguish performers along the learning and motor skill proficiency continuum are (1) knowledge structure and information processing, (2) how the goal of the skill is achieved, and (3) changes in coordination and improved movement efficiency and muscle activation changes.

Knowledge Structure and Information Processing

As learners progress through the learning stages, they process information faster and more accurately, know more information, and are able to use that information in different ways (McPherson & Vickers, 2004; Singer & Janelle, 1999; Starkes & Ericsson, 2003). Singer and Janelle (1999) specifically noted that experts have greater domain-specific knowledge, are able to detect more relevant information and find use for this information, can faster and more effectively store and access information, can better recognize patterns of play, and use circumstances and situations to predict or anticipate future actions, and overall make decisions that are more rapid and more appropriate. The ability to anticipate upcoming actions by opponents using past and current information enables experts to be less mentally clogged and less mentally burdened. Experts use concepts, not just independent pieces of information. They also relate information together better, a process called chunking. For instance, late in a soccer game, an offensive player may put together a series of "clues" about the game circumstances (e.g., score, fatigued defenders, defender tendencies developed over the course of the game) to decide and implement a particular tactical move (Baker et al., 2003a,b; McPherson, 1994). The importance of information processing in experts may be the key feature that distinguishes the highest-level performers (Singer & Janelle, 1999; Starkes & Ericsson, 2003).

Better knowledge structure of advanced performers is accompanied by different *visual search* patterns. Early learners typically look at only the most direct and immediately important cues, such as watching the ball, though they also may place visual attention on any number if irrelevant cues. Individuals later begin to learn to look for different stimuli or clues to help them anticipate and perform better (Abernethy, 1999; Helsen & Starkes, 1999). For example, experts watch the body language of opposing players in sports like tennis in order to anticipate where the player intends to hit the ball or move. Researchers have shown that general patterns of experts include more efficient searches and patterned searches, more time spent on important cues, and that these differences have been found across the athletic spectrum, from boxing (Ripoll et al., 1995) to field sports (Baker et al., 2003a). Helsen and Starkes (1999) even maintained that the smooth and efficient and highly effective movements of the advanced soccer players in their studies were a result of better knowledge structure factors like decision-making skills, and not physiological capabilities *per se*. Some may argue this point, but the

SIDE**NOTE**	**VISUAL SEARCH IN SURGERY**

Visual search is important in activities other than athletics. Wilson et al. (2010) examined the gaze characteristics of experienced surgeons versus novice surgeons in a computerized virtual reality surgical task. In the photos below, the experimental setup is shown. In the upper left photo the subject is manipulating mock surgical instrument controllers to interact with the virtual surgical task (A, and lower photo). She is wearing a pupil gaze-tracking device (B) to assess the location of her focal vision on the computer screen. The experimenter's computer screen (C, and right photo) monitors the gaze-tracking devise on the eye. The results of the study showed that experts completed the surgical task faster, moved the computer surgical controls more efficiently, and spent more time fixated on the target compared to the novices. The novices spent their visual search moving back and forth from tracking the surgical tool to the target, seemingly needing to continually double-check their progress.

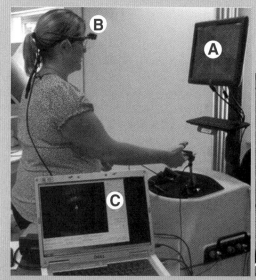
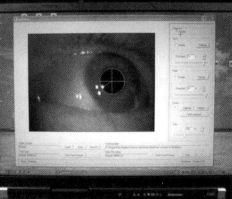

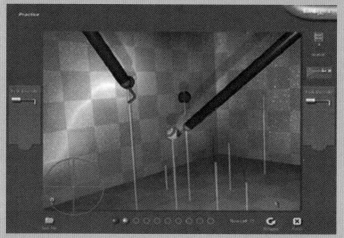

From Wilson, M., McGrath, J., Vine, S., Brewer, J., Defriend, D., & Masters, R. (2010). Psychomotor control in a virtual laparoscopic surgery training environment: Gaze control parameters differentiate novices from experts. *Surgical Endoscopy, 24*(10), 2458–2464, with permission from Springer.

message here is that physiological and neuromuscular capabilities are most effective when used or exploited at the appropriate times.

Better Skilled Persons Change How the Goal of a Skill Is Achieved

As learners improve, they change how they accomplish goals. For instance, beginning soccer players may emphasize kicking power when goal shooting, whereas more skilled players rely more on an accurate and deft touch. Beginners may drive the ball directly at the goalie; experts attempt to fool the goalie. In a similar manner, beginning and intermediate tennis players emphasize serve velocity as they improve. With more advancement, tennis players begin focusing on serve direction to force

SIDE**NOTE**	**INTERPERSONAL COORDINATION**

Dyads are groups of two individuals either working together or in opposition Tim against one another, representing a microcosm of team play through "interpersonal coordination." Athletic dyads are commonly observed as one-on-one situations and provide abundant data on decision-making processes. Athletes must play off one another, with offensive and defensive players keying in on different sources of information and matching them with different goals and tactics and situational circumstances. For example, Headrick et al. (2012) reported that dyad play in youth soccer players was affected dramatically by proximity to the goal. Duarte et al. (2012) reported that in developing 11-year-old players, the more successful offensive players used unpredictability as a weapon. The more successful defensive players used actions to actively constrain the offensive player's actions, that is, to limit their options. In the photo below, the soccer dyad is influenced by the proximity to the goal and the goalkeeper.

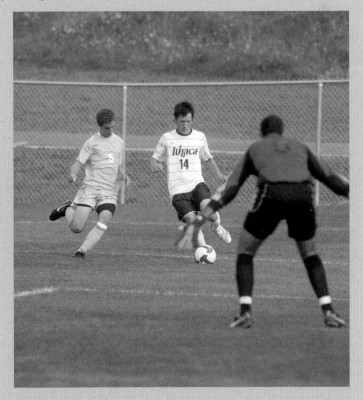

Photo courtesy Tim McKinney.

the opposing player into backhand or forehand returns. Ripoll et al. (1995) showed that expert box-ers compared to subelite boxers prioritized rejecting an attack by an opponent over taking advantage of a possible opening for their own attack. How the learner achieves the goal of the skill is very task dependent and is a combination of the learner's knowledge base and an already accumulated skill set.

Experts Have Better Coordination and Movement Efficiency

That experts have better coordination seems almost a definition of expertise. Coordination looks dif-ferent depending on the task, but there are some common characteristics of highly coordinated move-ments, some of which we examined in the motor unit behavior section of Chapter 3. Overall, experts tend to use less muscle activation for a given task, which produces smoother and more energy efficient movements (Lay et al., 2002). On the other hand, experts or well-trained persons often have the capa-bility to call upon more neuromuscular resources to maximize performance (Blackwell & Cole, 1994; Fimland et al., 2010; Gabriel et al., 2006).

 Whole-body coordination differences are often easy to spot. Novices tend to look stiff and jerky, which may be a result of them linking together limb segments to act as a single unit. Based on Bern-stein's (1967) original hypotheses, some authors have suggested that novices rigidly link limb segments in order to reduce the degrees of freedom (in this case mechanical degrees of freedom) and, as learning progresses to the expert stages, the mechanical degrees of freedom are released (Vereijken et al., 1992). This reduction in degrees of freedom by novices has certainly been observed, but is not universal. Kon-czak et al. (2009) found that expert violinists reduce shoulder movements (rigidly linking the shoulder to the trunk) compared to novices. What can be concluded from these observations is that as learning progresses one learns control body and limb segments differently in order to meet new challenges and new goals. Clearly, though, efficiency of movement by limiting unnecessary movements and muscle actions predominates in the acquisition of high-level motor skills.

Concepts in Action

Learning Skills in Response to Dysfunction

We often think that the learning process pertains only to children or perhaps adults learning new skills. But injury, disease, pain, and even the aging process itself are conditions that may cause one's motor skills to deteriorate, requiring new learning to maintain functional capabilities. Con-sider, for instance, a study by Patsika et al. (2011) who examined knee extension strength and coordination during a simple sit to stand task in middle-aged women with and without knee osteo-arthritis. The women with osteoarthritis displayed more EMG activation per unit of force exerted during strength tasks, and a slower and less muscularly efficient sit to stand movement. The authors concluded that the strength impairment in these women caused them to adopt different and less efficient muscle coordination strategies for rising out of a chair. These strategies centered on the use of hip muscles, perhaps as a way to avoid knee pain. The key point here is that the osteoarthritis sufferers had regressed in fundamental motor skill performance that was further contributing to neg-ative well-being. By identifying the faulty coordination mechanisms and cognitive strategies of these individuals, strategies for improvement were identified. One strategy could be to regain normal hip and knee coordination. This could only happen after strength was regained, pain was alleviated or managed, and the original coordination mechanisms relearned. The second approach would be to learn a new strategy and coordination mechanisms that accommodate and minimize the individuals' new reality of pain and discomfort. Either way, the need to relearn puts the individual back in the initial stages of the learning process.

| SIDE**NOTE** | **LEARNED COORDINATION AND PHYSIOLOGICAL CONSEQUENCES** |

The characteristics that describe one's progression through learning stages are not limited to learning motor skills. They are important even for progression in activities that many consider to be largely based on genetic physiological capacities. Consider the importance of muscle coordination and movement efficiency as they related to a study by Lay et al. (2002), who had fit persons practice on a rowing ergometer for just 10 practice days. The subjects practiced at an intensity level too low to elicit physiological adaptations. After the 10 days of practice, the subjects were able to exercise at a submaximal work level using less energy (e.g., VO_2 consumption) and less EMG activation than before practice. Other results found more tightly coordinated muscle activation patterns and movement patterns as revealed by biomechanical analysis. These authors concluded that coordination mechanisms were organized to minimize metabolic cost (or maximize efficiency). The figure below is a representative example of their EMG data from the biceps brachii, showing prepractice EMG (left traces) to be larger and less defined than the postpractice traces (right traces). These data show less muscle activation applied more precisely, giving a physiological rationale for how performance became more metabolically efficient due to practice.

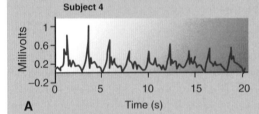
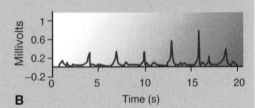

Reprinted from Lay, B., Sparrow, W., Hughes, K., & O'Dwyer, N. (2002). Practice effects on coordination and control, metabolic energy expenditure, and muscle activation. *Human Movement Science, 21*(5–6), 807–830, with permission from Elsevier.

INDIVIDUAL DIFFERENCES IN LEARNING AND THE USE OF LEARNING ASSESSMENTS

Using the concepts of measurement learned in Chapter 6 together with retention and transfer tests, it is possible to gauge learning progress. Progress, though, does not by itself classify the learner to a particular learning stage, nor does it mean the same practice techniques should continue to be used. Assessment is used as a tool to evaluate past learning, which then gives rise to understanding the learner's performance level and direction for future learning and practice goals. Assessment is also a tool to evaluate individual differences to particular instructional techniques.

Individual Differences in Learning

Most of us are familiar with someone who just seems learning things quickly while other struggle. Or someone who just cannot seem to grasp a concept until it is presented in a different way. These examples illustrate differences in **learning style**, which is defined as a learner's preferred way of responding to a learning task, in terms of how one learns and the quality of one's learning. Learning style may be specific to the environment and nature of what is being learned, meaning that individuals may have a different math learning style versus a motor skill learning style (Coker, 1995). Learning styles have come under much examination in the educational literature, where there is evidence to support the idea that matching instruction to the learning style improves learning (see Cassidy, 2004; Hayes & Allinson, 1993, for reviews). There are a number of learning style theories, but most of them center on what sources of information and sensory modalities best fit with the learner. Most prominent classifications are visual/verbal learners and tactile/kinesthetic learners, which is determined through the use of questionnaires. Visual/verbal learners are best served by listening and reading, and can make good use of charts and graphs. Tactile/kinesthetic learners key into hands-on experimentation, often in the form of lab experimentation.

Identifying learning styles for motor skills is a relatively unexplored area with scarcely any empirical research (e.g., Buell et al., 1987) available to support its use (Fuelscher et al., 2012). Moreover, at this point, there are no well-researched tools for assessing one's learning style in the motor skill domain. The VARK-Athlete test (Dunn & Flemming, 2012) has been used, but it has yet to undergo extensive reliability and validity studies. Nevertheless, there is a sufficient theoretical basis from other fields to suggest that matching a learning style with an instructional style may facilitate learning, and most seasoned coaches can provide anecdotal evidence that not all learners learn in the same way. Conceptually, it is reasonable that motor skill learners could have a verbal/visual or tactile/kinesthetic preference. The essential point to draw from this discussion is that a learner not learning or failing to progress through learning stages may be due to incompatibility between instruction and how the learner learns. Assessments revealing progress in one area but not another can prompt investigation into the underlying instructional techniques and may reveal more efficacious techniques.

Using Assessments to Guide Practice

Not only can assessments provide insight to the effectiveness of instructional techniques but also the rate and quality of learning of the performer. Assessments provide insight to what is learned and what is not learned, and hence the underlying mechanisms behind performance. Diligent use of learning assessments can thus provide a basis upon which to plan and structure practice. Consider an adolescent swimmer engaged in competitive swimming. She has well learned the basic freestyle stroke, and even at a relatively young age can be considered at a point of automaticity. Over the course of 2 years in competition, she strongly improves her performance times to a point of age-group subelite status. Most of her practice sessions emphasized learning and refining technical motor skills, like stroke mechanics, starting, flip turns, and fitness. Her stroke skill training fixated on refinement and underwater video records showed that her strokes were consistent and persistent, but they break down somewhat during fatigue (marginal stability). During her third year in competition, her performance times improve, but not to the extent of her competitors, that is, winning has plateaued. Assessments show that her fitness is sufficient, but her stroke mechanics not only remain unstable during fatigue but are different from what other swimmers are doing. In particular, she is adept at the propeller-like "sculling stroke," but her competitors have adopted the deep catch "paddling stroke," which is more effective (von Loebbecke & Mittal, 2012).

At this point, the swimmer can still be classified as subelite for her age group, but she is at a crossroads. Her coaches could continue to train her using the sculling stroke, hoping to make it better and keep it stable during fatigue. They could also focus on other aspects of the swimmer's performance, such as physiological fitness. Alternately, she could begin to learn the new paddling stroke, which would set her performance back further as she learned to master the technique. She and her coaches decide to learn the new technique, thus placing her in the cognitive phase of learning for the stroke, despite being at an automatic stage for other skills such as tactical skills, turns, and the start. Her prior learning of stroke mechanics may positively transfer regarding feel for the water, but the actual bilateral movement pattern of the old stroke may be so ingrained that negative transfer may result. Dry land and simple pool training of the new stroke will require continual transfer and retention tests to determine if the new stroke is being retained under complex and competitive environments. In sum, the use of tests to assess learning and the identification of learning stages provide a framework to evaluate progress and the effectiveness of practice, as well as help plan a roadmap to reach future goals.

SUMMARY

Motor learning is defined as an increased capability to produce motor skills as a result of practice or experience. Learning is inferred when motor skill performance increases over practice time, and this performance is persistent over time, more consistent, stable in the face of challenging environments, and flexible to changing situations. Assessing if changes in performance actually reflect learning is done using retention tests and transfer tests. Retention tests assess for persistence and consistency, whereas transfer tests assess for stability and adaptability.

During the learning process, a plateau in performance may occur. There are several reasons plateaus occur, but the most frustrating for learners is most often because the instruction is targeting the wrong aspects of the motor skill, or because the learner must begin learning entirely new components of the motor skill. Identifying plateaus and characteristics of performance that describe where a performer is at in the learning process provides insight to instructional techniques and those factors contributing to learner progression. Assessment of learning is an essential element in evaluating the nature of plateaus and overall instructional effectiveness.

An essential characteristic of the learning process is transfer of learning. Transfer enables motor skills learned in one context to apply in other contexts. Transfer is typically noted when highly learned simple skills are applied during the learning of more complex skills, or when skills learned in a closed environment are transferred to an open, real-game environment. Transfer thus enables skills to diversity and become more flexible. Instructors must be on the lookout, however, for skills that transfer negatively to new situations and may cause learning to be impeded.

The learning process progresses through stages; generally, new learning is highly cognitive as learners get the feel for movements. Well-learned movements are automatic and are performed with more consistency and fewer errors. Among the other characteristics that are learned over time include better coordination and better information processing. In many instances, higher-skilled performers are best distinguished from other performers by knowledge base and better and faster information processing. Identifying the stage a learner is at helps to identify weaknesses and strengths, assess the effectiveness of practice, and provide an overall guide for progress.

STUDY QUESTIONS

1. Which characteristics of performance indicate that learning has occurred?
2. In Fitts and Posner's learning stages, the third stage differs primarily from the second stage in what way?
3. In Gentile's 2-stage model of motor learning, the first stage is characterized by determining the proper stimuli. What does this mean?
4. In Gentile's 2-stage model of learning, the second stage is characterized by fixation and diversification. What does this mean?
5. What is an automatic motor skill and describe why or why not this defines expertise.
6. What are the three types of causes of a performance plateaus? Give examples of each and discuss those that are most often troubling for learners.
7. The better coordination of an expert versus a novice means what? Give examples.
8. Difference in knowledge structure is just one factor that characterizes performance at different stages of learning. How do beginners differ from experts in this regard? What other ways to experts differ from novices?
9. What two reasons are behind the transfer of skills phenomenon? What are the benefits of transfer? How does the specificity of learning principle play a role in transfer?
10. Rapid acquisition of a new skill by someone proficient at a similar skill is likely due to what?

11. Using the motor skill of your choice and yourself as the learner, outline an assessment plan (i.e., transfer and retention tests) to indicate the stage of motor skill learning. Describe changes in the assessment that would reveal that learning occurred over a period of practice.

12. Using any common educational learning style inventory (see two choices below), evaluate your own learning style and the recommendations for instruction based on this style. Do you think these results hold any validity for you and your performance of motor skills? Why or why not?
Index of Learning Styles: http://www4.ncsu.edu/unity/lockers/users/f/felder/public/ILSpage.html
DVC Learning Style for College: http://acenetwork.remote-learner.net/file.php/1/Program_Resources/finallearningstylemerged.pdf

Bibliography

Abernethy, B. B. (1999). The 1997 Coleman Roberts Griffith address movement expertise: A juncture between psychology theory and practice. *Journal of Applied Sport Psychology*, *11*(1), 126–141.

Abernethy, P. P., Wilson, G. G., & Logan, P. P. (1995). Strength and power assessment: Issues, controversies and challenges. *Sports Medicine*, *19*(6), 401–417.

Ausenda, C., & Carnovali, M. (2011). Transfer of motor skill learning from the healthy hand to the paretic hand in stroke patients: A randomized controlled trial. *European Journal of Physical and Rehabilitation Medicine*, *47*(3), 417–425.

Baker, J. J., Cote, J. J., & Abernethy, B. B. (2003a). Sport-specific practice and the development of expert decision-making in team ball sports. *Journal of Applied Sport Psychology*, *15*(1), 12–25.

Baker, J. J., Horton, S. S., Robertson-Wilson, J. J., & Wall, M. M. (2003b). Nurturing sport expertise: Factors influencing the development of elite athlete. *Journal of Sports Science and Medicine*, *2*(1), 1–9.

Bernstein, N. A. (1967). *The co-ordination and regulation of movements*. Oxford, England: Pergamon Press.

Blackwell, J. R., & Cole, K. J. (1994). Wrist kinematics differ in expert and novice tennis players performing the backhand stroke: Implications for tennis elbow. *Journal of Biomechanics*, *27*(5), 509–516.

Buell, C., Pettigrew, F., & Langendorfer, S. (1987). Effect of perceptual style strength on acquisition of a novel motor task. *Perceptual and Motor Skills*, *65*(3), 743–747.

Cassidy, S. (2004). Learning styles: An overview of theories, models, and measures. *Educational Psychology*, *24*(4), 419–444.

Coker, C. (1995). Learning style consistency across cognitive and motor settings. *Perceptual and Motor Skills*, *81*(3 Pt 1), 1023–1026.

Duarte, R., Araújo, D., Davids, K., Travassos, B., Gazimba, V., & Sampaio, J. (2012). Interpersonal coordination tendencies shape 1-vs-1 sub-phase performance outcomes in youth soccer. *Journal of Sports Sciences*, *30*(9), 871–877.

Dunn, J. L., & Flemming, N. (2012). The VARK-Athlete Questionnaire. http://www.vark-learn.com/english/page.asp?p=athletes

Fagard, J., & Corroyer, D. (2003). Using a continuous index of laterality to determine how laterality is related to interhemispheric transfer and bimanual coordination in children. *Developmental Psychobiology*, *43*(1), 44–56.

Fimland, M., Helgerud, J., Gruber, M., Leivseth, G., & Hoff, J. (2010). Enhanced neural drive after maximal strength training in multiple sclerosis patients. *European Journal of Applied Physiology*, *110*(2), 435–443.

Fitts, P. M., & Posner, M. I. (1967). *Human performance*. Oxford, England: Brooks and Cole.

Fuelscher, I., Ball, K., & Macmahon, C. (2012). Perspectives on learning styles in motor and sport skills. *Frontiers in Psychology*, *3*(69), 1–3, doi: 10.3389/fpsyg.2012.

Gabriel, D., Kamen, G., & Frost, G. (2006). Neural adaptations to resistive exercise: Mechanisms and recommendations for training practices. *Sports Medicine*, *36*(2), 133–149.

Gauthier, L. V., Taub, E., Mark, V. W., Perkins, C., & Uswatte, G. (2009). Improvement after constraint-induced movement therapy is independent of infarct location in chronic stroke patients. *Stroke*, *40*(7), 2468–2472.

Gentile, A. M. (2000). Skill acquisition: Action, movement, and neuromotor processes. In J. H. Car & R. B. Shepherd (Eds.) *Movement science: Foundations for physical therapy* (2nd ed., pp. 111–187). Rockville, MD: Aspen.

Hayes, J., & Allinson, C. W. (1993). Matching learning style and instructional strategy: An application of the person-environment interaction paradigm. *Perceptual and Motor Skills*, 76(1), 63–79.

Haywood, K. (1993). *Lifespan motor development*. Champaign, IL: Human Kinetics.

Headrick, J., Davids, K., Renshaw, I., Araújo, D., Passos, P., & Fernandes, O. (2012). Proximity-to-goal as a constraint on patterns of behaviour in attacker–defender dyads in team games. *Journal of Sports Sciences*, 30(3), 247–253.

Helsen, W. F., & Starkes, J. L. (1999). A multidimensional approach to skilled perception and performance in sport. *Applied Cognitive Psychology*, 13(1), 1–27.

Jones, A. M. (2006). The physiology of the world record holder for the woman's marathon. *International Journal of Sports Sciences and Coaching, 1*(2), 101–116.

Konczak, J., Vander Velden, H., & Jaeger, L. (2009). Learning to play the violin: Motor control by freezing, not freeing degrees of freedom. *Journal of Motor Behavior*, 41(3), 243–252.

Lay, B. S., Sparrow, W. A., Hughes, K. M., & O'Dwyer, N. J. (2002). Practice effects on coordination and control, metabolic energy expenditure, and muscle activation. *Human Movement Science*, 21(5/6), 807–830.

Mackrous, I., & Proteau, L. (2007). Specificity of practice results from differences in movement planning strategies. *Experimental Brain Research*, 183(2), 181–193.

McPherson, S. L. (1994). The development of sport expertise: Mapping the tactical domain. *Quest*, 46(2), 223–240, 247–262.

McPherson, S. L., & Vickers, J. N. (2004). Cognitive control in motor expertise. *International Journal of Sport and Exercise Psychology*, 2(3), 274–300.

Patsika, G., Kellis, E., & Amiridis, I. O. (2011). Neuromuscular efficiency during sit to stand movement in women with knee osteoarthritis. *Journal of Electromyography and Kinesiology*, 21(5), 689–694.

Proteau, L., Marteniuk, R., & Lévesque, L. (1992). A sensorimotor basis for motor learning: Evidence indicating specificity of practice. *Quarterly Journal of Experimental Psychology. Human Experimental Psychology*, 44(3), 557–575.

Ripoll, H. H., Kerlirzin, Y. Y., Stein, J. F., & Reine, B. B. (1995). Analysis of information processing, decision making, and visual strategies in complex problem solving sport situations. *Human Movement Science*, 14(3), 325–349.

Singer, R. N., & Janelle, C. M. (1999). Determining sport expertise: From genes to supremes. *International Journal of Sport Psychology*, 30(2), 117–150.

Soucy, M., & Proteau, L. (2001). Development of multiple movement representations with practice: Specificity versus flexibility. *Journal of Motor Behavior*, 33(3), 243–254.

Stark, A., Meiner, Z., Lefkovitz, R., & Levin, N. (2012). Plasticity in cortical motor upper-limb representation following stroke and rehabilitation: Two longitudinal multi-joint FMRI case-studies. *Brain Topography*, 25(2), 205–219.

Starkes, J. L., & Ericsson, K. A. (2003). *Expert performance in sports: Advances in research on sport expertise*. Champaign, IL: Human Kinetics.

Stöckel, T., & Weigelt, M. (2012). Brain lateralisation and motor learning: Selective effects of dominant and non-dominant hand practice on the early acquisition of throwing skills. *Laterality*, 17(1), 18–37.

Sutcliffe, T. L., Logan, W. J., & Fehlings, D. L. (2009). Pediatric constraint-induced movement therapy is associated with increased contralateral cortical activity on functional magnetic resonance imaging. *Journal of Child Neurology*, 24(10), 1230–1235.

Taub, E., & Morris, D. M. (2001). Constraint-induced movement therapy to enhance recovery after stroke. *Current Atherosclerosis Reports*, 3(4), 279–286.

Vangheluwe, S., Suy, E., Wenderoth, N., & Swinnen, S. (2006). Learning and transfer of bimanual multifrequency patterns: Effector-independent and effector-specific levels of movement representation. *Experimental Brain Research*, 170(4), 543–554.

Vereijken, B. B., Whiting, H. A., & Newell, K. M. (1992). Free(z)ing degrees of freedom in skill acquisition. *Journal of Motor Behavior*, 24(1), 133–142.

von Loebbecke, A., & Mittal, R. (2012). Comparative analysis of thrust production for distinct arm-pull styles in competitive swimming. *Journal of Biomechanical Engineering*, 134(7), 074501. http://dx.doi.org/10.1115/1.4007028

Wilson, M., McGrath, J., Vine, S., Brewer, J., Defriend, D., & Masters, R. (2010). Psychomotor control in a virtual laparoscopic surgery training environment: Gaze control parameters differentiate novices from experts. *Surgical Endoscopy*, 24(10), 2458–2464.

8 | Information Processing and Motor Skill Performance

PURPOSE, IMPORTANCE, AND OBJECTIVES OF THIS CHAPTER

The purpose of this chapter is to describe the mental attributes and behavioral elements necessary to maximize the learning and performance of motor skills. Specifically, this chapter focuses on memory, attention, and intention as the foundational elements of learning that must be a part of any successful training or practice situation. With this understanding the learner and instructor can develop practice and training programs and individual mind-sets to maximize learning and performance and avoid training pitfalls.

After reading this chapter, you should be able to:

1. Explain information processing concepts and multiple resource theory and their impact on learning and performance.
2. Explain motor memory and how to use various techniques to improve motor memory.
3. Explain attention, focus, and related concepts and how these concepts contribute to the learning and performance of motor skills.
4. Explain the techniques to improve attention skills and how to use these and other techniques to improve information processing accuracy and speed, overcome mental barriers like anxiety, and overall improve motor skill performance.
5. Explain the widespread influence played by mental intention in information processing, learning, motor skill performance, and physiological adaptations to practice and training.

In the previous chapter, we learned that key distinguishing traits of highly skilled performers are task-specific knowledge structure and better information processing. In this chapter, we explore these concepts more closely and particularly focus on those aspects of information processing critical to the learning process and provide the critical foundation for both learning and peak performance to occur. In particular, we look at the concepts of memory, attention, and intention and their relationships among one another and how to maximize the learning and use of these psychological characteristics to guide physiological performance.

INFORMATION PROCESSING AND MULTIPLE RESOURCE THEORY

The job of our central nervous system (CNS) is to process information. Information arrives from sources external to the body and internal to the body, and some is already contained within our own CNS. Everything we see, hear, taste, touch, and smell provides information. A vast number of physiological processes are monitored by visceroreceptors and somatoreceptors, all of which send information to the CNS. Some of this information is explicitly looked for, and some is implicitly gathered without conscious awareness. In the CNS, this information meets up with stored information in the form of memories, plans, and processes. This information is then processed in the form of identification, interpretation, and filtering, and is finally acted upon. These actions by our brain include reasoning, monitoring, storing and retrieving information, running the physiological processes of our body, producing emotional and rational behaviors, communicating, and making decisions.

But the brain cannot necessarily do all this at the same time. Our brain has limited capacities that, in turn, limit our performance. In this section we look at multiple resource theory as a model of our brain's information processing and then two information processing resources. These resources—memory and attention—factor prominently in the application of motor learning principles. Behind these mental processing resources, the dominant role of intention is discussed and applied.

The processing the brain does is widespread and varied. **Multiple resource theory** posits that we have a variety of processing resources. Though our brain has areas to process specific types of information, such as verbal output, auditory, olfactory, visual sensory processing, and emotional reasoning, these do not necessarily correspond to resources as identified by multiple resource theory. Nevertheless, the theory adequately describes that our brain has the capability to process different types and amounts of information, though there is redundancy in the system. All of these resources have limited but flexible capacities. Sometimes the resource capacities can be expanded and are often times shrunk. Factors such as arousal, fatigue, motivation, and health can alter the capacity.

The reason for processing degradation is because information tends to be handled by our brain in a *serial processing* manner (one after another) rather than in a *parallel processing* manner (side by side simultaneous processing). When simultaneous information needs to be processed, it gets jammed up in a bottleneck (Welford, 1952), waiting for one task after another to be processed (Fig. 8.1). When two tasks arrive simultaneously or closely spaced, one task needs to delay while the other is being carried out. This delay to get to the second task is called the **psychological refractory period** (PRP). The PRP is nicely illustrated in an offensive player's feint move on a defender. A simple head fake by a basketball player prior to a step to the right or left may be all that is needed to delay a defensive player. Even if the defender does not actually move to follow the head fake, mentally they may be processing the information. Even as the defensive player sees the step, they must finish processing the head fake first before going on to processing the step. This PRP delay may be as long as 80 to 100 ms, which is long enough for the offensive player to get the jump on the defensive player.

Information processing is typically degraded if two or more tasks require the same or similar resource. A single large processing requirement may also tax the resource capacity. If two or more different tasks are done, then different resources may be called upon; thus, capacity may not be as limited. However, capacities can be taxed easily while doing multiple tasks. Driving in heavy traffic and bad weather provides a good example of resources being stretched. Even as the driver slows down, there is a good chance the radio will be turned off and passengers told to quiet down. The need to concentrate on the environmental conditions is so demanding that all resources are diverted away from listening to music and carrying on conversations. Furthermore, there is a good chance that stress and anxiety will consume resources and divert attention. A sobering reality to the limitations we have in processing information is evidenced by the dramatic rise in driving fatalities attributed to texting while driving (Wilson & Stimpson, 2010).

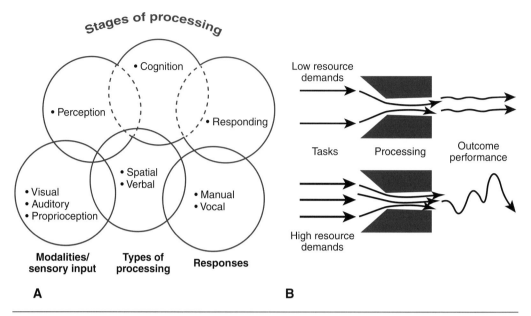

Figure 8.1 • Schematic of multiple resource theory based on concepts from Wickens (2008). **A**. In this model are three dimensions of resource use: (1) types of sensory input, (2) types of processing, and (3) types of responses. Each of these interacts with different stages of processing, creating another layer of interaction. The examples given in each dimension (circle) require different resources; for example, manual responses are processed different from vocal responses. The illustration implies that processing dimensions interfere with one another to different amounts. **B**. This diagram illustrates that more tasks, and tasks that use similar and interacting resources, will experience more degradation as revealed by poor outcomes. Multiple task processing tends to get bottlenecked, causing only one task to be processed at a time and/or task processing to interfere with one another. Note that any time dual tasks are processed performance will worsen (wavy lines); that is, there is no perfect sharing of resources.

MEMORY

Memory is a cognitive processing function that people tend to associate with facts and figures, and not motor skills. The simple ability to recall and repeat large numbers of motor skills over and over again even after long time periods indicates that we have a large capacity to remember motor skills we have learned, that is, **motor memory**. Certainly it is implied that a motor skill learned is a motor skill remembered, but motor and nonmotor memory also play a critical role during the motor skill learning process and during high-level performance. A soccer player, for instance, may scan the defense and instantaneously recall a previous pattern of play from earlier in the game or even from a previous year, giving the player information to anticipate an unfolding defensive strategy. Motor memory is sometimes mistakenly called muscle memory, a term that holds no real definition in the scientific literature.

Memory can be roughly broken down into **working memory** and **long-term memory**. Working, or short-term, memory is the temporary use and storage system for information. It is the active system for information processing, especially for the immediate situational needs, such as decision making, problem solving, movement production and evaluation, and storage and retrieval of long-term memory information. Information lasts only about 30 seconds in working memory. Capacity of working memory is about 7 (+ or − 2) words or digits. In movement, this translates to about 7 sequences in a movement, such as discrete gymnastic or dance movements (Starkes et al., 1987). Highly skilled people have larger working memory and long-term memory capacities that are skill specific.

SIDE**NOTE**

Cell phone use (including texting) during driving is an example of multitasking, that is, attempting to do more than one thing at a time. Much of what we know about multiple resources and information processing comes from multitasking experiments, specifically dual-task experimental paradigms. Dual-task paradigms have subjects engage in one primary task while concurrently attending to another secondary task. These experiments (e.g., Levy & Pashler, 2008) overwhelmingly demonstrate that multitasking as understood by most people is a fallacy. Our information processing speed and accuracy declines dramatically when we try to do more than one thing at a time, and this processing is degraded to a larger extent when the multiple tasks draw upon the same or similar resources, or when the resource demands are great. Studies have shown, for example, that dual-task processing is slowed when individuals engage in active-type listening (Gherri & Eimer, 2011) or when engaged in emotional conversations versus mundane conversations during cell phone use (Dula et al., 2011). Information processing will also degrade with the expectation of another task because attention is placed toward anticipation. This includes studying while having an active texting or tweeting session.

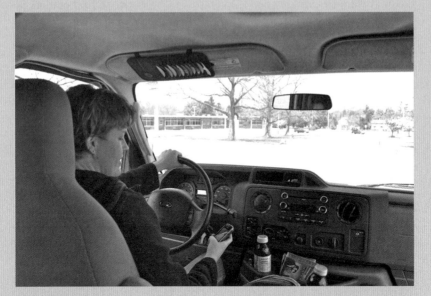

Photo courtesy Whitman R. Ives.

Multitasking in real life is largely accomplished by prioritizing tasks and attention switching. Accomplished "multitaskers" ignore unimportant stimuli and information, focus attention on a single thing at a time, and fully and rapidly switch attention at predetermined time periods. (See later in the chapter for a discussion of attention.)

There are, however, rare cases of *supertaskers*; persons who seem unaffected by multitasking. Watson and Strayer (2010) identified about 2.5% of their subject pool being supertaskers and noted, "our studies over the last decade have found that a great many people have the belief that the laws of attention do not apply to them (e.g., they have seen other drivers who are impaired while multitasking, but they themselves are the exception to the rule). In fact, some readers may also be wondering whether they too are supertaskers; however, we suggest that the odds of this are against them." These authors believe that the ability to supertask may come at the expense of other processing capabilities, though they did not identify what those could be.

Long-term memory is the "permanent" repository of information. Within long-term memory is stored *procedural, declarative, semantic*, and *episodic* information. Procedural information refers to how to do something whereas declarative information is what to do. Semantic information is a general knowledge of the world—facts and concepts—gained through experience, and episodic information are personally experienced events and the times they occurred. These different types of stored memory give support to the idea that various aspects of motor skill remembered differently, and thus, the how, what, and why of practice should be equally valued and practiced.

Strategies for Improving and Facilitating Memory Storage

There are three basic factors that must be taken into consideration regarding memory retention of motor skills. First, the characteristics of the movement itself influence what is remembered; second, remembering strategies influence retention; and third, the characteristics of practice influence what is remembered.

Movement characteristics are certain features or attributes of a movement that influence one's ability to remember that movement. For instance, continuous and rhythmic skills are more resistant to forgetting than discrete skills, probably because their repeated nature provides for more practice and the procedural requirements are often less complex than discrete skills. Location, position, and distance characteristics are important and thus more easily remembered features of a movement. Thus, pointing out important positions of the body is a good instructional method. Similarly, identifying the height for the ball toss in a tennis serve helps the remembering process. These terms are not altogether distinct, such that remembering a stance position could be described as the location of the feet relative to one another or distance apart (e.g., shoulder-width apart). Initial or starting positions give information on the movement to follow, and remembering a final position enables the learner to work through the movement that leads to the end position. First and last positions of a movement are naturally better remembered, as are proper or natural movement sequences. Consequently, middle portions of movement sequences tend not to be remembered as well, though they may be just as important and thus may require additional memory effort. For example, the middle stage of a golf swing with the club head back up over the head and the body cocked and ready to swing the club forward is a crucial position for an effective golf swing. Though it is in the middle of the movement, if this critical point is identified to the learner as important and made meaningful, then it is much better remembered.

Remembering strategies are vital to the long-term retention and learning of motor skills and should be incorporated insofar as feasible into the practice environment. There are a number of memory strategies that can be used depending on the appropriate circumstances. For motor skill learning, four strategies stand out: (1) repetition, (2) imparting meaningfulness and understanding, (3) learner self-control over how and what movements are practiced, and (4) fostering mastery and intention to remember.

Repetition is rehearsal of the movement again and again and again. This is a fundamental tenet of all of practice, but it does not necessarily mean that the exact same movement is repeated in a monotonous or rote manner. Even the most similar repetitive movements, like hitting tennis forehand drives off a ball machine, are coordinated in different ways as the nervous system continually refines the movement. According to Bernstein (1967),

> The process of practice towards the achievement of new motor habits essentially consists in the gradual success of a search for optimal motor solutions to the appropriate problems. Because of this, practice, when properly undertaken, does not consist in repeating the means of solution of a motor problem time after time, but in process of solving this problem again and again by techniques which we changed and perfected from repetition to repetition. It is already apparent here that, in many cases, "practice is a particular type of repetition without repetition" and that motor training, if this position is ignored, is merely mechanical repetition by rote, a method which has been discredited in pedagogy for some time. (p. 134)

Repetition designed to continually improve and find better solutions may result in memory storage of not only the refined movement but also the mechanisms by with the movement was refined and adapted. Hence, the process to alter and diversify the movement pattern may also form in memory storage.

Meaningful movements are better learned and remembered, and meaningfulness can be promoted when the learner understands how and why the skill needs to be done. Put differently, attaching meaning is more complex than simply stating that it is meaningful; the learner needs to understand why it is meaningful. It can be useful in attaching meaning to have the learner visualize the movement or attach a verbal label to a specific aspect of movement. A verbal label can be as simple as a grunt at the moment of ball impact or a self-talk instruction to bend the knees. Verbal labels may serve to provide sequencing remember, such as "tuck and roll."

Enabling learner self-control over what movements are practiced and how they are practiced empowers the individual to take charge of their own learning and enhances memory. Self-controlled practice may consist of the learner deciding when to get feedback or demonstrations, preselecting certain characteristics of the movement to individualize (e.g., self-defining important distances and body positions) (for a review, see Wulf et al., 2010b). Similarly, when the learner subjectively organizes facets of the motor skill learning process, particularly organizing large skill sets in a way that fits them, memory is also improved. This approach may appear undisciplined and disorganized, but only if unchecked. Fundamentally, if learners have a say in their own learning, it is likely that practice is more meaningful, they pay more attention, and they may devise their own methods of remembering. Movements then tend to be organized not only in a way that is meaningful but in a way that fits the way the learner learns. This does not mean that the learner is the only one responsible for practice and remembering, as this strategy may contribute to learning the wrong things. The instructor must help guide the learner's organization.

A focus on mastery and the intention to remember seem easy concepts, but they are often overlooked. Movements are best remembered when willful effort is given to try and remember the activities during practice, and when the intention is on mastery of the skills. Mastery provides a high goal for achievement and when done correctly, provides a tangible goal that is most relevant to the skill itself.

The *characteristics of practice* refers to what is learned during practice in comparison to what one is being tested on. In a broader context, this refers to the specificity of learning or practice principles explored in Chapter 7. Briefly, this means that memory and learning is specific to what was practiced, particularly in regard to the type and amount of sensory information. Consider a novice driver learning to use the clutch and brake and stick shift of an automobile with a manual transmission. On a protected track with no obstacles or dangers, learning and remembering may come easily. These same skills, however, may not be displayed on congested city streets; in fact the driver may freeze, "grind" gears, or select the wrong gear. In the practice situation, the shift and braking patterns were nicely sequential and corresponded to simple environmental cues that were stored in memory as sensory information. In a real world driving scenario of chaotic sensory inputs and out-of-sequence brake and shift patterns, previously learned skills and sensory cues may be inadequate. This is an example of the practice circumstances being different from the "test" circumstances and memory being specific to the characteristics of the learning environment. The more that practice is like the real life setting, the better the recall will be in the game or on the test. This does not, however, mean that the learning process should start off with complex, game-like practices. What it does mean is that eventually practice will need to address very challenging situations.

The remembering concepts are outlined with implementation strategies in Table 8.1. The applications described in the Table and in previous examples reveal that even when practice performance is high, good learning and retention of information may not follow. To optimize information

TABLE 8.1	Memory and Remembering Concepts	
Concept	**Explanation**	**Applications**
1. Characteristics of the movement	Some movement aspects are more easily remembered, namely, continuous or rhythmic movements, and specific locations or positions.	Identifying important body positions provides a basis for remembering the whole movement. If possible, make even discrete movements "rhythmical."
2. Remembering strategies	Four key strategies: rote repetition, meaningfulness, self-control over learning, intention to remember	Most of these can be applied in every situation. The learner must go into the situation with the intention to remember, and this is facilitated by enabling the learner some control over what is being learned, and by identifying why it is important and meaningful.
3. Characteristics of practice & specificity of practice	Remembering a movement is better when the movement is done in the same form and context as when practiced.	This is an element of functional training and specific practice. Practice should be game-like, even when practicing isolated skill sets like backhand drive in tennis. Under real-game stress, the proper form of a skill may break down because it was not stored in the context of a demanding high urgency situation.

processing and thus maximize memory and retention, there must be a balance between challenging practice conditions and practice performance. There are no hard and fast guidelines for this balance, but the *challenge point framework* (Guadagnoli & Lee, 2004) provides direction on how to approach the problem. According to Guadagnoli and Lee (2004), the amount of learning available depends on the information processing capabilities of the learner, the difficulty of the task, and the practice conditions contributing to the amount and nature of available information. At some point—the challenge point—cognitive processing is optimized, and thus learning and memory are maximized because the amount of information available is fully understandable and not overwhelming or uninterpretable. Figure 8.2 illustrates the interaction of these concepts, showing that a practice task too easy or too difficult (in comparison to the learner's skill level) does not provide a good learning environment because the amount of information is too little (task too easy) or overwhelming or hard to interpret (task too hard). At the same time there is a point in which the task performance during practice begins to suffer greatly because the task is too difficult. At the intersection point of potential learning and task performance is the point suggested by the authors to be optimal for learning and memory to occur. The summary point of this model is that task difficulty and environmental challenges during practice are essential for optimizing cognitive processing and learning. Identifying the optimal challenge point for each individual and his or her stage of learning follows a trial and error approach, starting with easier tasks and progressively adding more difficulty (Guadagnoli & Lee, 2004).

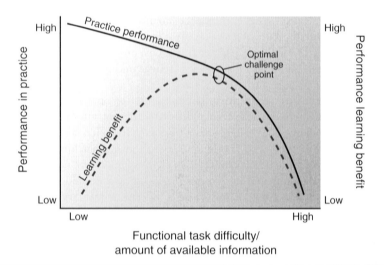

Figure 8.2 • The optimal challenge point is the point at which the potential learning benefit is maximized. As tasks become more difficult, practice performance sharply decreases. In addition, as difficulty increases, the amount of available information increases, but not all this information can be used. Learning is optimized—the challenge point—when practice performance is strong and when the available information is capable of being used. Too much information is overburdening and too little is insufficient. The shape of the curves and the location of the challenge point differ from novice to expert and from skill to skill.

ATTENTION

It is apparent from multiple resource theory that for optimal information processing to take place, the amount of information coming into the system cannot be overwhelming. Limiting the amount of information can happen in two ways; the first is to limit what actually comes into the CNS, and the second is for the CNS to filter out or ignore information before it is processed further. Both happen, but for our purposes, it is most useful to examine the process of limiting information before it reaches our CNS. We do this by altering our attention.

Attention is the mental process of concentrating on specific things, that is, an exclusive allocation of processing resources. Attention can be placed on the external environment, on the internal bodily environment, or on mental processes themselves. For example, mental math and daydreaming both place attention on mental processes. Attention can be a conscious or subconscious action. A conscious act, sometimes called an explicit act, differs from a subconscious (or implicit) act by the level of the individual's awareness. In conscious attention the individual is aware of where attention is being placed, but in subconscious attention the individual cannot identify when or where attention is being placed. This may sound like a contradiction, but in reality our sensory systems are never turned off, and the brain monitors sensory information and prioritizes this information even if we are not consciously monitoring these inputs.

Placing attention on something purposeful and specific is called **selective attention** and is one of the keys to avoid overburdening information processing resources. Selective attention implies that attention is placed on the most important, or most meaningful, things relevant to completing a task while ignoring other stimuli. Selective attention can be broadly considered to be either spatial or temporal. *Spatial attention* is placed on objects to identify and gather information from their spatial location. Vision and hearing provide the main sources of spatial attention, though touch provides a good source of information from objects close by (Vecera & Rizzo, 2003). *Temporal attention* is attention placed toward anticipation of upcoming events or the monitoring of information occurring over time. Music, speech, and motor skill production are key areas in which temporal attention is used in abundance (Correa et al., 2006). The ability to place attention on a proper point in time or the proper point in space is an essential anticipation skill that serves to reduce uncertainty and enable faster and more accurate reactions (Correa et al., 2006).

Focus of attention refers to the quality of our concentration on a stimuli or ongoing situation. With a poor focus of attention, our minds may drift to irrelevant information, thereby allocating information processing resources away from what is necessary. It is often necessary to **attention switch** from one stimulus or information processing resource to another. Switching may occur spatially or temporally. A long distance runner, for example, may place attention on a nearby competitor, shift to tactical decisions, shift again to monitor his internal physiological state, and then shift back to tactics. A quick and transient switch in attention switching is called a **momentary intention**. For example, while playing tennis the player can attend to the ball and then quickly switch attention to monitor the actions of the opposing player. Knowing where to attention switch means that attention can be placed on the most important things, as illustrated by the attention switching behavior of surgical nurses in Figure 8.3.

In sum, the ability to focus attention, switch attention, and select the most meaningful cues and information to concentrate on is necessary to avoid a cognitive meltdown. How we identify the most meaningful and important information, how we increase our focus, and how we learn to switch attention are learned through practice and are very much situation and context specific. These concepts are discussed next.

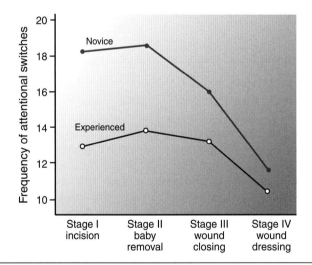

Figure 8.3 • Effective attention switching requires knowing the most efficient place to place attention and is a skill learned in many settings. The visual attention data shown here are from surgical nurses in actual surgeries of caesarean section births. Stages 1 and II progress from incision to removal of the baby and placenta, while stages III and IV progress from closing the wound to wound dressing. Attention could be placed on a variety of important areas, from observing the baby to visceral organs to vital signs to the surgical instruments to the needs of the physician. Experienced nurses' attention switched less during the surgery, especially during the states of highest workload and highest risk (stages I and II). The experienced nurses focused attention more on the body cavity and the physician's instruments needs, having developing what the authors' concluded was situational awareness. (From Koh, R., Park, T., Wickens, C., Ong, L., & Chia, S. (2011). Differences in attentional strategies by novice and experienced operating theatre scrub nurses. *Journal of Experimental Psychology: Applied, 17*(3), 233–246. Copyright © 2011 by the American Psychological Association. Adapted with permission.)

Concepts in Action

Attentional Focus, Change Blindness, and Deception

Maintaining a focus of attention has a downside in that we may miss events happening outside of our focus. Kevin O'Regan at the Paris Descartes Institute of Neurosciences and Cognition (http://nivea.psycho.univ-paris5.fr/) and Daniel Simons and his colleagues at the University of Illinois at Urbana-Champaign have done numerous studies on attentional focus and a phenomenon called change blindness. Change blindness occurs when we are so focused on one thing that we miss changes occurring around us, even if they are within our visual field. Among the well-known studies coming from Simons' lab is the "gorilla in the midst" study. To view this and other videos used by the researchers to assess change blindness and focus of attention, access the lab's Web page at http://www.simonslab.com/. Click on to the "videos" link and run the gorilla video and the other videos they have made available.

Change blindness and diverting of attention through visual misdirection are essential to magicians, who use these phenomena to create illusions. See the video on the PBS Web site for more on how these concepts are used in action to deceive viewers: http://www.pbs.org/wgbh/nova/body/psychology-magic.html. These same concepts are used by athletes to deceive opponents by diverting attention with visual misdirection. Athletes can be affected by change blindness within fields of view related to their expertise, though they are less affected when the change is meaningful and relevant to the context of the action versus something nonrelevant (Werner & Theis, 2000). A left-handed pitcher's pick-off move to first base (e.g., Andy Pettitte) and the basketball no-look pass are prime examples of misdirection taking advantage of change blindness.

Broad versus Narrow and Internal versus External Attention

The direction of our attention has been broadly categorized on a two-dimensional scale of view (internal versus external) and width (broad versus narrow). This two-dimensional classification was developed by Nideffer (1976, 1990) and is illustrated in Figure 8.4. Although Nideffer originally developed

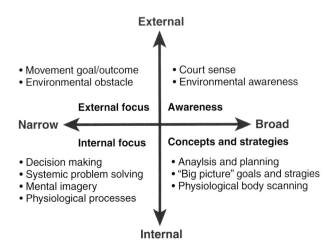

Figure 8.4 • Nideffer's attentional profile based on view and width. View concerns internal versus external and width refers to broad versus narrow. See text for more explanation.

this test to evaluate the traits of individuals, the concepts have become more universally applied to understanding the basic relationships between the type of activity or information processing needed and where attention is placed.

External broad is attention placed on the environment as a whole, whereas external narrow is attention placed on a specific environmental feature or specific movement goal or outcome. Internal attention can be placed on internal physiological processes or mental processing. An internal narrow focus is on specific decision making or problem solving, including imagery use. Internal narrow can be placed on specific physiological processes, such as pain/discomfort or heart rate. Internal broad attention placed on the "big picture," whether that is of the bodily environment or thinking. The mental big picture pertains to planning and outcome goals, and physiological big picture is a general sense of how one is doing. Normally, the physiological big picture is evaluated by a brief body scan of signs and symptoms, such as a runner evaluating multiple body symptoms to provide a rating of perceived exertion. This latter case reveals that a broad attention is not the ability to focus on many things at once, but the ability to attention switch and mental processes cued into data gathered by implicit attention mechanisms.

In the past 15 years, an abundance of research reports, notably from Gabriele Wulf and her colleagues (e.g., Freudenheim et al., 2010; Wulf & Prinz, 2001; Wulf et al., 2010a,b), have shown that motor skills across the spectrum, from gross to fine and open to closed, are learned and performed better when attention is placed externally. It is believed that focusing on a specific movement outcome simplifies the brain's movement planning and essentially enables the brain to organize the most effective solution to the movement problem. For example, Wulf et al. (2010a) found that focus during vertical jumping placed on the jump measurement tool versus an internal attention on the fingertips resulted in not only greater jump height but less muscle activation, indicating much greater efficiency (Figure 8.5).

Despite the robust findings supporting the use of an external focus of attention, like many concepts, there may be exceptions, such as an interaction between learner expertise and the type of motor skill (Beilock et al., 2002). In particular, it may be beneficial for new learners to periodically focus internally on movement dynamics to establish a fundamental movement pattern or movement "approximation" (Peh et al., 2011). Perhaps the most common exception concerns vigorous endurance activities. Though focusing externally, also called a *dissociative focus* in the research literature, has been shown to reduce exercisers' ratings of perceived exertion in endurance activities and improve swimming sprint speed (Freudenheim et al., 2010) and running metabolic efficiency (Schücker et al., 2009), an internal focus of attention may be associated with better performance in high-level endurance athletes. High-level endurance athletes, runners, and swimmers in particular tend to adopt an internal focus of attention. Also called an *associative focus*, these athletes attend to their own physiological processes, like heart rate or fatigue. Masters and Ogles (1998) in their comprehensive review, and recently confirmed by Hutchinson and Tenenbaum (2007), noted that self-monitoring enables these athletes to regulate their effort appropriate to the environmental challenges and their own race strategies. At high levels of effort, it becomes extremely difficult to ignore the overwhelming physiological signals of fatigue, pain, and stress, but even then high level athletes are able to attention switch to external factors such as competitors and environmental circumstances. This associative strategy differs in some respects to the internal focus shown to reduce motor skill performance. The internal focus during motor skill execution may disrupt procedural information processing, whereas the associative focus may simply be information gathering related to tactics and strategies.

Attention Demands and the Type of Motor Skill

The attention requirements of motor skills are quite varied. Furthermore, for a specific motor skill, the attention requirements may change depending on the situation or circumstances surrounding the execution of the skill and may differ from person to person. One of the most noticeable aspects of attention is that the demands of attention (i.e., those things that require our attention) change over practice. In particular, some tasks demand less attention as skill level improves. As tasks become automatic, the

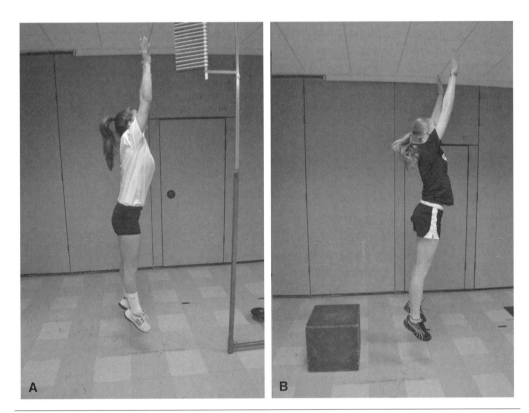

Figure 8.5 • Two jumping situations are presented that give rise to different focuses of attention. **A.** On the left the player has an external focus on the measurement tool, effectively placing in her mind a movement outcome goal. Though obscured by her arms, she is looking at the target vanes on the jump device. **B.** On the right the player is doing a depth jump to vertical jump with no overt attention instructions and no outcome target to jump to. She is in the middle of the vertical jump portion and is looking high on the wall across from her. In most cases the athlete will focus on internal body actions such as absorbing the landing impact from the box drop and the stretch-shorten reversal rather than an external movement outcome. A teaching strategy here would be to explore different attentional targets, including the need to switch attention from box drop portion of the movement to the vertical jump portion. (Photo courtesy Jeffrey C. Ives.)

need to place attention on actual movement execution is reduced. This automaticity, though, does not mean that our minds are free to wander. What it means is that resources are freed up to be used elsewhere. Yogi Berra, Hall of Fame catcher for the NY Yankees, once remarked that "you can't think and hit at the same time." More specifically, Yogi was succinctly stating that one cannot think about the swing while placing attention on the ball at the same time.

The concept of automaticity illustrates that attention requirements change over learning stages. With improving skills the learner is freed to place attention on other cues, has an increased capability to place attention on new cues, and learns what information is important to process and the irrelevant information to ignore. With these new attention skills comes improvement in motor skill performance.

Explicit and Implicit Learning of Attention Skills

Attention skills are generally not explicitly taught, save for the exception of instructional comments like "keep your eye on the ball" or "watch the other player." Such limited instruction in attention is not an oversight because attention skills are learned both explicitly and implicitly. Specific practice at attention

| SIDE**NOTE** | **POINT LIGHT DISPLAYS AND BIOLOGICAL MOTION PERCEPTION** |

Picking up useful information from the environment is a skill learned from infancy. Among the earliest information learned involves the identification of people and their movements. Researchers have made significant use of videos to examine aspects of the perception of human motion. Pinto and his colleagues (e.g., Pinto & Shiffrar, 1999) were among the first to examine biological motion perception using point light displays (PLDs). PLDs are biomechanical "stick figure" objects (mostly people) that show only points of light placed on aspects of the object in motion, such as at joints of the human body. The illustrations below show sample PLDs during walking: (a) two sequenced frames during normal walking, (b) inverted image, (c) ipsilateral limbs only, and (d) upper limbs only, and (e) limbs and trunk are separated and placed randomly, albeit in their normal orientation. Still images are hard to decipher, but during motion the relative orientations and sequencing of the limbs and joints make identification of walking a simple task. Manipulating the image such as in b, c, d, or even e only slightly interferes with identification because the basic object motions are still intact (see Pinto & Shiffrar, 1999). These data have provided insight into what features of movement, whether it is specific limb features or whole-body sequencing, we pay attention to when observing others.

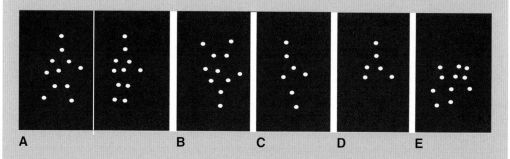

A   B   C   D   E

Niko Troje and his colleagues at the Queen's University in Ontario used video PLDs in a similar manner. The researchers have compiled a PLD database of human and animal motions from which individuals are asked to identify features, such as gender and the emotional state of a PLD actor walking. Troje's work has revealed how behavioral characteristics are carried out in motor actions ranging from anger to the actions of a sporting opponent to social intentions to the fertility of women. Try out these videos for yourself by accessing the lab's Web page at http://www.biomotionlab.ca/.

skills, like watching the ball, are explicit, whereas incidental learning that comes without an awareness of what is being learned is called implicit. High-level athletes will often talk about picking up movement cues from opposing players, like shoulder rotation during a volleyball serve, but can rarely say when or how they learned it. Rather, they just "picked it up along the way." According to Magill (1998) these regulatory and environmental cues are probably better off left to be learned implicitly.

Consider, for example, the elegant experiment by Farrow and Abernethy (2002), in which video visual occlusion techniques were used to train the anticipatory skills of tennis players returning the serve. One group was taught explicitly where to place attention—on racquet and body mechanics of the server—and another group was simply told to anticipate how fast the serve was going to be. For the latter group, it was the purpose to see if they could implicitly learn where to place attention and use that to improve return of serve performance. The results showed that

Concepts in Action

The Quiet Eye

Joan Vickers, a researcher at the University of Calgary, has coined the term "quiet eye" to explain the attentional focus characteristics of the high-level performers in her research. Using gaze-tracking equipment, Dr. Vickers noted that the best performances by athletes, for example, golfers putting and basketball players shooting free throws, occurred when their gaze and attention was external on the target for just a second or two (the quiet eye), and then let their bodies go without much thought. Even in very rapid and unstable environments, such as a hockey goalie stopping a shot, it was found that most stops are made when the goalies tracked the stick of the shooter and then made a final fixation on the target (puck) before making a motor action (Panchuk & Vickers, 2009). Panchuk and Vickers (2009), using gaze-tracking devices (see images below) and visual occlusion techniques, noted that elite hockey goalies fixated on the puck strike with a quiet eye right before initiating the motor action; using that information to predict the path of the puck and generate an interceptive movement pattern. This did not prevent changing the movement pattern (called a movement reversal) while the puck was in mid flight, but such changes are not consistent with the best success. On the left photo is the point of gaze (small circle) of the goalie as recorded by the gaze-tracking equipment. On the right is a view of the experimental setup with shots on goal.

These authors have taken their research to the field, helping to improve hockey performance and free-throw shooting of basketball players. For more on these applications, see the "Scientific American Frontiers" videos on the "Quiet Eye" and "Brainy Putting" at http://www.pbs.org/saf/1206/video/watchonline.htm.

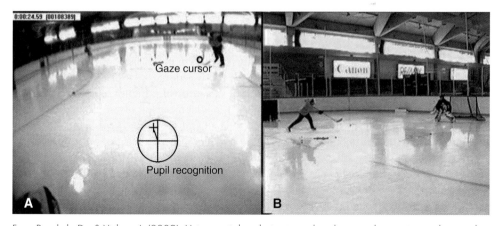

From Panchuk, D., & Vickers, J. (2009). Using spatial occlusion to explore the control strategies used in rapid interceptive actions: Predictive or prospective control? *Journal of Sports Sciences, 27*(12), 1249–1260. Reprinted by permission of the publisher Taylor & Francis Ltd; http://www.tandf.co.uk/journals.

the implicit group learned the return of serve better than the explicit group and a control group, and demonstrated their better performance both in the video occlusion testing and in real on-court return of serve. The authors suggested that by simply providing an objective (anticipate serve speed) that the players were able to explore the best solutions to the problem, which in this case must have been an "implicit understanding of the association between racquet head motion, spin and service speed, this group also implicitly acquired an understanding of the relationship between racquet head movement and resultant ball direction, thereby facilitating their anticipatory performance

(p. 483)." This study demonstrated that attention switching and selective attention are often learned through a trial and error approach. Over time and trials, learners figure out which cues are important and should be attended to, and which cues are irrelevant and should be ignored, particularly depending on the situation.

Using Attention as an Instructional Technique

Attention skills are not only a component of motor skill performance, but are skills that can be exploited from an instructional standpoint. These instruction tips below emphasize movement initiation, prioritizing movement components, and focusing on external cues.

The initiation of the movement generally requires more attention than the rest of the movement, and without a good start, the rest of the movement may suffer. Particularly for new learners, not only does movement initiation demand attention, but by placing attention on the initiation of movement, the whole movement may be better influenced. In a similar manner, not all components of the movement require the same amount of attention. Movements can be broken down and separated into parts, and some parts may require more attention because of their complexity or importance to the overall movement. Sometimes these important components are not obvious or meaningful to the learner, and so the instructor can highlight them by having the learning focus attention on these components. For example, the single leg take-off during a layup in basketball is a critical transition from dribbling to shooting and sets the stage for coordinated shot making. Placing attention on the take-off rather than the actual shot will facilitate the learning of this skill to a point of automaticity, after which the actual shot making can then be emphasized.

One of the most important ways an instructor can use attention as an instructional technique is to emphasize an external focus of attention (Wulf et al., 2010a,b). As stated previously, focusing on external cues rather than internal cues appears to facilitate performance and learning. For example, instead of focusing on the hands or "feel" in a golf swing, the focus should be on the club head or a movement outcome. New learners, however, have a difficult time doing this, believing that they must be "in-tune" with their bodies and monitor every action. Many instructional techniques reinforce this type of internal focus by emphasizing particular body positions or muscle actions. Creative instructors find ways to give an external focus that promotes proper body action.

Consider, for instance, minor biomechanical flaws in throwing. Figure 8.6 illustrates a young pitcher with his bent elbow too far forward compared to a biomechanically efficient throw, and his stride is too short. It almost looks like he is behind the ball and pushing it. Giving an athlete verbal instructions on how the arm motion should look, even after studying their own video performance, generally serves to confuse the athlete as they dwell on arm position during throwing. A different strategy involves a movement goal with an external focus of attention that requires the athlete to correct the problem in order to meet the goal. A couple of strategies could be used to help the pitcher in Figure 8.6. One would be to mark a point on the ground for a longer stride, which may improve the arm action. If this does not correct the arm action, a more arm-specific task may be in order. For instance, he could use a ball with a "tail," with the instructions to snap the tail at a far off target. The target location gets set through trial and error to force thrower to adopt a motion that is biomechanically sound. Such a teaching strategy may not work every time for every learner, but this example shows that using an external focus can be used to modify internal processes.

HOW PRACTICE IMPROVES ATTENTION SKILLS AND INFORMATION PROCESSING

Even with effective attention skills, there remain situations capable of overtaxing attention and information processing resources, particularly with limited time to prepare for movement. When these resources are taxed, we react and respond slowly, movement quality suffers, and our movement choices

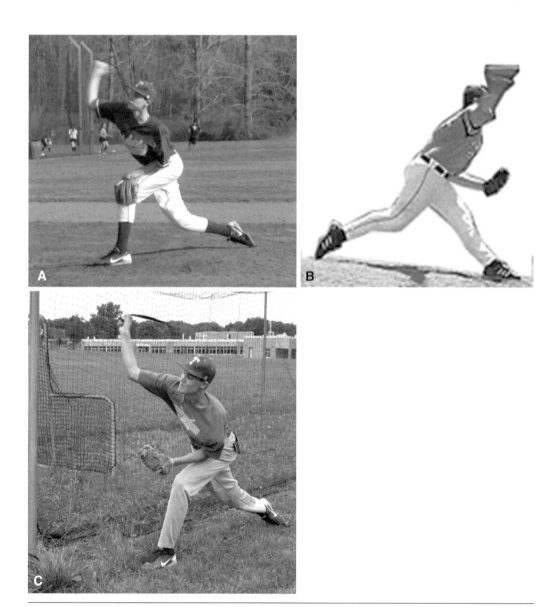

Figure 8.6 • External focus technique to improve body mechanics. **A.** This high school pitcher is obviously a mature thrower but has a flaw in his throwing mechanics. At this point in the throwing motion, his arm should be more extended. Attempting to correct these mechanics by simple verbal instruction having the pitcher focus on straightening out his arm is unlikely to work. Another strategy would be to devise a task that forces a correction in mechanics. **B.** Correct pitching mechanics showing proper shoulder to elbow to hand orientation. (From Fleisig, G., Chu, Y., Weber, A., & Andrews, J. (2009). Variability in baseball pitching biomechanics among various levels of competition. *Sports Biomechanics*, *8*(1), 10–21. With permission from Taylor & Francis Ltd.; http://www.informaworld.com.) **C.** Using a ball with a tail, the pitcher is instructed to snap the tail onto an external target; in this case the pole of a batting cage. By manipulating the target location and initial position of the player, biomechanical changes can be developed. The pitcher's arm is now more extended. See text for more details.

may be poor. One element of practice should be to enable information processing to be challenged in order to develop both faster and more appropriate decision making.

Faster and more accurate information processing largely comes via anticipation and simplifying the situation. Anticipation enables the performer to predict or provide a mental probability estimate of an upcoming situation, effectively narrowing down response choices. Anticipation is largely a product of using warning signals and other situational cues, such as body mechanics of the opposing tennis player to predict the direction of the shot. Back in Chapter 6, we saw that complex situations, which may include multiple and complex stimuli and complex response choices, negatively affects information processing speed and accuracy. Practice enables the performer to discriminate among important cues and stimuli, and pair those stimuli with effective response choices. Though high-level performers have a greater repertoire of movement choices, they are rapidly able to narrow down and select the most effective response for a given situation.

Is it possible to train these information processing skills? The answer is yes, and it is probably simpler than first might appear. As we saw earlier, much of what we can learn regarding attention, visual search, and so forth is learned implicitly. Plainly put, with more practice come faster RTs and better movements. This is especially true in complex movements or situations with multiple RT choices. Practice introduces the individual to warnings and reduces situational complexity and uncertainty. Practice also helps the learner synthesize important information so that anticipation can be used. There are four particular strategies, however, that promote the learning of information processing during practice. The first and overarching strategy is that attention and information processing must be practiced in situations that specifically challenge information processing resources, including chaotic, emotional, and fast-paced environments. It sounds simple, but in our experience little time is devoted to this type of practice in sport environments.

The second strategy is alertness and attentiveness. It is difficult to squeeze out milliseconds of time saving unless the learner is alert and focused. Third, the learner should adopt a **sensory set** focus rather than a **motor set** focus. A sensory set is when focus of attention is placed on the stimuli and reacting as fast as possible to the stimuli, in contrast to a motor set in which focus is placed on the movement response. Consider a swimmer on the starting platform. Her attention may be on the starting gun (sensory set) or on the forceful leg drive response (motor set). Improving RT in this setting should include practice with a sensory set in addition to a motor set. Finally, it has been suggested that mental practice to plan tactics to particular events can help speed up processing during actual events (Vealey & Greenleaf, 1998). More on mental practice is discussed in Chapter 9.

Concepts in Action

Practicing for Worst-Case Scenarios

Practice under chaotic worst-case scenarios enables information processing to be ready if and when these scenarios occur. Capt. Chesley "Sully" Sullenberger, the Hero on the Hudson in 2009 after successfully landing a commercial jetliner on the Hudson River and saving every life, noted his training when he stated, "The physiological reaction I had for this was strong and I had to force myself to use my training and force calm on the situation." This training went far back to his Navy fighter pilot days to his continued practice on simulators according to Federal Aviation Administration rules. This simulator training focuses on dire situations and worst-case scenarios against near impossible odds, and provides a sober look into the necessity of practice for decision making and controlling emotional states.

■ Thinking It Through 8.1 Focus of Attention and Reaction Speed

Access the Web page "CognitiveFun.net." Open the link to "Tests" and then "Attention Tests." You will perform the auditory RT under two different conditions of focus of attention: a sensory set and a motor set. First, take a few practice trials to get familiar with the test. Keep the volume of the auditory stimuli loud and use the space bar as your response. Rest your fingertips on the space bar. Next, perform 20 trials of the auditory RT tests while adopting a sensory set. For these close your eyes and focus attention on the sound, and do not worry about how hard or fast you press the space bar. You will need to open your eyes between trials to reset for the next trial. Record your mean RT after the 20 trials. Next, perform the experiment again, but this time you are going to adopt a motor set in which you will concentrate on making a fast and precise movement. For these 20 trials, keep your eyes open and attend to your fingers and spacebar and respond with a precise spacebar press that does not bottom out the spacebar. In other words, react as fast as you can to the stimulus sound and press the spacebar as fast as you can, but do not bottom out the spacebar. Record your RTs after 20 trials.

How do the sensory set and motor set RTs differ? Why?

INFORMATION PROCESSING, STRESS, AROUSAL, AND ANXIETY

Information processing is highly susceptible to both internal and external influences. Among the most common disruptors of effective information processing is poorly managed stress and competitive anxiety. *Stress* (or stress response) is defined as the physiological and psychological changes that happen in response to changing conditions or stressors. Stress is often thought of as something negative or harmful, but stress is a normal process that often has positive consequences. For instance, the response to exercise is a stress response that is positive and promotes good health. When stress levels get high or uncontrolled, particularly psychological stress, resources may be challenged and functioning may begin to break down. Too much stress may lead to distracting negative or irrelevant thoughts, and may further contribute to anxiety and nervousness. In contrast, some individuals may "shut down" in response to excessive psychological stressors. Too little stress, which may be seen as a highly relaxed state or apathy, may result in low arousal levels that then decreases alertness and attentional focus, and may lower resource capacity.

Arousal refers to the activation level of the emotional, mental, and physiological systems, but in practice is evaluated by physiological measurements such as heart rate, blood pressure, and sweating. The arousal level, before and during motor performance, affects movement quality and movement preparation time and is commonly manipulated by athletes and nonathletes alike to get into a state of readiness. Arousal can be lowered through relaxation methods or increased by "psyching up." *Anxiety* is sometimes understood to be at the high end of the arousal spectrum, but anxiety refers to the emotional or cognitive sense of worry.

Stress, anxiety, and arousal should not be confused. Under high states of stress, the body and mind may become highly aroused, such as during a fight or flight response. Stress may be accompanied by arousal of systems that can impede motor skill performance, like distracting memories and poorly controlled emotions. Alternately, sometimes the response to stress can be to shut down mental and physiological systems, resulting in physiological and psychological lethargy or depression. For optimal motor skill performance, it is necessary to overcome too much or too little of a stress response, and manage arousal to levels that are optimal for action and information processing.

The optimal level of arousal for motor performance is specific to an individual but is influenced by the motor skill type and the context under which the motor skill is performed. Different motor skills and different situations may require different levels of arousal. For example, football linemen may need more aroused than golfers during putting, but this should not be mistaken to think that putting

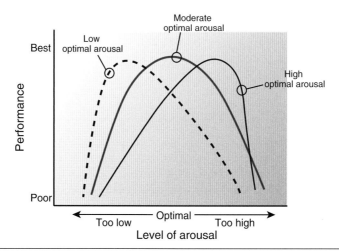

Figure 8.7 • Inverted-U principle. The optimal level of arousal for best performance is situation, motor skill, and individual specific.

requires extreme calmness. For instance, expert golfers are able to use and manage competitive stress and increased arousal to improve performance (Cooke et al., 2011). The optimal level of arousal for a given skill is related to the quantity of things that need to be done and the complexity of what needs to be done. Generally, if a task is more complex, then less arousal is necessary. But the level of muscular activation must also be factored in. Higher levels or arousal may enable a higher level of neuromuscular activity and thus force output. Individuals can learn to keep appropriate, including high, mental arousal while maintaining neuromuscular relaxation if that is what is necessary.

The relationship between arousal and performance can be generally understood by examining the **inverted-U principle** of arousal in Figure 8.7. Though this figure oversimplifies the relationship, it does illustrate that when arousal is too high or too low, performance suffers, but there is a large range of optimal. The arousal curve may differ depending on the characteristics of the performer, the situation, and the motor skill.

The optimal level of arousal for the performer to match the movement situation is individual specific, but for each individual there appears to be levels that are too high and too low around *individual zones of optimal functioning* (*IZOF;* Hanin, 2000). Hanin's IZOF model further described that individuals not only have specific arousal needs but also an overall emotional bearing that is specific to them for a given situation. Researchers have found that negative emotions, including fear and nervousness, lead to negative performance (Cottyn et al., 2012; Robazza et al., 1999). Positive emotions such as excitement, hope, and happiness may lead to high arousal but also better performance (Robazza et al., 2008). The IZOF model posits that the level of negative and positive emotions will be situation specific depending on the individual. That is, some persons may be able to succeed despite more negative emotions, or may need lower levels of positive emotions.

Arousal and anxiety level of the individual can be dependent on the situation where the skill is being performed. In general, the importance of the situation and the uncertainty of the situation increase performer arousal, even to a state of anxiety. In these cases the level of arousal may be excessive for the situation, and if stress and anxiety are involved, then irrelevant or negative resources may be aroused.

Attention Control, Arousal, and Performance

Extreme arousal or anxiety can reduce attentional capacity and can distract an individual with negative thoughts or an inappropriate attentional focus. In extreme cases anxiety can lead to "choking," which is suboptimal performance under competitive pressure. Current theories of choking point to athletes overfocusing on skill execution or on being worried about performance failure (see Hill et al., 2010;

Jackson et al., 2006, for reviews of these theories). While both scenarios likely contribute to choking, high-level athletes are less prone to overfocus on skill execution. For instance, using verbal reports, Oudejans et al. (2011) evaluated the focus of attention of 70 expert athletes in 19 different sports during high stress times. Of these athletes, 25% stated that their mind wandered to performance failure, and only 4% stated they monitored skill execution. Over 50% stated that they purposefully turned their mind to positive thoughts or regaining concentration.

The psychophysiological outcomes of stress and anxiety leading to poor performance are emerging. Wilson et al. (2009) found that under stressful conditions that poor goal shooting among expert soccer players was associated with poor gaze control, such as hasty gaze fixations and focusing on the goalkeeper too long during penalty shots. The authors suggested that attention control breaks down, resulting in the athletes being too influenced by distracting stimuli and threat. In this case the threat was the goalkeeper, and the more the athletes focused on the keeper, the more they kicked the ball at the keeper. These results coincide with Vickers and Williams (2007), who noted that under high physiological and cognitive arousal that the rifle shooting performance of biathletes who did not choke under pressure was highly associated with maintaining a quiet eye on the external target. Consider also an experiment by Gage et al. (2003), who had people walk on a normal surface and on an elevated walkway that created a falling threat and anxiety. Physiological data from galvanic skin responses indicated anxiousness during elevated walking. During walking the subjects had a reaction time task to respond verbally to a buzzer. As the threat increased, reaction time slowed, indicating that anxiety took attention resources away from reacting to the buzzer. Walking speed also slowed under the threat, showing the effects of anxiety on movement. Walking could have slowed due to the subjects being more careful or because attention was also drawn away from walking in addition to buzzer anticipation. Either way, anxiety reduced attention to the important tasks, resulting in slower reactions and slower walking.

These experiments demonstrate that performers may need to change attention demands by either reducing the width or direction of attention. Under anxiety conditions it is generally recommended to reduce the width of attention in order to focus on the most immediate and pressing needs. Selecting what these needs are and avoiding a wandering attention span is not easy. Moreover, maintaining a very narrow focus should not be seen as the solution to all high anxiety and stress situations. If a broad external focus is necessary for success, such as scanning the environment for cues, maintaining

SIDE**NOTE**	**AROUSAL, GENDER DIFFERENCES, AND MOTOR SKILL PERFORMANCE**

Individual differences in arousal responses are nicely illustrated in research by Noteboom et al. (2001). These authors found that steadiness on a pinch force task declined following high arousal and anxiety induced by electric shock, but not by high arousal and anxiety induced by doing mental math problems. Male and female subjects in this study had to maintain a constant pinch force, but when electric shock (or threat of shock) increased, their steadiness got worse. The level of arousal was determined by physiological signs of heart rate, blood pressure, and electrodermal activity, and anxiety measure on a visual analog scale. In contrast, when "forced" to do difficult math under time constraints, the level of arousal increased just as with the shock, but motor performance on the pinch force steadiness test was only minimally affected. That is, the source of arousal influenced the subsequent performance on the motor skill. While both sexes were negatively affected by the shock treatment, females were significantly more affected than the males. The authors speculated that the females may have had a greater neuroendocrine response leading to greater arousal and/or anxiety that was not detected by the experimental methods, or that the arousal/anxiety led to a different level of motor output by the females.

a narrow focus may be a detriment to performance. In addition, some internal cues (e.g., thoughts, plans, activities, sensory info) that are desirable for good performance may be ignored when the focus is too narrow.

■ Thinking It Through 8.2 Getting "Psyched Out"

Competitors commonly take advantage of other players' inability to focus attention and control arousal or anxiety in order to cause them to choke. Consider the real case of Dave, who was a 6'4", 240-lb pitcher for a community college baseball team. He was a highly regarded draft prospect who could throw an unhittable 95+ mph sinking fastball but with a touch of wildness. He was also known as bit of a "head case." At every game he pitched were major league baseball scouts with radar guns. In one game against a nonconference rival, he came on in the 9th inning with a one-run lead to close out the game. After walking the first batter on some close pitches, his opponents began razzing and jeering him from the bench, trying to raise his anxiety level and distract him. Over the next four batters, he did not come close to throwing a strike and walked all four to lose the game. The sportsmanship of jeering aside, the opposing players played the mental game to "psych out" the pitcher. The other side of this story is that his coaches left him in the game for the purpose of allowing him to work through his emotional states. If you were the coach, what would you have done to get the pitcher on track? Using the concepts discussed in this chapter, speculate where you think the pitcher's mental focus was placed and where it should have been placed.

Training and practice can help one to learn to focus attention, select appropriate cues, and be able to switch attention. It might seem that relaxation training is a good way to overcome anxiety and therefore eliminate the need to rely on a narrow focus. However, relaxation training is essentially practice of focusing attention on relaxation. Unless it is in some sort of rehabilitation or clinical setting, having attention placed on relaxation takes away from attention on the important task at hand, like shooting the free throw, selecting a good pitch to hit, and so forth. The point is that relaxation training may not be effective unless attention control to the goal of the task is also practiced.

INTENTION AND EFFORT AND ATTENTION

The importance of attention control cannot be overstated. The nature and quality of our attention contributes directly to the quality of motor performance and even more, the *physiological adaptations that arise* from motor performance training. Attention skills are among the first motor learning skills that should be emphasized to learners, having an impact on most every other aspect of motor performance. Attention skills, however, do not stand alone. Useful attention skills cannot be learned or carried out with **intention** and **effort**.

Intention is primarily a psychological process; it provides a goal or a plan of action that includes the what, why, and how of a movement. On a large scale, it provides a purpose and an outcome goal for training or practice. Intent can include easily identifiable goals like overcoming a specific motor skill weakness or improving relaxation while shooting free throws. Intention can also include very specific physiological outcomes, such as training to cause maximal motor unit activation.

Of direct relevance to exercise, science and allied health practitioners is that intention drives neurophysiological processes and biomechanical outcomes, and subsequently, neurophysiological and physiological adaptations. To suggest that intention by itself is an important training and practice factor may seem an exaggeration, but research bears this out. Consider work by Bonnard et al. (2003) in which their subjects performed rhythmic wrist flexion and extension movements. The movements were periodically and unexpectedly perturbed by magnetic brain stimulation over the motor cortex. Instructions to the subjects were to either do nothing or to resist the perturbation. When told to resist, there was no change in the flexor or extensor muscle activity before the perturbation, but after the perturbation, there was a marked change in the muscle response. These authors found that simply by having a specific intention (resist or not resist) that the corticospinal excitability was increased. Even more, these authors concluded that intention was so important that it was critical in determining if a motor plan was actually executed, or in other words, help to bind the cognitive and motor processes. Latash and Jaric (1998) also looked at varying movement instructions combined with unexpectedly perturbed movements and found that muscle activation patterns may differ even when the biomechanical outcomes are the same. These authors concluded that the individual's intention behind the motor act drives muscle coordination. Put differently, intention is used to overcome the problem of motor redundancy.

Almosnino and his colleagues (2011) examined isokinetic knee flexion torque curves under conditions of maximal, submaximal, and feigned effort, finding that the feigned effort often had a markedly different torque curve (Fig. 8.8). These data prompted the authors to suggest that cognitive intent may be evidenced in the biomechanical outcome. In another study, Behm and Sale (1993) determined that movement intention gave rise to motor plans, which further gave rise to physiological adaptations during training (see accompanying Concepts in Action box for more information on this study).

Intention helps select specific muscle coordination patterns and on a larger scale provides the larger reasoning or rationale for doing acts. This rationale provides the why and how of attention and is behind motivation and guidance for self-regulation (Shapiro & Schwartz, 2000). For example, a child may have motor skill goal to ride a bike, but the intention may be either to escape bullies or go to the store. Without a specific purpose, meaning and importance are lost, and knowing where to place attention becomes uncertain. In previous sections the importance of a movement being meaningful were highlighted. Intention also gives rise to how a plan is to be accomplished. Part of this is technical, for example, practice scheduling and using specific biomechanical techniques.

To illustrate, consider a competitive time-trial cyclist. Of course the cyclist wants to get better, but what will it take to do so? Should the cyclist go out every day with maximal effort in order to fatigue her physiological systems? Perhaps, but it might be a better idea to have the intention to ride on the cusp of the anaerobic threshold for as long as she can in order to better force a shift in the threshold

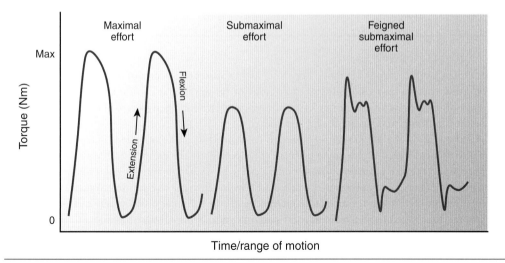

Figure 8.8 • Different isokinetic knee extension/flexion torque curves based on data from Almosnino et al. (2011). The maximal and submaximal efforts produce stereotypical smooth curves. In contrast, some subjects produced a jerky curve when told to feign an injury, prompting the authors to suggest that the information regarding cognitive intent may be contained in the biomechanics of movement.

Concepts in Action

Intentional Training and Physiological Adaptations

Can intention really change the results of training? Consider the seminal experiment by Behm and Sale (1993) in which they had persons train ankle dorsiflexion on an isokinetic dynamometer. One group trained at high isokinetic speed and another group trained isometrically. However, the isometric group tried, or intended, to produce rapid ballistic actions. At posttest the isometric group improved as much or more in high-speed isokinetic strength than did the isokinetic group. Despite actually training in an isometric fashion, the isometric group had minimal improvement in isometric strength. Results from electromyography (EMG) and muscle contraction properties confirmed that the isometric group had neuromuscular changes consistent with high-speed strength. The authors concluded that more important to the specificity of training principle than the actual movement was the intention of the contraction. The motor commands that led to muscle action and subsequently, physiological adaptations were based on the intent of the contraction, and thus the training process should start there.

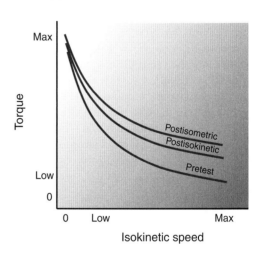

Schematic illustration of the changes in strength across the force–velocity curve reported by Behm and Sale. The pretest scores are the mean of both groups, which did not differ from one another. After training the high-speed isokinetic training group (postisokinetic) had the greatest strength gains specific to their high-speed training regimen. The isometric training group (postisometric) had their greatest strength gains not at the speed they trained at (isometric), but at the speed they intended to train at (high speed/ballistic).

value. Or she could focus on rhythmic breathing and consistent velocities in an attempt to train efficiency. Either option may differentially train inter- or intramuscular coordination. Alternately, she could hop off the road bike and engage in specific resistance training designed to improve force sharing among the hip flexors and among the hip extensors.

Another part of the intention process has to do with effort and motivation. In other words, how much effort one decides to give must be planned, especially if the effort required is maximal, as is often necessary. Effort is often erroneously considered to be mostly a physiological term, meaning how much time and energy one devotes to the task, and how much vigor one puts into practice or training. Yet psychological effort must come before physiological effort. Preparation, cognitive effort, alertness and arousal, time taken to plan training, and studying game films, all these require a degree of mental effort. Concentration requires mental effort. Overcoming fear or anxiety requires mental effort. Without full mental effort during practices or games, one may drift off and loose attention, and motor performance suffers.

In summary, intention gives rise to purposeful effort, and both set the foundation for effective attention. Maintaining intention, effort, and attention on a short-term basis (e.g., one game or week) may be relatively simple, but the outstanding performers do it month after month and year after year.

SUMMARY

Information processing is defined as the essential the job of the CNS. Taking in information; interpreting and making sense of information; storing, categorizing, and recalling information; and making decisions and executing plans are all part of the brain's role. The brain, however, is limited in its ability to process a lot of information or simultaneously process multiple types of information. Though the brain has multiple processing resources, when faced with multiple demands, the ability to process information diminishes. This leads to slow and inaccurate processing and decision making. There are a number of factors that influence the speed and effectiveness if information processing, particularly in situations that tax resources. Among these are memory and control of attention.

Memory is an important resource that factors into high-level performance and is one cognitive processing resource with clearly identifiable strategies for improvement. One of the memory strategies is to make movements meaningful, which also plays a role in attention. Attention control is arguably most important way to regulate resource use and may be the best first strategy to use to improve the information processing aspects of motor skill performance. Knowing where to place attention, the quality of attention, and the ability to switch attention dictates the amount and type of information being received by the CNS. Attention, based on Nideffer's theories, falls on a two-dimensional scale of narrow to broad, and internal to external. Though individuals may have innate traits that give rise to a particular attentional style, individual must adopt attention styles to meet situational needs. For instance, in sport-related stress conditions, attention control to be narrow and external is often suggested to be ways to combat the negative effects of improper arousal and anxiety. Learning the appropriate attention control strategies is often an implicit process, but explicit attention can be directly instructed and learned. Among the important attention strategies is that an external focus of attention may aid in the learning and performing of many motor skills.

Optimal arousal levels are important to maximize information processing and motor skill performance. The best level of arousal is individual specific, but the situation and motor skill will influence the amount of arousal. Stress and anxiety may lead to inappropriate levels of arousal and contribute to diminished information processing and performance through distracting and negative thoughts. Overcoming these negative influences begins with changing attention to positive and meaningful factors, such as the task goal.

Underlying attention control is intention. Without the proper intention, our selective and focused attention are uncertain, and our ability to maximize mental and physical effort is limited. Intention serves to filter the incoming information and provides purpose to outgoing commands. Intention not only modifies attention and effort but in doing so directly influences the nature of physiological performance and physiological adaptations arising from training and practice. Specifically, intent and effort influences motor unit recruitment and other characteristics of intramuscular coordination, dictates muscle activation schemes for whole-body coordination, and motivates us. The take-home message is that all training and practice, from individual exercises to year-long plans, must be intentional for maximum benefits.

STUDY QUESTIONS

1. Why do the demands of attention change with different skill levels?
2. Define selective attention, focus of attention, and attention switching.
3. What is the psychological refractory period and what does it reveal?
4. Which techniques are used to help remembering motor skills?
5. Discuss the role of attention in multiple resource theory and the truth in "multitasking."
6. A boxer tends to twitch his eye at some point before throwing a punch, thereby giving his opponent a preliminary warning. Discuss why this may help and hinder his opponent.

7. A golfer is so anxious that he is shaking. He performs some relaxation techniques and reduces the physiological indices of anxiety (i.e., muscle tension). Why might this relaxation not enhance his performance?

8. Excessive levels of arousal may negatively affect performance in what manner?

9. How might practice be structured to improve information processing?

10. A beginner and an expert are playing tennis against one another. The expert is able to talk to her opponent and the crowd while playing—without a noticeable decrement in performance. If the novice talks and plays at the same time, her playing suffers greatly. Why? Use concepts from this chapter and Chapter 7 to answer the question.

11. Dick and Jane are in a driver's education class practicing using a manual transmission, that is, coordinating the clutch, brake, accelerator, and stick shift. Jane does the sequence over and over again—repeatedly doing clutch in, accelerator off, shift, clutch out, and accelerator on. Dick repeats the sequence a few times, adds in imagery of each gear location and how the engine sounds, tries to figure out the best sequences by himself, and works toward being in a drag race. Who will remember how to use the manual transmission better and why?

12. What is the difference between implicit and explicit attention? Discuss.

13. Discuss internal versus external and narrow versus broad with respect to attention and the benefits and downsides of each.

14. Describe the importance of the intention—attention—effort relationship.

Bibliography

Almosnino, S., Stevenson, J. M., Day, A. G., Bardana, D. D., Diaconescu, E. D., & Dvir, Z. (2011). Differentiating between types and levels of isokinetic knee musculature efforts. *Journal of Electromyography & Kinesiology, 21*(6), 974–981.

Behm, D. G., & Sale, D. G. (1993). Intended rather than actual movement velocity determines velocity-specific training response. *Journal of Applied Physiology, 74*(1), 359–368.

Beilock, S., Carr, T., MacMahon, C., & Starkes, J. (2002). When paying attention becomes counterproductive: Impact of divided versus skill-focused attention on novice and experienced performance of sensorimotor skills. *Journal of Experimental Psychology: Applied, 8*(1), 6–16.

Bernstein, N. (1967). *The Co-ordination and regulation of movements.* Oxford, England: Pergamon Press.

Bonnard, M., Camus, M., de Graaf, J., & Pailhous, J. (2003). Direct evidence for a binding between cognitive and motor functions in humans: A TMS study. *Journal of Cognitive Neuroscience, 15*(8), 1207–1216.

Cooke, A., Kavussanu, M., McIntyre, D., Boardley, I., & Ring, C. (2011). Effects of competitive pressure on expert performance: Underlying psychological, physiological, and kinematic mechanisms. *Psychophysiology, 48*(8), 1146–1156.

Correa, A., Lupiáñez, J., Madrid, E., & Tudela, P. (2006). Temporal attention enhances early visual processing: A review and new evidence from event-related potentials. *Brain Research, 1076*(1), 116–128.

Cottyn, J., De Clercq, D., Crombez, G., & Lenoir, M. (2012). The interaction of functional and dysfunctional emotions during balance beam performance. *Research Quarterly for Exercise and Sport, 83*(2), 300–307.

Dula, C., Martin, B., Fox, R., & Leonard, R. (2011). Differing types of cellular phone conversations and dangerous driving. *Accident: Analysis and Prevention, 43*(1), 187–193.

Farrow, D., & Abernethy, B. (2002). Can anticipatory skills be learned through implicit video-based perceptual training? *Journal of Sports Sciences, 20*, 471–485.

Freudenheim, A., Wulf, G., Madureira, F., Pasetto, S., & Corrêa, U. (2010). An external focus of attention results in greater swimming speed. *International Journal of Sports Science & Coaching, 5*(4), 533–542.

Gage, W., Sleik, R., Polych, M., McKenzie, N., & Brown, L. (2003). The allocation of attention during locomotion is altered by anxiety. *Experimental Brain Research, 150*(3), 385–394.

Guadagnoli, M., & Lee, T. (2004). Challenge point: A framework for conceptualizing the effects of various practice conditions in motor learning. *Journal of Motor Behavior, 36*(2), 212–224.

Gherri, E., & Eimer, M. (2011). Active listening impairs visual perception and selectivity: An ERP study of auditory dual-task costs on visual attention. *Journal of Cognitive Neuroscience, 23*(4), 832–844.

Hanin, Y. L. (2000). Individual zones of optimal functioning (IZOF) model: Emotion-performance relationships in sports. In Y.L. Hanin (Ed.), *Emotions in sport*. Champaign, IL: Human Kinetics.

Hill, D. M., Hanton, S., Matthews, N., & Fleming, S. (2010). Choking in sport: A review. *International Review of Sport & Exercise Psychology, 3*(1), 24–39.

Hutchinson, J., & Tenenbaum, G. (2007). Attention focus during physical effort: The mediating role of task intensity. *Psychology of Sport & Exercise, 8*(2), 233–245.

Jackson, R. C., Ashford, K. J., & Norsworthy, G. (2006). Attentional focus, dispositional reinvestment, and skilled motor performance under pressure. *Journal of Sport and Exercise Psychology, 28*, 49–68.

Latash, M., & Jaric, S. (1998). Instruction-dependent muscle activation patterns within a two-joint synergy: Separating mechanics from neurophysiology. *Journal of Motor Behavior, 30*(3), 194–198.

Levy, J., & Pashler, H. (2008). Task prioritization in multitasking during driving: Opportunity to abort a concurrent task does not insulate braking responses from dual-task slowing. *Applied Cognitive Psychology, 22*, 507–525.

Magill, R. A. (1998). Knowledge is more than we can talk about: Implicit learning in motor skill acquisition. *Research Quarterly for Exercise and Sport, 69*, 104–110.

Masters, K. S., & Ogles, B. M. (1998). Associative and dissociative cognitive strategies in exercise and running: 20 years later, what do we know? *Sport Psychologist, 12*(3), 253–270.

Nideffer, R. M. (1976). Test of attentional and interpersonal style. *Journal of Personality and Social Psychology, 34*(3), 394–404.

Nideffer, R. M. (1990). Use of the Test of Attentional and Interpersonal Style (TAIS) in sport. *Sport Psychologist, 4*(3), 285–300.

Noteboom, J., Fleshner, M., & Enoka, R. (2001). Activation of the arousal response can impair performance on a simple motor task. *Journal of Applied Physiology, 91*(2), 821–831.

Oudejans, R. D., Kuijpers, W., Kooijman, C. C., & Bakker, F. C. (2011). Thoughts and attention of athletes under pressure: Skill-focus or performance worries? *Anxiety, Stress & Coping, 24*(1), 59–73.

Panchuk, D., & Vickers, J. (2009). Using spatial occlusion to explore the control strategies used in rapid interceptive actions: Predictive or prospective control? *Journal of Sports Sciences, 27*(12), 1249–1260.

Peh, S., Chow, J., & Davids, K. (2011). Focus of attention and its impact on movement behaviour. *Journal of Science and Medicine in Sport, 14*(1), 70–78.

Pinto, J., & Shiffrar, M. (1999). Subconfigurations of the human form in the perception of biological motion displays. *Acta Psychologica, 102*(2–3), 293–318.

Robazza, C., Bortoli, L., & Nougier, V. (1999). Emotions, heart rate and performance in archery. A case study. *The Journal of Sports Medicine and Physical Fitness, 39*(2), 169–176.

Robazza, C., Pellizzari, M., Bertollo, M., & Hanin, Y. (2008). Functional impact of emotions on athletic performance: Comparing the IZOF model and the directional perception approach. *Journal of Sports Sciences, 26*(10), 1033–1047.

Schücker, L., Hagemann, N., Strauss, B., & Völker, K. (2009). The effect of attentional focus on running economy. *Journal of Sports Sciences, 27*(12), 1241–1248.

Shapiro, S., & Schwartz, G. (2000). Intentional systemic mindfulness: An integrative model for self-regulation and health. *Advances in Mind-Body Medicine, 16*(2), 128–134.

Starkes, J. L., Deakin, J. M., Lindley, S. S., & Crisp, F. F. (1987). Motor versus verbal recall of ballet sequences by young expert dancers. *Journal of Sport Psychology, 9*(3), 222–230.

Vealey, R. S., & Greenleaf, C. A. (1998). Seeing is believing: Understanding and using imagery in sport. In J. M. Williams (Ed.) *Applied sport psychology: Personal growth to peak performance* (pp. 237–269) . Mountain View, CA: Mayfield Publishing Company.

Vecera, S., & Rizzo, M. (2003). Spatial attention: Normal processes and their breakdown. *Neurologic Clinics, 21*(3), 575–607.

Vickers, J., & Williams, A. (2007). Performing under pressure: The effects of physiological arousal, cognitive anxiety, and gaze control in biathlon. *Journal of Motor Behavior, 39*(5), 381–394.

Watson, J., & Strayer, D. (2010). Supertaskers: Profiles in extraordinary multitasking ability. *Psychonomic Bulletin & Review, 17*(4), 479–485.

Welford, A. T. (1952). The "psychological refractory period" and the timing of high speed performance—A review and a theory. *British Journal of Psychology, 43*, 2–19.

Werner, S., & Thies, B. (2000). Is 'change blindness' attenuated by domain-specific expertise? An expert–novices comparison of change detection in football images. *Visual Cognition, 7*(1–3), 163–173.

Wickens, C. (2008). Multiple resources and mental workload. *Human Factors, 50*(3), 449–455.

Wilson, F., & Stimpson, J. (2010). Trends in fatalities from distracted driving in the United States, 1999 to 2008. *American Journal of Public Health, 100*(11), 2213–2219.

Wilson, M. R., Wood, G., & Vine, S. J. (2009). Anxiety, attentional control, and performance impairment in penalty kicks. *Journal of Sport & Exercise Psychology, 31*(6), 761–775.

Wulf, G., Dufek, J., Lozano, L., & Pettigrew, C. (2010a). Increased jump height and reduced EMG activity with an external focus. *Human Movement Science, 29*(3), 440–448.

Wulf, G., & Prinz, W. (2001). Directing attention to movement effects enhances learning: A review. *Psychonomic Bulletin & Review, 8*(4), 648–660.

Wulf, G., Shea, C., & Lewthwaite, R. (2010b). Motor skill learning and performance: A review of influential factors. *Medical Education, 44*(1), 75–84.

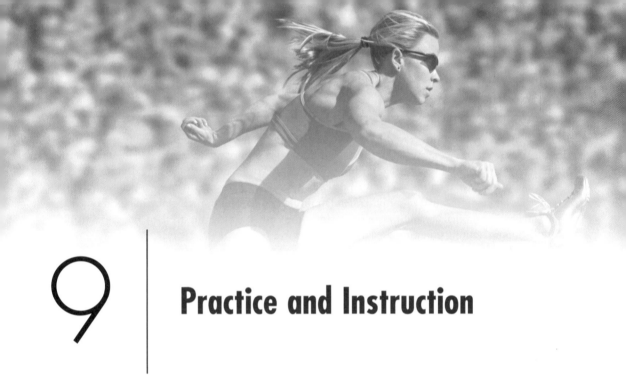

9 | Practice and Instruction

PURPOSE, IMPORTANCE, AND OBJECTIVES OF THIS CHAPTER

The purpose of this chapter is to describe the fundamental features and strategies that make for effective practice and the instructional techniques necessary to implement and maximize practice effectiveness. Specifically, this chapter focuses on constraints-led learning, discovery learning, and deliberate practice models that provide the essential characteristics of practice. With this understanding, the learner and instructor can develop practice and training programs and individual mind-sets to maximize learning and performance, avoid pitfalls, and overcome setbacks.

After reading this chapter, you should be able to:

1. Explain how practice differs from training.
2. Explain the characteristics of discovery learning, constraints-led learning, and deliberate practice.
3. Explain each of the five essential features of effective practice and how to implement each feature from an instructional standpoint.
4. Explain when, why, and how to use augmented feedback to improve communication and improve the learning environment.
5. Explain how to engage the learner in his or her own motor skill learning, and why doing so improves learning.
6. Explain the role of observation and imagery in the learning process, and the basic neurophysiology of observation and imagery.

There are two components to practice, the learner and the instructor. In Chapters 7 and 8, we looked at the learning process and characteristics of high-level performers. We specifically examined memory and attention and other information-processing factors of the learner that are essential components in learning and performance. How these factors are exploited and used to improve instruction and optimize the learning environment is the focus of this chapter. In particular, we look at the nature of practice and strategies to maximize the benefits of practice.

WHAT IS PRACTICE?

Practice is defined as dedicated effort toward improving upon a skill or task. It is often used inter-changeably with training, but in kinesiology and exercise science, it is useful to define these terms differently based on what is targeted for improvement. Practice is aimed at learning decision-making skills and motor execution skills, or more precisely, improving mental performance, tactics, strategies, team play, and motor skills. On the other hand, **training** is aimed at improving physiological function-ing and physical proficiency abilities. In this chapter, the term practice is mostly used, but the principles for developing training programs are largely the same.

Contrary to popular notions, effective practice is not repetition after repetition until "perfect." If we recall back to the systems model in Chapter 4, movement emerges from an interaction of the task, the individual, and the environment. Put simply, effective motor skills are highly situation dependent, and the requirements for effective movement may change instantly. Effective practice enables the learner to have a wide and adaptable movement repertoire to effectively overcome situational challenges and take advantage of situational opportunities.

The nature of practice must vary depending on the needs of the learner. A child learning to ride a bike has different needs than a world-class athlete training for the Olympics or a stroke sufferer learn-ing to walk. Given these vastly different needs, can there exist fundamental characteristics of practice that apply across the board? Based on experimental data gathered over the past 80 years, the answer is yes. This research reveals that there are five essential features of practice, whether it is an individual practice session (practice microstructure) or an entire time frame over which motor skills are devel-oped (practice macrostructure). These characteristics are (1) *a specific intention to improve and master the skill*, (2) a *strong motivation and effort*, (3) *individual-based practice and learner input into practice*, (4) *effective communication and information*, and (5) *overlearning with variation*. How these characteristics are implemented varies widely with a number of techniques and instructional strategies and depends on the nature of the learner and the microstructure or macrostructure of practice. In this chapter, we emphasize instructional strategies and learning for healthy individuals across the spectrum from novice to expert.

PRACTICE PARADIGMS

Though the practice and instructional strategies discussed here are based on decades of research, they emphasize recent research involving information-processing skills such as memory and attention (see Chapters 7 and 8), experimental work with discovery learning paradigms, systems theories with constraints-led approaches, and research work underscoring the development of expert performance through deliberate practice. We provide a brief overview of these paradigms first before detailing the five essential features of practice.

Systems Theories, Constraints-Led Approaches, and Discovery Learning

In Chapter 5, we examined the systems model that posited that movement emerges from an interaction of individual, task, and environmental factors. Each of these factors imposes limitations or *constraints* to how movement can emerge and thus requires the nervous system to look for ways to accommodate or take advantage of the situation (Newell, 1986). Constraints include game rules and time, muscle strength, fatigue, emotional state, and playing surface traction. These are all factors that constrain or influence what movement can be executed and how it can be executed.

To reiterate from Chapter 5, constraint-based information from the environment continually merges with internal sensory information and task-based constraints. Perceptual systems interpret the nature of these constraints and determine ways to take them into account for movement planning and execution. This process is known as searching for *affordances* and ties together what is perceived by an individual and what action subsequently takes place. Affordances, according to Gibson (1977), are qualities or clues in the environment that inevitably lead to specific action responses that require minimal sensory processing. For instance, a four-foot-high rock wall provides information whether the wall can be scaled by jumping or climbing. Qualities of the wall permit either solution depending on other factors. A child approaching the wall is constrained by stature and strength, and therefore, the wall affords no qualities for being jumped (or even climbed). In contrast, a fit hurdler with no obvious physical constraints can jump the wall with ease. This example illustrates that affordances emerge based on interactions of task and individual constraints. While some affordances are universal across populations (e.g., the qualities of keyboard keys lead to being pressed and not pulled), others are highly specific to each individual based on the individual's own characteristics and capabilities, and often require discovery by the learner after much practice (Fajen et al., 2009; Greeno, 1994; Renshaw et al., 2009).

In order to guide learners to overcome constraints, detect and understand affordances, and overall direct learners toward better technical skills, instructors lead the learner by controlling constraints. In the constraints-led approach, instructors manipulate constraints to have the learner discover affordances that further lead the learner to discover solutions to movement problems (Hristovski et al., 2011; Renshaw et al., 2009). Figure 9.1, based on Newell's (1986, 2007) concept of interacting constraints and instruction, shows that individual, task, and environmental constraints merge, forcing the system into perception and action coupling in order to organize an effective movement. It is at the interaction of these constraints that practice and instruction is critical to develop the most effective movements and motor skills.

Constraints can be physical barriers, rules or instructions, or any number of other factors that are manipulated as part of the practice microstructure. They may be as simple as adding stress or time pressure, or setting up situations in which a player is forced to move only in one direction. Constraints are not presented haphazardly but are specifically introduced to give the learner an opportunity to creatively overcome game-like challenges. Consider the case of a child learning to climb high on a climbing structure as shown in Figure 9.2. The fear of falling is a common constraint to climbing, so learning to jump and land safely from heights is a first step. In the figure, the girl is first learning to land from higher and higher heights, which gives her confidence to climb higher on the climbing structure.

In a constraints-led setting, it is important to have available the perceptual information that is present in game settings. For instance, coordination during cricket batting is developed differently off a bowling (pitching) machine and from video virtual reality images than from a real bowler because the information offered is different (Pinder et al., 2011a; Renshaw et al., 2007). These differences in

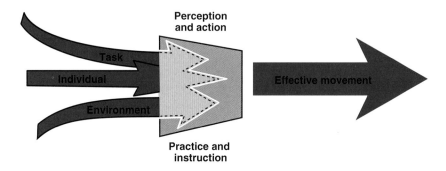

Figure 9.1 • Task, individual, and environmental constraints are viewed as interacting factors that perception and action processes need to untangle or decipher in order for effective movements to emerge. The role of practice and instruction is to facilitate the untangling such that affordances are uncovered and effective movement emerges that satisfies the constraints of the situation.

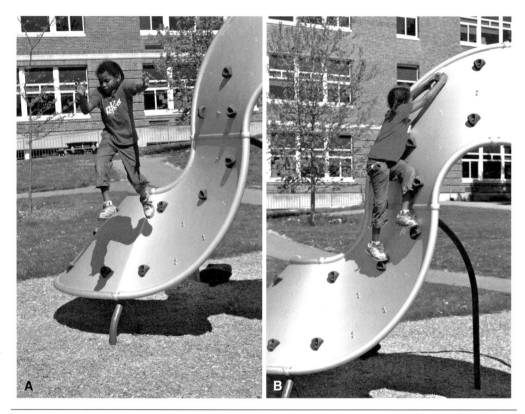

Figure 9.2 • One of the constraints to climbing is fear of falling. **A.** Here a girl practices jumping and landing from higher and higher heights. **B.** Once she feels comfortable that she can land safely from a height, she progresses to climbing higher and onto more challenging holds. (Photo courtesy Jeffrey Ives.)

information change perception, which thus changes the perception–action coupling (see accompanying Concepts in Action box). From an instructional standpoint, coaches should be wary of overly breaking down movements into small constituent components and practicing the components separately, as critical perceptual information may be lost. Instead, coaches should consider basic simplification strategies in which the movements are kept relatively whole. Further, to implement effective constraint-led instruction, coaches must have knowledge of how the environment, task, and individual interact. This is particularly important during childhood and development as physical constraints, such as muscle strength and hand size, not only influence movement control but may change rapidly over time.

When used properly, the constraints-led approach requires the learner to figure out on their own the best movement solutions. The process, known as **discovery** or **exploratory learning**, is fundamentally rooted in an individual trial and error approach to learning. It requires the learner to search for optimal strategies to do a task, given the constraints of the task. This process includes finding the best perceptual cues or variables to produce motor responses that are specific to the environment and task constraints, and fit within the individual's own physiological and psychological makeup (Vereijken & Whiting, 1990; Vereijken et al., 1992).

In discovery learning, explicit skills are not taught, but rather, the learner is taught or led how to learn the skill by himself or herself ("guided discovery"). The instructor's role is critical in this process. Instead of providing prescriptive instructions or precise modeling, the instructor leads the learner through a progression of problems using limited feedback in the traditional sense, and thus emphasizes implicit learning processes over explicit processes. One of the first strategies of the instructor is to reduce the degrees of freedom and provide the optimal environment to learn. Consider, for example,

Concepts in Action

Batting off a Machine or Live Pitching?

The use of batting machines in baseball, softball, and cricket is widespread, yet many have questioned their use as not providing a real-life experience. The photos below from Pinder et al. (2009) illustrate that body movements during batting vary markedly between a throwing machine (left photo) and live pitching (right photo), in part due to the advance information and readiness afforded by the live throwing. Pinder et al. (2011b) have recently discussed this issue and noted that there is a trade-off between quality (live pitching) versus quantity (throwing machine) that has even the expert national level coaches disagreeing as to their use. In their look at cricket batting, these authors summarized that the development of interceptive action within a constrained environment (throwing machine) enables developing players to refine movement dynamics. On the other hand, more advanced players need the perceptual cues of the real bowler (thrower) and the variation of real-life actions to develop a more diverse and adaptable skill set. This is not to say that throwing machines have no role for training expert batters, but their use needs to be evaluated closely. The summary point here is that pitching machines are best used for a specific purpose and with the understanding that they do not replace live pitching as a tool. Coaches faced with a shortage of effective practice pitchers may be better served to modify live hitting drills rather than use a pitching machine. Using nonpitchers in small-games play with soft baseballs is one way to enable young players to see live pitching in a safe environment.

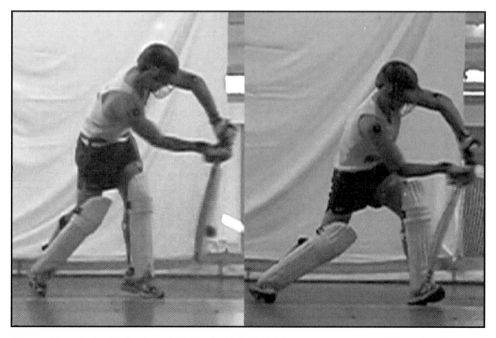

(Reprinted from Pinder, R., Renshaw, I., & Davids, K. (2009). Information-movement coupling in developing cricketers under changing ecological practice constraints. *Human Movement Science, 28*(4), 468–479, with permission from Elsevier.)

a child learning to walk. Children see the parents and others modeling walking, which encourages them to walk and gives them basic movement ideas. The parents' main role is to create a learning environment. Verbal encouragement, hand holding (provides confidence and reduces the degrees of freedom by enabling balance), and providing a safe environment like walking on a rug are several ways parents optimize the learning environment. The child discovers for himself what movements he should make, how to make them, why make them, and the obstacles and constraints to walking. Instructors get inside the learning situation to uncover obstacles and constraints, but do not necessarily provide explicit information on how to proceed. In their examination of 10 elite coaches, Nash et al. (2011) found that a common theme among the coaches was to create an individualized learning environment. The coaches did this by engaging the athletes into their own learning by guided discovery, describing themselves as facilitators more than coaches.

Discovery learning has been shown to be effective in learning a host of motor skills (Orrell et al., 2006; Smeeton et al., 2005), but this should not be interpreted that explicit and prescriptive instructions have no role (Raab et al., 2009). If the learner cannot be coaxed or constrained into discovering an effective way to execute a motor skill, there may be need for more direct approaches. In cases in which the learner has no idea how to proceed, or safety is an issue, direct instructions may be necessary.

Deliberate Practice

Since the early 1990s, Ericsson et al. (e.g., Ericsson et al., 1993; Ericsson, 2007) have investigated the practice characteristics of expert performers. From these investigations, these authors have concluded that high-level performance is an outcome of 10 years or 10,000 hours of **deliberate practice**. Deliberate practice is a specific term describing practice activities with specific features, namely, high levels of motivation and effort, activities based on knowledge and characteristics of the performer, immediate and continual feedback, a large amount of repetition, and intent to improve. Some of these features may look different based on the task (e.g., sports vs. nonsports, individual vs. team activity), but the general concepts are robust across many disciplines.

The 10-year rule appears to be a bit variable, ranging from 4,000 to 10,000 hours by age 20, depending on the activity (sport, nonsport) and team versus individual sports (Baker et al., 2003a,b). Côté et al. have more recently noted that early years are marked by sampling, middle years by specialization, and then investment in later years (e.g., Côté et al., 2003, 2007). The sampling years are marked by what might be termed "deliberate play," and though this seems to counter the idea of deliberate practice, this type of play has been suggested to not only develop fundamental skills and abilities but also the motivation to pursue more rigorous practice activities (Ward et al., 2007) or develop creativity (Memmert et al., 2010).

Regardless of the exact number of practice hours and the nature of early exposure, there is an overwhelming consensus that expert athletes spend more time in on-field practice, more time in challenging activities, and more time in off-field practice–related activities such as video reviewing and weight training (see Baker et al., 2003b; Ward et al., 2007, for reviews). Ericsson (2007) noted that improvement over time was not a linear process, and is prone to stall once a comfortable level of automaticity was reached. He noted this "arrested development" would continue even with accumulations of practice, because the practice is not effortful toward improvement and change.

■ Thinking It Through 9.1 Barriers to Expertise

Ericsson et al. (1993) noted four barriers prevented individuals from engaging in deliberate practice and achieving expert levels. These barriers were time, resource availability, motivation, and effort. Data on Olympians dropping out of their sport coincide with these barriers (Gibbons et al., 2002). Individuals not starting early enough, or not having enough time to engage in rigorous practice over 10 years, are disadvantaged. Likewise, without resources of money, access to facilities and coaches, willing parents, and

continued on following page

even cultural expectations, it is difficult to attain high levels. The motivation and effort constraints relate to one's willingness to be single-minded over a long time and be physically capable (including injury-free) of going through such effort.

One potential barrier to performance achievement not held in high regard by Ericsson and other supporters (e.g., Côté et al., 2003), but widely believed by other researchers and laypersons alike, is genetics. The deliberate practice supporters suggest that genetics may offer some domain selection, but that expertise may be gained without some sort of genetic superiority. On the other side of the debate are many that argue that genetics play a decisive role in trainability and capability for achievement (Ahmetov & Rogozkin, 2009; Bouchard et al., 1997; see also Davids & Baker, 2007; Wackerhage et al., 2009, for reviews). Read through the literature listed here and come to your own conclusions. If genetics are found to be determining factors in expertise, should genetic testing be used to match individuals with activities? If you were a parent, would you genetically test your children?

THE ESSENTIAL FEATURES OF PRACTICE

The fundamental concepts of discovery learning, dynamic systems with constraints-led approaches, and deliberate practice, give rise to the five essential features of practice and the instructional strategies to implement them. Again, these features are (1) a specific intention to improve and master the skill, (2) a strong motivation and effort, (3) individual-based practice and learner input into practice, (4) effective communication and information, and (5) overlearning with variation. Each of these is discussed below with implementation strategies for instructors and coaches.

Intention toward Improvement and Mastery

As we saw in the last two chapters, intention is essential to the attention process and to provide goals and motivation. Ericsson et al. (1993) noted early on that the specific intention to improve was one of the defining elements of the deliberate practice strategies of experts. In its most basic form, each practice microstructure and the practice macrostructure must include specific and general goals. These goals may be to overcome weaknesses, maximize strengths, or change techniques. The goal of practice is not simply the overarching goal to get better, but each practice session must aim toward some improvement in some factor. Even if the learning process results in a performance decrement (e.g., plateaus and progression through learning stages), there must be a specific outcome and process goal to direct the course of practice and the performer's mind-set. Put differently, the intent of practice is not to play, not to work hard, not to have fun, but all effort is focused toward improvement and, ultimately, skill mastery.

Learners generally adopt two types of achievement goals: mastery or performance. The intention in **mastery goals** is to improve and learn, and comparisons are made to oneself regarding achievement. In contrast, the intention of **performance goals** is to be better than others or norm-referenced standards (Skjesol & Halvari, 2005). Learners across the age, disability, and skill continuum variously may adopt either or both types of achievement goals with success, but in the long term, an overarching focus toward mastery increases learning outcomes, provides for more flexible and adaptive behaviors, and improves the "motivational climate" (Elliot & Church, 1997; Roberts et al., 1997; Valentini & Rudisill, 2004). Furthermore, this may lead to greater persistence following failure, greater self-efficacy, more effort, and a greater likelihood of taking on challenging tasks (Roberts, 2001; for review see Skjesol & Halvari, 2005).

Identifying specific intentions or goals must be a combined effort of the instructor and learner, and based on the learner's level of skills and abilities, and the identification of a pathway to mastery performance. This pathway necessarily includes the practice of activities that are the most challenging, the most aversive, or that have the most room for improvement. Experts continually strive to learn the next step or overcome the next obstacle rather than continually practice what they already know. Elite soccer players, for instance, were found to differ from subelite players not only in the total amount of dedicated practice time but also in the percent time spent in challenging decision-making drills, which are understood to be among the defining attributes of the best performers (Ward et al., 2007). Expertise of an instructor or coach in matching the individual to a practice roadmap is a mark of successful coaching and cannot be underestimated (Nash et al., 2011).

In order to overcome weaknesses and identify focus areas for practice, individuals need to engage in a variety of activities to identify these areas and improve upon them. Helsen et al. (1998) noted that soccer players and field hockey players engaged in individual training such as weight lifting and video analysis, team practice, and sport-specific learning like journaling, imaging, and coaching and tailored everyday life activities (e.g., sleep and study) around their sport. Each practice activity, as varied as strength training and journaling, had a specific and well-thought-out purpose.

One of the hallmarks of successful coaches is thoughtful planning and organized practice sessions with precise goals and objectives that may be based on individual skills or team strategies (Baker et al., 2003b). In their review, Baker et al. (2003b) noted that the best coaches of the highest level athletes made use of limited practice time by maximizing player involvement (i.e., no standing around) and simulated game stress and physical and mental effort as often as possible. These authors also noted that expert coaches, like expert athletes, have more domain-specific knowledge and use that to provide more advanced instructional feedback to guide learners through problem areas. Interviews with elite coaches support these data, revealing further that practice quality designed with skill learning, intensity, high expectations, and competitive specificity was paramount (Nash et al., 2011). Figure 9.3 illustrates a common practice setting in which players are neither physically nor mentally engaged. Put differently, the consensus is that it is more effective to have a short, intense, purposeful, and highly organized practice than a long, carefree, and poorly organized practice.

The focus of practice and of instructional strategies should differ across the continuum of the learning process, particularly as it relates to children and novices. For instance, technical instruction is

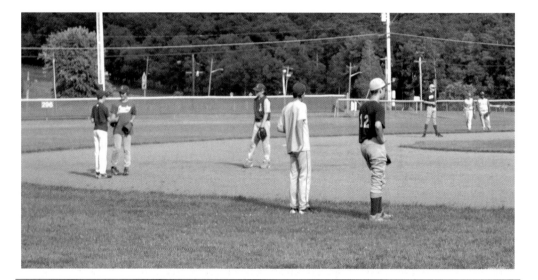

Figure 9.3 • A lack of practice organization coupled with unclear goals leads to poor motivation and effort, and subsequently, enthusiasm and enjoyment suffer. In this photo, there are no fewer than eight players doing nothing, while a single coach hits infield ground balls. None of the shortstops are even looking at the coach. Practice time could be much better spent by engaging the players that are standing around, even if it requires players to practice drills on their own or have players serve as coaches. (Photo courtesy Jeffrey Ives.)

important for novices, and an emphasis on enjoyment and social interaction is important for children. In later stages, team tactics and responding to game-like chaos and pressure may become the emphasis of practice (see Baker et al., 2003b for review).

Motivation and Mental and Physical Effort

The intention described above is necessary to motivate the effort required of deliberate practice. Achieving a high level of performance is a long and hard road filled with setbacks, and teasing out the smallest amount of improvement may take years of tedious concentrated effort. Without maximal effort, maximal improvement cannot be achieved. From previous chapters, we know that effort is both a psychological and physiological process. High physiological effort is necessary for maximal physiological adaptations, such as improving anaerobic threshold and maximal motor unit activation. From our discussion in Chapter 4, we know that this level of physiological effort cannot happen without concentrated mental effort, particularly focused attention. Effort must be maximal day in and day out, and year in and year out, with the caveat that rest is vital for both physiological and psychological recovery and adaptation. Elite coaches, that is, coaches continually turning out elite athletes, repeatedly make use of highly intense, effortful, and stressful practices (Nash et al., 2011). These characteristics are designed to not only mimic the competitive environment for better transfer but also create a more cognitively and physically involved environment for learning and physiological adaptations to take place.

According to deliberate practice models, effort during practice is directed differently than effort during work or play, based on intentionality (Ericsson et al., 1993; Ericsson & Lehmann, 1996). Effort during work is designed to produce a quality product reliably, and automaticity and efficiency are desired. Oftentimes, learning is stalled because the well-entrenched methods that produce reliable results are favored and new methods of unknown outcome are rejected. Effort during play is largely placed on what brings most enjoyment. According to Ericsson and Lehmann (1996), motivation to continue putting time and effort into practice that may be unenjoyable and without immediate benefits may be the biggest obstacle to obtaining expert performance. Effort during deliberate practice, however, should be intentful and effortful toward improvement, and thus reliability, automaticity, and enjoyment are not emphasis points.

| SIDE**NOTE** | **MOTIVATION, EFFORT, AND DROPOUT** |

The findings that large amounts of time and effort in deliberate practice are necessary for the development of expertise must be tempered by the potential to cause dropout. Parents and coaches have more influence over dropout of younger athletes compared to older athletes, thus they should be aware of dropout risk factors. Researchers investigating dropout have noted that early specialization that includes year round off-field training for fitness may be one key risk factor (Wall & Côté, 2007). Wall and Côté (2007) suggested that off-field fitness training may lack sufficient enjoyment for children (ages 6–13) to remain motivated. With increasing age, the need for fun becomes less of a factor, but other factors contributing to the athlete's satisfaction and the value they place on the activity become more important. Boiché and Sarrazin (2009), for instance, reported that both satisfaction and value were related to the athlete's perceived competence, teammate interactions, and the climate set by coaches and parents. When the athletes' goals or priorities conflict with those of teammates, coaches, and parents, and mastery not emphasized, then satisfaction diminishes and dropout increases. These authors suggest that to maintain balance among motivation, high effort, and satisfaction, it is imperative that parents and coaches be educated on these issues. Ongoing communication is instrumental, and children need to be encouraged to speak openly about what motivates them.

Motivation is necessary to drive strong effort, but a full discussion of motivational strategies of the scope of this text. It is sufficient, however, to note that many of the essential features of practice also serve to motivate. These include mastery achievement goals, learner-oriented and controlled practice, and feedback and effective communication from coaches. In particular, communication from coaches on expectations is critical in motivating athletes and engaging them in the practice and learning process (Nash et al., 2011).

Learner-Based Practice and Learner Input into Practice

One of the fundamental tenets of deliberate practice is that practice is set up for the individual based on the individual's prior knowledge and existing skills and abilities. These abilities may include physiological or psychological characteristics, and may involve learning style differences (Fuelscher et al., 2012). One of the most important strategies cited by elite coaches is that they take a long-term approach in developing individual athletes. Athlete age, maturity, and other individual characteristics are used to guide the microstructure and macrostructure of the practice environment (Nash et al., 2011). The performer and the instructor must be able to recognize this previous knowledge and build upon it, requiring the instructor to get inside the learning situation and match the performer's abilities, needs, and wants with the practice environment. This concept also applies to team sports, in which team practice is designed around the collective team abilities and attributes. Team sports pose a challenge to practice, because individuals must not only improve their individual skills but must integrate these skills within the team (Helsen et al., 1998; Memmert et al., 2010; Ward et al., 2007).

In conjunction with practice based on the learner's capabilities, practice is most effective when the learner has some control over the practice environment. When learners are allowed to select their own schedules and specific aspects of what they choose to practice, performance and learning are more solidly retained (Post et al., 2011; Wu & Magill, 2011). Enabling the learner some control over when they receive feedback and instruction is another strategy for empowering the learner. When learners are provided some control over when and how feedback is provided, performance and learning are better compared to a strict instructor-based schedule (Janelle et al., 1997; Sheaves et al., 2012). Giving the learner some control over the practice environment and feedback appears to enhance meaningfulness and motivation, enables the user to extract the most relevant information, and thus facilitates more complete information processing (Wulf, 2007). The beneficial effects of self-controlled practices have been reported across the motor skill learning continuum, including basic skills in children, complex skills in adults, and rehabilitation patients (see Wulf, 2007, for review).

From an instructional standpoint, setting up a learner-based and controlled practice environment is among the most difficult things to do. Discovery learning using a constraints-led approach provides practical implementation strategies for this type of practice microstructure. One instructional approach enabling discovery learning emphasizes implicit learning through an external focus of attention and constraints (Williams & Ford, 2009; Wulf et al., 2010). The external focus emphasizes movement goals and not processes so that learners must work their way to solving the movement problem. The constraints-led process is one in which the learner is progressively provided with obstacles or challenges to overcome, and in the process of overcoming these obstacles, movements emerge. Such obstacles might be as simple as putting a mitt on a basketball player's dominant hand to force nondominant hand dribbling. The discovery learning environment requires a much preparation and thought by instructors. In this type of practice, the coach may appear to be "hands-off," but only because successful coaches exhibit patience in allowing trial and error by the athlete. If the learner begins progressing off track, for example, inefficient form in a squat exercise, it is the coach's role to bring them back by altering constraints and instructional focus. According to researchers and practitioners, this type of implicit learning creates more adaptable and resilient learning (Davids et al., 2008; Williams & Ford, 2009).

Understanding how the characteristics of an individual interact with the task and environmental constraints is an essential aspect of good coaching. Team sport coaches are faced with particular challenges in making individual-based practices. There are simply too many athletes and too few coaches. In such cases, one strategy is to partition learners by proficiencies, shortcomings, and abilities.

This can work two ways. The first is to group players needing similar instruction or needing to overcome similar weakness. In this way, instructor time can be made more efficient. The second way is to group learners with specific deficiencies with learners with proficiencies in those areas, and then turn the proficient performers into instructors.

The reader should not mistake discovery learning as never containing precise and prescriptive instruction and modeling, that is, the "do it this way" approach. There are times for explicit learning, an internal focus of attention, and other instructional strategies that may not leave much room for exploration. One mark of a successful coach is to know when this type of instructional strategy is necessary, and when it is not.

■ Thinking It Through 9.2 Instruction in Basketball

Jim is the tallest player on his middle school basketball team. His coach needs him to play down low in the center position to grab rebounds, score from in close near the basket, and guard the other team's big man. This will require Jim to physically battle and jostle with other large players, something he is timid in doing. Using the concepts of constraints and learner-based instruction, devise a plan to help Jim overcome his timidity and be a more assertive basketball player. In particular, provide strategies by which Jim can take control over the learning environment to feel a sense of empowerment and motivation.

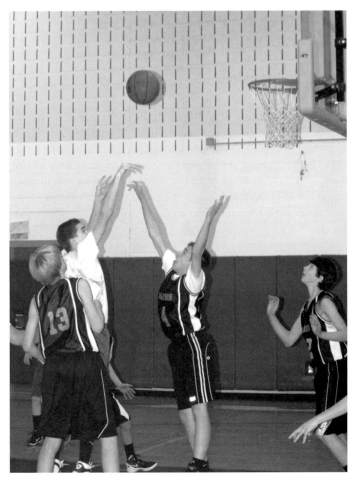

Photo courtesy Jeffrey Ives.

Communication and Information

The sport psychology literature has demonstrated convincingly that strong communication between learner and coach is critical to learning and performance (e.g., Passmore, 2010). In one survey of over 800 Olympic athletes, the athletes cited teaching ability, ability to motivate and encourage, and sport/training knowledge as the most important characteristics of coaches (Gibbons et al., 2002). Effective communication is behind each of these traits as it fosters trust, encourages and motivates, and transmits knowledge and information. Communication is a two-way street in which the learner and instructor must reveal their needs, thoughts, struggles, victories, plans, and intentions (Nash et al., 2011). Communication is thus necessary to foster intention and effort and create the environment for learner-based practice and control. Mike Krzyewsky, the winningest men's basketball coach in NCAA history, noted that "effective teamwork begins and ends with communication." Of particular relevance to the practice environment is the exchange of movement-relevant information in the form of pre-movement instructions and postmovement feedback. Outstanding coaches not only have the ability to motivate and teach but also have high levels of technical skill knowledge from which to provide teaching materials (Gibbons et al., 2002).

INSTRUCTIONS

Instructions largely consist of verbal or written information provided before physical practice takes place, but demonstration or modeling of motor skills can also be considered a form of pre-practice instructions. Modeling is discussed in detail later in this chapter and is not considered here. Instructions should, first and foremost, be appropriate for the skills and abilities of the learner. This includes avoiding disclosing high level or critical information that is beyond the capability for the novice learner or child to understand (Hodges & Franks, 2002). For instance, instructing beginning tennis players to pay attention to the body dynamics of the opposing player would be incompatible with the novice's visual search and information-processing capabilities.

Instructions often center on identifying the goal of the movement, but even this apparently simple instruction may prove confusing in regard to the type of task, particularly as it relates to open and closed skills. Hodges and Franks (2002) noted that a specific set of instructions regarding movement dynamics could work well in a closed skill activity, but a similar set of instructions for an open skill would be inconsistent with the variability required of performance and could result in confusion for the learner. This suggestion can be expanded to more general terms in that there appears to be no single optimal movement template for a given movement, only what is optimal for a given person. Therefore, explicit instructions on what to do and how to do it are less effective, and providing explicit knowledge of processes and perceptual information that tend to be learned implicitly may be a detriment to performance and learning (Hodges & Franks, 2002). In their extensive review, Hodges and Franks (2002) noted that there are too many learner and practice variables mediating the effects of instructions to make definitive and specific conclusions. Individual learner personality characteristics, habits, and prior experiences may influence instruction interpretation. Table 9.1 outlines some general guidelines that may be implemented across situations.

FEEDBACK

Providing timely feedback to the learner regarding performance is one of the characteristics of deliberate practice (Ericsson et al., 1993). Feedback is also essential in the discovery learning process, as well as to the goal of making the learning process tailored to the individual. Yet, the nature of effective feedback is not always clear.

Information passed from instructor to learner regarding aspects of performance is properly defined as **augmented feedback** (**AFB**), because the information is value added. That is, the feedback has enhanced, modified, or revealed information that the performer would not ordinarily receive. Note, however, that AFB is also given to motivate a learner, and not simply pass along information.

TABLE 9.1	Guidelines for Providing Instructions
Concept	**Explanation and Applications**
1. Instructions should convey goals appropriate to the learning situation.	The information conveyed must be appropriate to the learning goals, for instance, improving movement outcomes or movement dynamics. In most learning situations, particularly for novices, instructing on movement outcomes that also direct the learner to an external focus of attention is a good starting point.
2. Instructions should lead learners to learn on their own based on individual characteristics.	Instructions should lead learners to their own movement optimization rather than a generic optimization movement template. Instructions should be used to direct the learner's attention or guide discovery of movement solutions or overcome bad habits by identifying errors. Instructors should be cautious—but not to the point of exclusion—about providing explicit instructions on movement dynamics.
3. Instructions must be understandable within the cognitive and physical capability of the learner.	Higher skilled performers have a much richer movement experience and can understand more information regarding movement nuances. The learning goals of experts will differ from novices in what is learned and how things are learned.
4. Instructions should encourage exploration and discovery of movement solutions.	Particularly during early phases of the acquisition of new movement skills, instructions should encourage exploration. But this is not the only time exploration is encouraged. Instructions that foster maintenance of preexisting stable movement patterns without exploring potentially better solutions may cause the learner to get entrenched in poor movement habits and limit the learner's movement repertoire.
5. Instructions should take into account that they will influence the learner's focus of attention.	This attention, whether internal or external, centered on movement dynamics or movement outcome, should be considered as part of the instruction process.

AFB is nearly always provided by an instructor, although technology enables electronic devices such as digital video and software to provide AFB. Another form of AFB is augmented sensory feedback, or more commonly known as **biofeedback**, which is the use of electronic devices to amplify biological processes to make them noticeable to the learner. See the accompanying Concepts in Action box for more information on biofeedback.

AFB has been researched in great depth over the past 40 years. From these works, we know that instructors must make decisions on the feedback's content, complexity, type, instructional nature, and frequency and timing. A brief overview of these concepts is provided here, followed by recommendations for providing AFB in a deliberate practice and discovery learning framework.

The *content of AFB* is essential to the type of information being passed along. Feedback content can be based on the response outcome or the response production, respectively known as knowledge of results (KRs) or knowledge of performance (KP). KR is information about the outcome of the motor skill, such as running time, jump height, or the location of a tennis serve. KR is the most common

Concepts in Action

Using Biofeedback Devices

Common biofeedback devices include heart rate and blood pressure monitors, respiratory rate monitors (pneumobellows), electrodermal monitors like galvanic skin response devices, electroencephalography (neurofeedback), and electromyography (EMG). Most biofeedback devices, heart rate monitors included, can be used to monitor physiological calming during relaxation training. In clinical settings, EMG biofeedback is also used to help in muscle retraining, and neurofeedback has been used for a number of cognitive training exercises (see photo). There is some evidence that neurofeedback may improve concentration and attention in persons from children with attention deficit disorder to Olympic athletes, and improve some physical abilities, but at this time, the evidence for improving motor skill proficiency is lacking (Gruzelier et al., 2006; Vernon, 2005). The most common biofeedback devices are heart rate monitors to evaluate exercise intensity. Telemetered HR devices are used in settings from cardiac rehabilitation to high-level athlete training and require little expertise to use (see photo). Activity monitors in the form of pedometers and accelerometers, and HR monitors are being used to motivate and promote user self-discovery. For example, Segerståhl and Oinas-Kukkonen (2011) found that adults who wore personal HR monitors at home and tied into a web monitoring service engaged in more exploratory exercise behaviors were more inclined to meet target exercise behaviors (e.g., exercise intensity) and were more motivated.

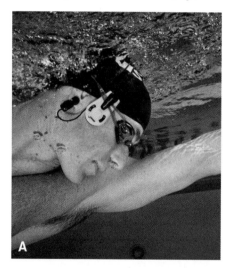 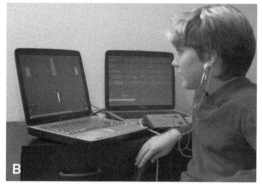

Biofeedback devices. **A.** This waterproof heart rate monitor uses infrared pulse technology to detect heart rate in the earlobe and then provides HR biofeedback verbally from the upper jawbone to the inner ear via what the manufacturer calls bone conduction technology. (AquaSport®; Photo courtesy of Finis Inc. and Jason Lezak.) **B.** Neurofeedback devices monitor EEG brain wave activity and provide biofeedback on the patterns of activity by translating them into computer graphics. Often these graphics are in the form of games that by changing the brain activity the user can interact with the computer game. (From Coben, R., Linden, M., & Myers, T. E. (2010). Neurofeedback for autistic spectrum disorder: A review of the literature. *Applied Psychophysiology and Biofeedback, 35*(1), 83–105, with permission from Springer.)

form of AFB and is generally the simplest to gather and provide. KP is often more complex than KR and provides information on how the movement was made, such as verbal indication of arm position during swimming, video assessment of leg position during hurdling, or a graphical biomechanical assessment of gait kinematics.

The content of AFB must also take into consideration which aspect(s) of movement receives feedback, which is one reason why the best content for AFB comes only after careful, critical, and continued assessment of performance. Put differently, AFB is only effective if it reflects aspects of performance needing change, and directs the learner to making appropriate changes.

For KP especially, the skill must be evaluated by its most important and least important parts, that is, the components must be prioritized. Determining what aspect of movement receives AFB requires an instructor with knowledge of the motor skill and knowledge of the performer. Intuitively, it would seem that the poorest aspect of a motor skill should receive feedback, but this is not always the case. Sometimes a poor movement component is the result of glitches in prior components, causing a sequential worsening of movement performance over the progression of the movement. For example, poor ball control and shooting during a basketball layup is often the result of uncoordinated footwork and leaping. In this case, feedback and instruction should be placed on footwork, and not shooting.

The *complexity of AFB* can vary from highly complex and detailed, or as simple as statements commenting as "good" or "bad." Determining the level of complexity begins with setting a *performance bandwidth*, that is, the amount of error that prompts a feedback correction. In general, beginners need a larger bandwidth or margin of error before AFB is provided, and experts need a smaller bandwidth. Complexity is also related to the qualitative or quantitative nature of the feedback. *Quantitative AFB* provides numerically objective information that is often precise regarding movement KP or KR. *Qualitative AFB* addresses the "quality" of movement and involves subjective statements such as "Too slow" or "Need more velocity." Quantitative AFB is generally better because it is more precise, but the level of experience and practice time must be taken into account. The novice needs, or sometimes can only use, simpler AFB such as qualitative or simple quantitative. With more experience, the AFB can get more complex and precise.

The *type of AFB* refers to the method of delivery, generally being categorized as verbal, physical guidance, modeling, video, and graphic. Verbal AFB, in the form of simple verbal communication, is the easiest and most common for both KR and KP. Perhaps the second most common form of AFB, particularly in exercise and sport science settings, is physical guidance. The instructor physically leads the learner through the motion or physically corrects an improper position or movement. Modeling AFB is the instructor mimicking the performance of the learner, essentially illustrating good or poor performance.

Video, such as game films or high-speed biomechanical analyses, is similar to modeling except the learner serves as their own model. Video AFB effectiveness is largely dependent on the performer's skill level and not so much the skill itself, perhaps in part because video provides not only specific performance feedback but also a larger view of the task requirements and demands (Hodges et al., 2003). For instance, novices may not benefit as much from video AFB as skilled players, perhaps because rhythm and timing nuances available in video are only picked up by skilled players (Bertram et al., 2007). Generally verbal AFB is used with video, but again, performer skill level and motor skill type may influence this effect (Bertram et al., 2007). A single video AFB session may provide a single revelation moment for the learner that can have lasting influences (e.g., Parsons & Alexander, 2012), but it generally needs to be used for more sessions for most effectiveness (e.g., Rucci & Tomporowski, 2010).

Graphical AFB methods tend to involve high technology, such as graphical displays of biomechanical information (Fig. 9.4). Biomechanical information, such as power curves during rowing strokes, is probably best reserved for the most skilled performers (Smith & Loschner, 2002). There are of yet only limited data regarding the effectiveness of biomechanical KP, but the data do show promising results (Rucci & Tomporowski, 2010).

The *instructional nature of AFB* directs the learner to how the feedback is used to alter performance. Feedback processing is manipulated by either providing descriptive AFB or prescriptive AFB. *Descriptive AFB* is just that, a KR or KP description of what was done in the movement. This type of AFB may prompt the learner into self-discovery over what they did wrong and what they need to do to correct their mistakes. In some cases, though, description provides no useful information for the

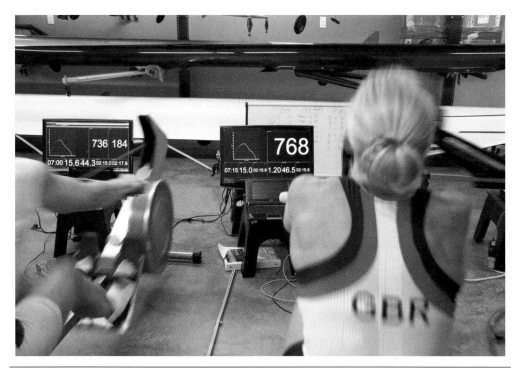

Figure 9.4 • Side-by-side instrumented rowing machines provide AFB on power output and force curves. These athletes may also receive AFB on their teammates to synchronize rowing mechanics among teammates. (Photo courtesy of RowPerfect3, http://www.rowperfect3.com/)

learner as they have no background to interpret its meaning. *Prescriptive AFB* does not provide information on the past movement, but rather, provides information on what needs to be done next time for a correct movement. Prescription takes away some of the problem-solving needs of the learner, but can help the learner progress along the correct path. There is a growing recognition that good coaching needs to move away from the "time-honored" prescriptive nature and more into learner-based self-discovery (Reid et al., 2007).

The *frequency of AFB* refers to how often feedback is given over the course of a practice session, ranging from after every motor skill trial to once at the end of a practice session. There is no precise answer to how much is sufficient, but there is consensus that too much feedback could lead to "information overload" or direct the learner to rely solely on the AFB as a crutch in place of self-knowledge. The detrimental effect of too much AFB is called the *guidance effect* (Salmoni et al., 1984). Though the guidance effect is relatively robust, it may not apply to all cases (Buchanan & Wang, 2012; Sidaway et al., 2012), and therefore, it is appropriate to look at the "right" amount of AFB for the best learning from a different perspective. The challenge point framework (Guadagnoli & Lee, 2004) introduced in Chapter 8 provides this perspective.

Using the challenge point framework, it can be seen that the optimal amount of AFB depends on the information-processing capabilities of the learner, the difficulty of the task, and the amount of afferent information available during practice. When large amounts of afferent information are available in challenging tasks, but are uninterpretable or overwhelming, then a relatively large amount of AFB may be needed to filter and simplify the information. In such cases, the instructor can provide *summary AFB*, which is a selection of the most important performance information given after a group of trials. When information is available but the task is simple, then less AFB may be needed. In essence, the nature of AFB should supplement the naturally occurring information to optimize cognitive effort. It should be kept in mind, though, that giving AFB in practice that is not available during regular competitions (such as practicing lifting techniques in front of a mirror; see Tremblay & Proteau, 1998) could have detrimental effects on actual performance. Eventually the learner will need to be weaned off the AFB.

The *timing of AFB* concerns when feedback is provided in relationship to the execution of a motor skill. AFB could be provided just before skill execution, during, or right after. If given just before or just after, there should be a time period to enable the learner to process the AFB with their own afferent information and movement plans. AFB given concurrently with skill execution may be distracting, but does have a useful place during continuous movements. For instances, ongoing KP of running kinematics while on a treadmill has been shown to improve running mechanics in both healthy (Crowell et al., 2010; Halvorsen et al., 2012) and injured (Noehren et al., 2011) runners, and concurrent KR has been shown to improve endurance performance (Metsios et al., 2006).

The numerous ways and reasons for administering AFB, coupled with some ambiguous data, give rise to confusion over when and how to provide AFB. With this in mind, Reid et al. (2007) have consolidated fundamental usage guidelines. These authors, using tennis as an example, suggested that coaches moderate their AFB to motivate and aid in performance, but not stifle independent thought or the development of individual strategies. Generally, novice learners need more AFB, but coaches and instructors must work toward lessening feedback or changing the nature of feedback as learners progress. As motor skill performance increases, the nature of AFB can be more precise or complex, and less prescriptive, but the purpose to foster self-discovery is still the same as with new learners. Of course, the specific content of the feedback may change as learners progress through learning stages. That is, the type, content, complexity, and frequency of AFB will differ among learners, but should emphasize learner problem solving and motivation toward specific goals. Perhaps the most effective way to determine when feedback should be given and in what form is to rely on the learner. As noted earlier, AFB is most effective when the learner has control over when and what information is provided (Wulf, 2007).

When used correctly, AFB enhances the self-discovery process. In the place of the all-pervading prescriptive AFB in motor skill instruction, AFB should be used to actively engage learners in their own learning to better develop them into independent self-learners (Williams & Ford, 2009). For instance, AFB could take the form of an instructor asking questions of the learner about the learner's performance. In addition, AFB can be provided on a timing schedule set by the learner when they feel it most necessary, such as when summary AFB is provided. Furthermore, AFB is most effective when learners direct where they receive it, and on what component or aspect of movement. Thus, providing AFB falls directly in line with learner-based control of the learning situation. These guidelines for providing AFB are more flexible for novices (especially children) because of their diminished problem-solving skills and ability to recognize and correct errors. Nevertheless, the goal of AFB for novices should also be problem solving and exploration.

Peh et al. (2011) suggested that AFB be in the form of facilitative feedback, in which information is used to channel the learner to explore a narrower or broader range of movement options. The information provided is largely in the form of constraints that are placed on the movement process that provides the learner with immediate feedback on ineffective movements. Consider, for instance, the use of training wheels for a child learning to ride a bike. The wheels simplify the movement, but also provide feedback when they engage with the ground. With the wheels in their lowest and safest position, the new rider has minimal balance requirements. As the training wheels are raised, the bike is free to lean, providing the beginning rider with more sensory feedback, which is also associated with an unstable bike and an abrupt jerk when the bike leans so far as to engage the training wheels. By changing the height of training wheels (changing feedback bandwidth), or by riding on a downhill slope (easier to pedal), or riding on grass (fear of falling reduced), the instructor has manipulated constraints to provide the best learning environment for the child's particular needs. Figure 9.5 illustrates this concept, in which the instructor is teaching the learner boxing punches. In one photo, the instructor is providing prescriptive feedback on positioning of the arm. In the other photo, the instructor is providing a constraints-based environment to lead the boxer to discover the best way to punch.

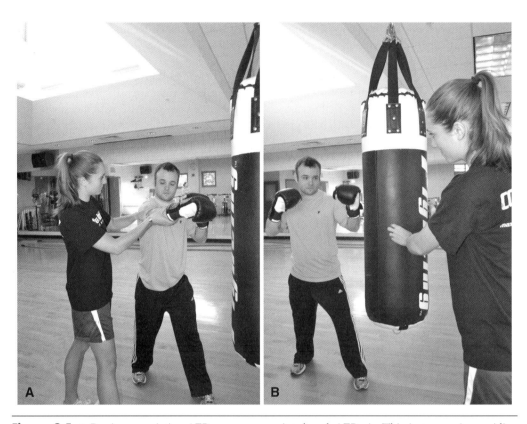

Figure 9.5 • Precise prescriptive AFB versus constraints-based AFB. **A.** This instructor is providing physical guidance AFB and precise prescriptive instructions on the orientation of the shoulder and elbow during a right cross punch. In the subsequent trial, the learner will likely be placing attention on his arm. **B.** The instructor is behind the bag instructing the learner to drive the punch through the bag to hit her hand, thus providing a movement goal with an external focus of attention. Constraints are the bag itself and the target location. The movement goal will require the learner to do a full extension and shoulder/torso rotation to accomplish the task of driving the punch through the heavy bag, even without consciously thinking about movement mechanics. (Photo courtesy Jeffrey Ives.)

SIDE**NOTE**	USING AFB TO MANIPULATE EXPECTANCY

Can false AFB be used to manipulate the learner into better performance? In particular, what if the instructor gave false AFB that the learner's performance was better than it really was? How might the learner respond? Consider an experiment by Stoate et al. (2012) in which experienced runners ran on a treadmill at 75% of their maximal oxygen consumption for 10 minutes. One group of runners was given fabricated feedback that their biomechanical movement efficiency was better than it actually was. These runners were told that their efficiency leads to better running performance; thus, the AFB led to an expectancy of better performance. Compared to a control group that did not receive such feedback, the fabricated AFB group had decreased oxygen consumption, perceptions of easier running and less fatigue, and better pre- to post mood states. In a similar manner, having subjects exercise for longer than they expected has been shown in increase ratings of perceived exertion without an increase in physiological effort (Eston et al., 2012). The effects of increasing expectations by manipulating AFB clearly can have powerful effects, but deceptive AFB may not work during high-intensity exercise when the innate afferent signals are strong (Hampson et al., 2004). Nevertheless, the idea of providing deceptive AFB raises a host of questions for coaches and trainers, ranging from the best method to manipulate AFB to ethical questions.

Overlearning and Practice Variation

The macrostructure and microstructure of practice should be set up to get to a point of **overlearning**. Overlearning is continual practice even past a point where performance seems to have peaked. The benefits of overlearning include modifying brain structures to be more resistant to forgetting and to enhance movement adaptability and flexibility (Magill, 2007). These benefits are not simply gained by doing more, but also by doing different in order to maximize learning. There is, though, a point of diminishing returns. In other words, instructors need to balance out the cost (practice time) to benefit (improvement) ratio. It is important to understand that the amount of practice is secondary to the quality of practice.

The microstructure of practice set up to maximize overlearning centers on a large number of repetitions done under variable practice situations. According to deliberate practice tenets, experts engage in repetition after repetition. Ericsson et al.' (1993) data from musicians revealed that practice was highly repetitive, repeating the same music sets over and over again with little apparent change. This should not be interpreted to mean there was no variation or attempt to do things differently. The nature of instrument playing makes it look like the repetition is consistent, but expert performers are constantly modifying their intentions, emotions, techniques, and approaches to playing.

Nikolai Bernstein (1967) commented that repetition is not repeating the movement solution, but repeating the process of solving the movement or finding a movement solution. Each movement, for example, each stroke of a tennis forehand drive off a ball machine, is a unique movement in that it attempts to be a better movement than the one before it. This can only happen effectively, of course, if the individual is intentionally attempting to do so. Bernstein's research on blacksmiths found that these highly skilled individuals produced very precise patterns of hammer head movement, but that the movements of the associated limbs and joints varied a great deal (Fig. 9.6). He observed that this was repetition without repeating, and highlights that the nervous system is continually striving to modify and adapt the large number of degrees of freedom to solve the movement problem. Variation in movement, in particular variation in how the nervous system organizes and executes movements, is understood to be an

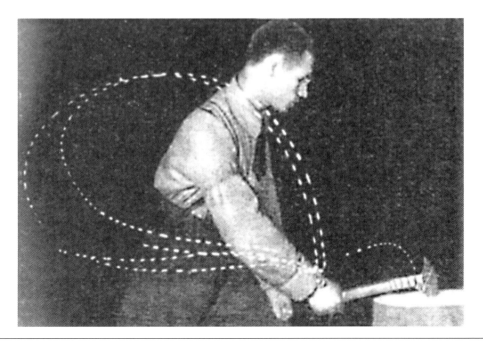

Figure 9.6 • Bernstein's cyclogram measurement method helped reveal that the process of hammering could vary greatly even in an expert blacksmith. Cyclograms revealed that even as blacksmiths repeatedly hitting a small target with astonishing accuracy, the trajectory of the hammerhead varied greatly throughout the motion, particularly at the movement midpoint.

indicator of high-level performance (Davids et al., 2003). This should not be confused with unstable and highly variable performance of novices. Instead, variability in the movement system enables adaptability and flexibility to new challenges. According to Davids et al. (2003), this variability enables those with less favorable genetic dispositions to adapt to individual-specific training environments and still succeed.

Manipulating the schedule of practice enables the instructor to manipulate the number and variation in repetitions in regard to a practice macrostructure. *Massed practice* is a practice structure in which practice is compacted into intervals with long durations and limited breaks between practice sessions. Conversely, *distributed practice* is when practices are spread out over longer time intervals because of more rest periods and/or shorter practice sessions. As a general finding, distributed practices are thought to be more effective, but both massed and distributed should be used to vary the practice schedule. According to Magill (2007), it is a good principle to first consider shorter but more frequent practice to be more effective than longer and less frequent practices.

The practice microstructure is essential to providing repetition with variation. An individual practice session can be set up varying from a *blocked practice* to a *random practice* schedule. Blocked practice is practicing a single motor skill completely, and then moving to the next motor skill and so forth. Random, or variable practice, has skills being practiced at variable times and occurrences over the course of a practice session. Generally variable practice has been shown to improve retention, probably because the learner is more actively engaged and attentive, leading to their own self-discovery of movement patterns (Handford et al., 1997)

Variable practice may aid in the retention of motor skills by promoting **contextual interference**. Contextual interference occurs when a skill is practiced in the context of another task, or when randomly changing from practicing one thing to another (see Magill & Hall, 1990, for early review). This would include rapidly changing from one offensive drill to another, or forcing a switch from offense to defense. Varying the movement context, especially when done rapidly and even unexpectedly to the learner, causes interference in the performance of the target skill and may result in poorer practice performance but better retention and transfer. The contextual interference effect may be dependent on the motor skill, learner characteristics and skill level, and practice scheduling (Jones & French, 2007; Magill & Hall, 1990; Travlos, 2010), but it is sufficient to suggest here that coaches should purposefully use the contextual interference effect, particularly with adults, to promote attention switching and complex problem solving. Over the long term, this may improve retention, transfer of skills, and game performance (Hall et al., 1994; Williams & Ford, 2009). Because contextual interference and variable practice may result in poorer practice performance, both coaches and learners must be encouraged to persist with this type of practice (Reid et al., 2007).

Regardless of the practice scheduling, it is important to understand that eventually movement patterns need to be stabilized and then destabilized via variation and diversification (Handford, 2006; Passos et al., 2008). Consider a basketball team practicing half court offensive plays. At first the drills are run without defenders to enable the players to get the overall idea of movement patterns and purposes. Eventually variation, in the form of constraints, is added. Initially this could be different movement outcomes (e.g., different scorers) or the addition of defenders. Over time defensive set variations, differently skilled defenders, quickening the pattern of play, and running the drill from a full court would enable diversification. Further diversification would include varying the offensive movement patterns and adding flexible movement patterns based on defensive sets. Other variable practice can be illustrated by a golfer at the driving range switching clubs every few balls, a baseball player seeing different pitches every couple of pitches, or a football team offense practicing offensive plays randomly as opposed to running the same play over and over again. Figure 9.7 illustrates practice scheduling and drills for tennis based on level of practice variability and contextual interference. The most complex situation is actual game play.

It may seem counterintuitive that new learning, particularly in novices and children, can occur in a variable practice setting. But new learners may have preexisting undesirable movement patterns that need to be destabilized to enable new and effective learning (Hodges & Franks, 2002). In the case of new learning of complex actions, it may be necessary to simplify the skill by breaking the skill down into its constituent components and practice the components separately. This method of simplification,

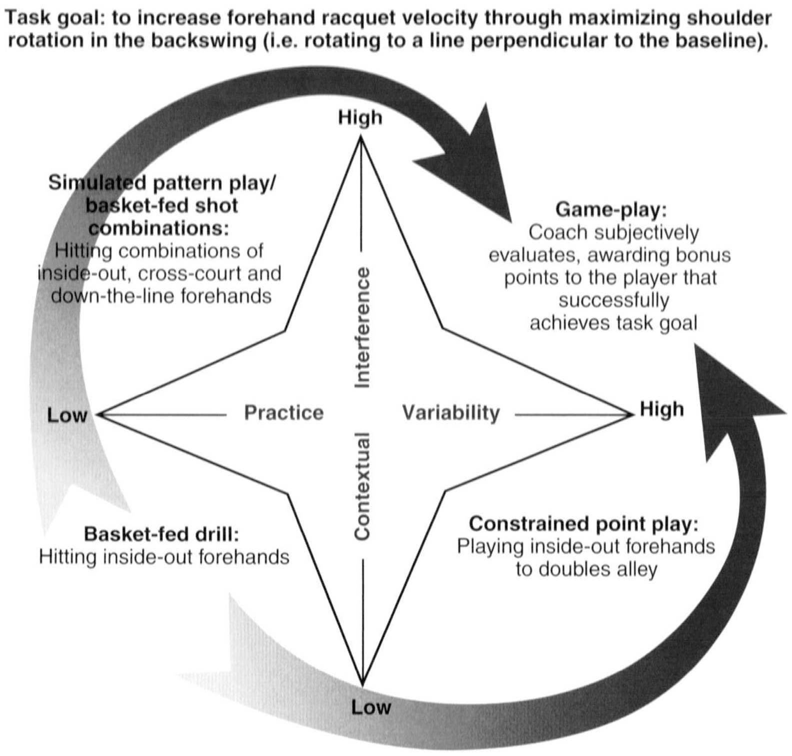

Figure 9.7 • A schedule of tennis drills based on difficulty in practice variability and contextual interference. Low variability includes the coach hitting ball after ball from a hopper (basket-feeding) to the player to force one type of stroke. High variability involves game play. Low contextual interference is simply rote repetition; high contextual interference involves more variability in strokes. Note that all drills are designed toward a single goal of increasing shoulder rotation and stroke velocity. (Reprinted from Reid, M., Crespo, M., Lay, B., & Berry, J. (2007). Skill acquisition in tennis: Research and current practice. *Journal of Science and Medicine in Sport*, *10*(1), 1–10, with permission from Elsevier.)

called **part practice**, requires breaking down the skill based on the task complexity and organization. In general, tasks low in complexity but high in organization (the movement parts fit well together) should be practiced as a whole. Tasks high in complexity, but low in organization, should be practiced in parts (e.g., tennis serve). In reality, skills lie in a continuum between complexity and organization, and complexity and organization are often defined by the learner. Overlearning and practice variation in these situations would have the individual sometimes practicing movement components separately, sometimes in proper sequence with one another, and sometimes even randomly if feasible. Renshaw et al. (2009) warned, however, against too much decomposition and reducing the skill into unintegrated parts because too much movement information is lost. These authors suggest coaches look first to an overall simplification of the task for new learners rather than resort to gross decomposition.

The goal of overlearning coupled with the need to put in full effort during practice often results in fatigue. Fatigue, by definition, affects performance, but it does not necessarily affect learning. If fatigue depletes mental resources and lowers attention, then practice may be ineffective. In addition, if the fatigue is task specific and leads to faulty movement patterns, then it may be better to avoid fatigue. For example, if one does an upper body weightlifting program before practicing free-throw shooting, arm and whole body coordination may be poor and lead to poor learning. However, if one does the free-throw practice after running, and thus practices with leg and "general" fatigue, then the practice

Concepts in Action

The Practice Philosophies of John Wooden

John Wooden is among the finest basketball coaches of all time, leading the UCLA men's basketball team to 10 NCAA championships in 12 years. Some of his basic principles of practice are listed below, with explanatory notes using contemporary terminology. Note that Coach Wooden had daily lesson plans for practice.

1. Fundamentals first. Basic skills need to be learned so they are executed quickly, automatically, and flawlessly. Knowing the fundamentals provides a foundation from which imagination and initiative emerge and grow.
2. Practice with variation. The basic framework of practice was the same, but variation and surprises kept attention and enjoyment. It is better to have more drills of shorter duration and very difficult drills with simple drills. In addition, use competitive drills and imitate game conditions as much as possible.
3. New material should be taught during the first half of practice. This enabled full attention and then application during the latter half.
4. Quick transitions from activity to activity. Quick and intense transitions not only mimic real-game transitions, they promote efficient use of time and increase motivation.
5. Increasing complexity of learning. Drills began simple and move to complex. Each aspect of progression from simple to complex was planned.
6. Conditioning and improvement. The overarching philosophy was to improve a little every day and make perfection (i.e., mastery) the goal. Conditioning was part of this improvement, as players were pushed to exhaustion, and then pushed a little more each day.
7. End on a positive note. The last 5 minutes was a break from the routine to have something new, fun, or interesting.
8. Avoid altering a plan during the lesson. Though not every drill was successful, breaking away from the day's plans would lead to haphazard practices. Drills and other practice activities were evaluated for effectiveness and then modified for the next time they were used. Practices always ended on time so that players knew exactly what was expected of them and could maintain the right intensity level.

may be like a real-game situation. Fatigue, thus, becomes a practice variable that may promote contextual interference and better retention of motor performance.

Table 9.2 summarizes the five essential features of practice. Working these features into practice takes time, thought, and patience, but the outcome promises to be worth it.

MENTAL PRACTICE

Among the practice techniques found in high-level performers is regular mental practice. Some associate mental practice solely with imagery or visualization techniques, but we also include relaxation and stress control, positive self-talk strategies, observational learning, and concentration improvement as components of mental practice. In this section, we examine only observation and imaging techniques as they are common techniques employed in the practice microstructure.

Modeling and Observation

The most common method of instruction, particularly for new learners, is **modeling**, otherwise known as demonstration or observational learning. In modeling, the instructor or model demonstrates the skill in person or on video, and the learner then mimics the skill. Modeling generally improves

TABLE 9.2	Summary of the Five Essential Characteristics of Effective Practice
Practice Concept	**Explanation and Applications**
1. A specific intention to improve and master the skill	Intention leads to purposeful practice. Mastery goals increase learning outcomes, provide for more flexible and adaptive behaviors, and improve motivation. This may lead to greater persistence following failure, greater self-efficacy, more effort, and a greater likelihood of taking on challenging tasks. Intention and mastery lead to better practice organization, more effective use of practice time.
2. Strong motivation and effort	Motivation leads to high mental effort, and high mental effort leads to high physiological effort. All are necessary for maximal motor skill and physiological improvement. Effort must be directed toward specific goals and not simply working hard. Intentionality and learner self-control over aspects of the learning process contribute to motivation.
3. Individual-based practice and learner input to the practice environment	Practices should be designed around individual or team needs and based on the individual/team knowledge, experience, skill level, strengths, and weaknesses. Learners should have some control over the learning process, such as the nature of feedback, to increase motivation, meaningfulness, and information retention. Constraints-based learning, set up by coaches, can be used to implement these goals.
4. Effective communication and information	Communication in the form of instructions and feedback transmits knowledge, fosters trust, encourages, and motivates. Instructions and feedback should be intentional and lead the learner to problem solving and self-discovery of better movement solutions. Too much prescriptive feedback, in particular, can lead to reliance on the feedback and inhibit problem solving.
5. Overlearning with variation	Practice should be aimed at learning the skill beyond a point of automaticity. Many repetitions are necessary to do this, but repetitions should vary to improve problem solving and movement flexibility to be adaptable to different situations. Practice variation forces more cognitive involvement and better learning.

the effectiveness of physical practice alone, but the effects of modeling are related to who models, the type of skill being modeled, what is measured as the outcome of the learning process, as well as the intentions and observational tactics of the learner (Ashford et al., 2006; Hodges et al., 2007). Because observation itself, not physical mimicry, is the critical component of the learning process, observational learning is considered mental practice.

Modeling is generally more effective with proficient and prominent modelers. Not only is the demonstration more likely to be correct, but learners are likely to pay more attention and ascribe meaning to what is being learned. It may be, however, that the expert model is too advanced, confusing novice learners (particularly children) by the complexity of the movement or by using intrinsic movement actions that the younger learners do not possess (Ashford et al., 2007; Hodges & Franks, 2002). It can be useful to have learners observe other novices learning a motor skill. The observers pick up strategies that work and do not work, and in doing so engage in problem solving to a much greater extent than simply observing an expert model. Modeling also works better when verbal cueing is added, probably because attention becomes more focused and information processing is sharpened (Janelle et al., 2003).

Not all motor skills or movement characteristics can be equally learned from modeling. Observers learn more from serial and continuous movement modeling compared to discrete movements (Ashford

| SIDE**NOTE** | **DEVELOPING EXPERT COACHES** |

The quality of coaching plays an important role in delivering effective practice, but how are expert coaches developed? Ford et al. (2009) noted that coaching cannot really be practiced unless one is actually coaching. For this reason, any intentful activity aimed at improving coaching ability may be considered experiential and deliberate practice. Gilbert et al. (2006, 2009) found that the pathway to successful coaching was not as clear as for athletes, but there were some similarities. Successful coaches tended to be successful athletes themselves, participating in multiple seasons of competition. Successful coaches also amassed thousands of hours of time in development as a coach, accumulating time as a part-time assistant or working in low-level leagues. Paradoxically, successful coaches spent little time in actual coaching training and educational activities. In fact, other researchers have noted that high-level coaches question the effectiveness of coaching educa-tion programs, and instead, depend more on informal information networks and mentoring (Nash et al., 2009). Depending on the coaching level (e.g., high school vs. college), the variation of coaching experience may play a role. For example, Gilbert et al. noted that successful high school coaches were more likely to have played and coached multiple sports, whereas successful NCAA Division I coaches tended to have specialized in one sport. Overall, the current research reveals that there has been very little systematic research on the developmental activities of successful coaches.

et al., 2006). Exactly what is best learned during observation may depend on the learner age, experience, or maturation level (Ashford et al., 2006, 2007; Hodges et al., 2007). It is clear that the learner's visual system picks up basic movement actions and constraints and task purposes, but children may benefit only with better movement outcomes, whereas adults may learn better movement dynamics (Ashford et al., 2007).

Hodges et al. (2007) reviewed numerous forms of observational learning and modeling and con-cluded that while some coordination information (e.g., timing and sequencing of limb movement) may be learned, the observer largely picks up constraints (including goals) that influence the task. Learners also tend to focus on end point or distal effector actions and outcomes, as these provide the most infor-mation regarding the overall movement and can be sufficient by themselves to enable reproduction of the entire movement. Thus, observational learning appears to follow the same principles as an external focus of attention in that it appears beneficial for the learner to focus attention on the movement goal or outcome rather than specific movement features (Hodges et al., 2007; Williams & Ford, 2009), which fosters self-exploration of movement solutions. However, it is important at times for modelers to direct the intention of the learner toward learning movement form versus movement outcome (Hodges et al., 2007). Coaches thus need to set up modeling situations to convey the appropriate information to the learner, and make this skill and age appropriate.

THE NEUROSCIENCE OF OBSERVATION

Observation has direct neurological consequences. A particular group of visuomotor neurons, called **mirror neurons**, work in a system called the **motor resonance system**. Figure 9.8 illustrates that the motor resonance system is activated when movements are observed (live, photo, or video) and when they are executed (see Holmes & Calmels, 2008, for review). The motor resonance system acts differently depending on the motor actions being observed. The system is less active when observing nonhuman actors, or when the movement is impossible, or when the observer is entirely unfamiliar with the task. When the motor resonance system is active, it appears to have four main functions (1) to understand the action, (2) to understand the intention, (3) to enable imitation, and (4) to understand behavioral state. In other words, parts of the motor system are active when watching motor behaviors in order to help the brain comprehend exactly what it is seeing, understand why (intention) the movement is being carried out, to help the brain later imitate or mimic the movement, and last, to help understand the emotions of the one being observed.

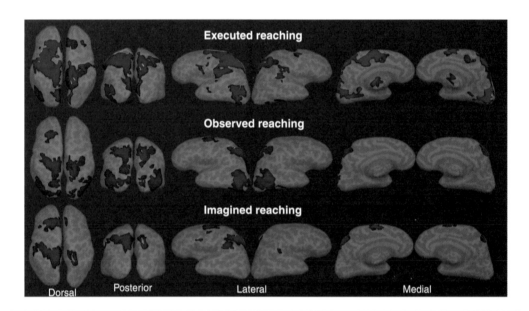

Figure 9.8 • A comparison of motor imagery and observation to actual movement. Each fMRI represents a pooled set of data from 15 subjects who are reaching for an object, with the lighter areas representing areas of brain activation. On the **top** are fMRI images during the actual reaching movement. In the **middle** traces, the subjects are watching the reaching movement being performed. In the **bottom** traces, the subjects are only imaging the movement. The active areas that overlap across the three conditions are suggested to be areas where mirror neurons are housed. (Reprinted from Filimon, F., Nelson, J., Hagler, D., & Sereno, M. (2007). Human cortical representations for reaching: Mirror neurons for execution, observation, and imagery. *Neuroimage*, *37*(4), 1315–1328, with permission from Elsevier.)

Imagery

Imagery is most often thought of as the mental or cognitive rehearsal of a skill, generally in the form of visualization (seeing the skill in one's mind) or imagery (imagining multiple sensory aspects of the skill, not just the visual). Imagery is used for two general purposes, (1) skill acquisition and (2) performance preparation. Skill acquisition typically involves the learner modeling the motor skill in their own mind over and over again. Learners may emphasize certain problem areas or emphasize the look or feel of the movement, depending on what is meaningful to them. Imagery without physical practice is only marginally successful, whereas physical practice with imagery is generally better than physical practice alone (Anwar et al., 2011; McEwen et al., 2009).

Imagery used for performance preparation is either rehearsal for a sequence of events (e.g., a gymnastics routine) or arousal modification. Rehearsal may include going over the entire performance, as in seeing the whole pattern of tactics and strategies during a game, or may emphasize one particular point in a discrete skill, like ball contact during baseball batting. Arousal modification can be some form of psyching up to increase arousal or relaxation to lower arousal. Using imagery as a stress control technique should include some form of problem solving, which is one way to focus attention on important matters while reducing anxiety. Whether using imagery for rehearsal or arousal, the result may be enhanced confidence, anxiety reduction, and more focused attention.

TECHNIQUES FOR IMAGING

There are three general characteristics that are a part of the imagery process. They are the *perspective* (internal, external), the *viewing angle*, and the *dominant sensory modality* (e.g., kinesthetic vs. visual). In the internal perspective, the person views himself in the first person as he would in real life. In the external, or third-person, perspective, the person views himself from out of body. The viewing angle is what is actually included in the mind's picture, for example, from the top or from the back in a third-person view, or the view of what the first-person image is looking at. Viewing angle appears to be largely dependent on the motor skill being imaged. The third factor in imagery is the dominant sensory modality. Imagers tend to emphasize either visual or kinesthetic information, even if sound and other sensory information is included. Regardless of which combination of perspective, angle, or sensory modality is imaged, there is growing belief that "agency" is critical as to how the brain is activated. Agency refers to the identity of the actual imaged person. Imagers may see themselves or others performing. Even if the imager takes on a first person perspective, but takes on the identity of someone else (e.g., a popular athlete), then the imager may not be in full control of her actions.

Holmes and Calmels (2008) summarized that identifying the best way to image, or the imaging characteristics of expert performers, has proven difficult due to methodological problems and the lack of consistent results. In particular, image perspective, view, and agency, as well as imagery clarity and vividness, may differ widely even in high-level athletes. These authors assert that imagery is generally so focused on the precise motor behavior of the performer that the social context is lost, which compromises the neural functional equivalence. Imagery scripts, thus, must have contextual information with intent for the most effectiveness.

THE NEUROSCIENCE OF IMAGERY

Like observational learning, mental imaging of motor actions has direct neurological implications. The same areas of the brain are active in similar manners during imaging a task as when actually performing the task. Magnetic resonance imaging and other brain scanning methods have shown that real and imagined movements share a common physiological substrate, but changing agency, perspective, viewing angle, and sensory modality changes areas of the brain that are active. Some researchers have shown that reflex excitability is increased when imaging a muscle or movement, suggesting that thinking about movements causes a spinal cord facilitatory effect on muscle activation. Care must be taken in interpreting these data, however, as the relationship between actual and imagined movements differ between skilled and unskilled performers and with an uncertain rationale for why (see Fig. 9.9). Holmes and Calmels (2008) cautioned that brain activity due to real or imagined movements may not be functionally equivalent.

Intention as the Basis for Mental Practice

From the prior sections, it is evident that the characteristics of imaging and observation activate the brain in ways that are profound and specific. A summary comparing observation and imagery characteristics is presented in Figure 9.10. These findings imply that to receive the desired physiological or motor response, the nature of the mental activity should be specific toward that response.

A number of studies support this view. Albeit somewhat controversial, there are studies showing that weeks of mental imaging of weight lifting improves muscle strength. Studies showing effective mental strength training (Ranganathan et al., 2004; Yue & Cole, 1992) have used a first-person perspective with external focus imagery in which the movement outcome, like moving an attached force transducer or lifting a table, is the intention. Such improvements have been ascribed to better central commands that are able to provide more activation and more efficient inter- and intra muscle coordination. The key finding from these imagery studies is that the essential ingredient to the mental training is intention.

■ Thinking It Through 9.3 Psyching Up

"Psyching up" is as a mental preparation strategy used right before and during games, practice, or training. Psyching up generally refers to increasing mental and physical arousal, but may also refer to any action designed to ready the mind (with or without the body) with a situation-appropriate mental state. Thus, psyching up may include some measure of relaxation, focused attention, or a change in thought processes with positive self-talk. With your understanding of information processing, intentionality, and mental practice, outline a psyching up strategy for soccer goalkeeper facing a penalty shot, a quarterback going on the field during a 2-minute drill, and a high school student taking her driver's test.

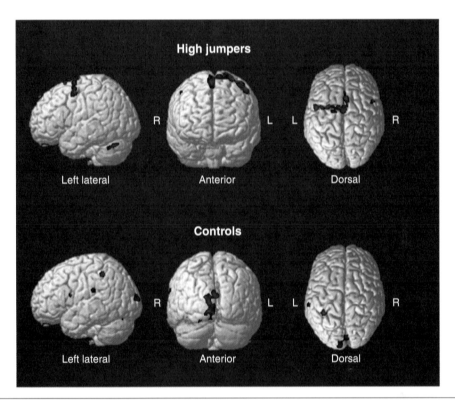

Figure 9.9 • Motor imagery and experience. In these fMRI images, experienced high jumpers and novice subjects were imaging a high-jump task. The experienced jumpers displayed vastly different areas of brain activation, primarily by activation of motor and sensory areas versus the novices whose activation mostly in the visual areas. These data demonstrate that practice and experience have contributed to the experts doing the task in vastly different manners. (Reprinted from Olsson, C., Jonsson, B., Larsson, A., & Nyberg, L. (2008). Motor representations and practice affect brain systems underlying imagery: An FMRI study of internal imagery in novices and active high jumpers. *The Open Neuroimaging Journal, 2,* 5–13, with permission.)

CREATING THE ENVIRONMENT FOR PRACTICE AND TRAINING

Knowing how to create a training environment based on dynamic systems theory, discovery learning, and deliberate practice seems to be a daunting task. Yet, some authors have laid out straightforward guidelines to implement these programs. Passos et al. (2008) introduced a four-stage "nonlinear peda-gogical methodology" to develop tactical and decision-making skills. These stages are (1) identifying the problem, (2) setting out a strategy, (3) creating an action model, and (4) building an exercise for practice. Ives and Shelley (2003) previously laid out a similar four-step process they termed *psychophysi-cal training*, specifically designed for the development of sport-specific strength and power training (see Chapter 12). The goal of psychophysical training is to maximize the transferability of physiological adaptations to sport settings. These guidelines focus on the functional training goal of bringing the sit-uational needs and constraints of real-life activities into the training environment to enhance training effectiveness. Some researchers (Bobbert & Van Soest, 1994; Voigt & Klausen, 1990) have reported that simply improving strength may not lead to enhanced power or speed of complex movements unless an athlete undergoes task-solving practice with their newly enhanced muscle strength. Thus, the athlete must blend the training with the right environmental and task constraints. This environment includes

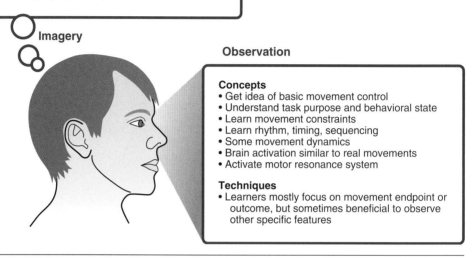

Figure 9.10 • Schematic illustration comparing imagery and observation.

many psychophysical elements that are specific to individual sports. According to the tenets of psychophysical training, altering movement intent and attention elements is a starting point for manipulating the cognitive environment necessary for enhancing the opportunity for sport-specific physiological adaptations to take place.

A number of researchers have used similar guidelines with a high level of success. For example, Hewett et al. (1996) reported remarkable improvements in teenage girls' (volleyball players) jump height and power. These authors, using basic plyometric and jumping type exercises, emphasized biomechanical form over maximal physical effort. To improve jumping form, they used verbal cues, feedback, and mental preparation of the athletes. Following training, these researchers found changes in neural coordination that they linked to improvements in injury prevention mechanisms. These improvements were far more than what is normally seen after a standard training program, and can likely be attributed to the unique training method used. Their plyometric training was more than just physiological effort. They used structured jumping and landing practice, emphasized on technique, and used verbal and visual cues.

SUMMARY

In this chapter, the basic guidelines for organizing the practice environment and ways to provide instruction to learners were presented. Based on the principles of dynamic systems theory, constraints-led instruction, discovery learning, and deliberate practice, five essential features of practice were identified. These features are (1) a specific intention to improve and master the skill, (2) a strong motivation and effort, (3) individual-based practice and learner control over practice, (4) effective communication and information, and (5) overlearning with variation.

Combining discovery learning tenets with deliberate practice provides a strong theoretical and practical framework for conducting practice based on focusing practice toward individual needs while promoting individual exploration of movement solutions. Movement solutions must be relevant to environmental, task, and individual constraints as indicated by the systems theory. The role of the instructor in creating the most effective learning environment is essential to this process, and is very difficult.

Mental practice, in the form of observation and imagery, is an important aspect to the structure of practice. When done with intentionality, observation and imaging result in neurological activity that is suggested to promote direct physiological adaptations necessary for improved performance.

The ideas presented in this chapter, particularly discovery learning and deliberate practice, are not new. Performers, coaches, and instructors for centuries have used these principles, which have now been formalized and streamlined based on research findings. These principles apply not only to improving motor skill performance but also in improving the fundamental physiological abilities through training. The concepts of feedback, intention, attention, effort and motivation, scheduling, and competent instruction are just as applicable in the training setting.

STUDY QUESTIONS

1. Define, and briefly describe, the basic concepts of discovery learning, constraints-led instruction, and deliberate practice.
2. Define, describe, and compare constraints and affordances.
3. Describe the five essential features of effective practice. Provide examples how an instructor might implement these features in the practice microstructure.
4. Describe the differences between mastery and performance goals. Which is better to guide the learning process and why?
5. Motivation and effort are considered feature of effective practice. Describe.
6. Give examples of a learner-based practice environment.
7. Define the ways and methods in which AFB can be provided. Summarize the basic guidelines for providing AFB.
8. According to Ericsson's deliberate practice theory, what are the barriers working against engaging in deliberate practice and obtaining expert levels of performance?
9. According to deliberate practice theory, what are the critical elements of the deliberate practice microstructure?
10. What does Bernstein's statement "repetition without repeating" mean? Use this concept to describe why variability is a trait of high-level performers. Explain why variable practice and contextual inference result in better learning than blocked practice.
11. What is biofeedback, and what are the most popular forms of biofeedback?
12. Describe and discuss the four steps to psychophysical training. As part of your answer, select a motor skill, which can be a specific skill component in a sport, and complete the steps to psychophysical training.
13. Discovery learning is understood to provide the best way for learning to occur. If this is the case, why is the instructor important? As part of your answer, detail what makes for a good instructor or coach.
14. Name five components of mental practice.
15. What should be the purposes of imagery and observation?
16. What do brain scans during imagery reveal?
17. Explain the motor resonance system and observation. What information is picked up during observation?

Bibliography

Ahmetov, I., & Rogozkin, V. (2009). Genes, athlete status and training—An overview. *Medicine and Sport Science*, *54*, 43–71.

Anwar, M., Tomi, N., & Ito, K. (2011). Motor imagery facilitates force field learning. *Brain Research*, *1395*, 21–29.

Ashford, D., Bennett, S., & Davids, K. (2006). Observational modeling effects for movement dynamics and movement outcome measures across differing task constraints: A meta-analysis. *Journal of Motor Behavior*, *38*(3), 185–205.

Ashford, D., Davids, K., & Bennett, S. (2007). Developmental effects influencing observational modelling: A meta-analysis. *Journal of Sports Sciences*, *25*(5), 547–558.

Baker, J. J., Cote, J. J., & Abernethy, B. B. (2003a). Sport-specific practice and the development of expert decision-making in team ball sports. *Journal of Applied Sport Psychology*, *15*(1), 12–25.

Baker, J. J., Horton, S. S., Robertson-Wilson, J. J., & Wall, M. M. (2003b). Nurturing sport expertise: Factors influencing the development of elite athlete. *Journal of Sports Science and Medicine*, *2*(1), 1–9.

Bernstein, N. A. (1967). *The co-ordination and regulation of movements*. Oxford, England: Pergamon Press.

Bertram, C. P., Marteniuk, R. G., & Guadagnoli, M. A. (2007). On the use and misuse of video analysis. *International Journal of Sports Science and Coaching*, *2*, 37–46.

Bobbert, M., & Van Soest, A. (1994). Effects of muscle strengthening on vertical jump height: A simulation study. *Medicine and Science in Sports and Exercise*, *26*(8), 1012–1020.

Boiché, J. S., & Sarrazin, P. G. (2009). Proximal and distal factors associated with dropout versus maintained participation in organized sport. *Journal of Sports Science & Medicine*, *8*(1), 9–16.

Bouchard, C. C., Malina, R. M., & Perusse, L. L. (1997). Genes and high-performance sports. In *Genetics of fitness and physical performance* (pp. 365–371). Champaign, IL: Human Kinetics.

Buchanan, J., & Wang, C. (2012). Overcoming the guidance effect in motor skill learning: Feedback all the time can be beneficial. *Experimental Brain Research*, *219*(2), 305–320.

Côté, J., Baker, J., & Abernethy, B. (2007). Play and practice in the development of sport expertise. In G. Tenenbaum & R. C. Eklund (Eds.) *Handbook of sport psychology* (pp. 184–202). New York: Wiley.

Côté, J. J., Baker, J. J., & Abernethy, B. B. (2003). From play to practice: A developmental framework for the acquisition of expertise in team sports. In J. L. Starkes & K. A. Ericsson (Eds.) *Expert performance in sports: Advances in research on sport expertise* (pp. 85–87, 89–113, 414–416). Champaign, IL: Human Kinetics.

Crowell, H., Milner, C., Hamill, J., & Davis, I. (2010). Reducing impact loading during running with the use of real-time visual feedback. *The Journal of Orthopaedic and Sports Physical Therapy*, *40*(4), 206–213.

Davids, K., & Baker, J. (2007). Genes, environment and sport performance: Why the nature-nurture dualism is no longer relevant. *Sports Medicine*, *37*(11), 961–980.

Davids, K., Button, C., & Bennett, S. (2008). *Dynamics of skill acquisition: A constraints-led approach*. Champaign, IL: Human Kinetics.

Davids, K., Glazier, P., Araújo, D., & Bartlett, R. (2003). Movement systems as dynamical systems: The functional role of variability and its implications for sports medicine. *Sports Medicine*, *33*(4), 245–260.

Elliot, A. J., & Church, M. A. (1997). A hierarchical model of approach and avoidance achievement motivation. *Journal of Personality and Social Psychology*, *72*, 218–232.

Ericsson, K. (2007). Deliberate practice and the modifiability of body and mind: Toward a science of the structure and acquisition of expert and elite performance. *International Journal of Sport Psychology*, *38*(1), 4–34.

Ericsson, K. A., Krampe, R. T., & Tesch-Romer, C. C. (1993). The role of deliberate practice in the acquisition of expert performance. *Psychological Review*, *100*(3), 363–406.

Ericsson, K., & Lehmann, A. (1996). Expert and exceptional performance: Evidence of maximal adaptation to task constraints. *Annual Review of Psychology*, *47*, 273–305.

Eston, R., Stansfield, R., Westoby, P., & Parfitt, G. (2012). Effect of deception and expected exercise duration on psychological and physiological variables during treadmill running and cycling. *Psychophysiology*, *49*(4), 462–469.

Fajen, B. R., Riley, M. A., & Turvey, M. T. (2009). Information, affordances, and the control of action in sport. *International Journal of Sport Psychology*, *40*(1), 79–107.

Ford, P., Coughlan, E., & Williams, M. (2009). The expert-performance approach as a framework for understanding and enhancing coaching performance, expertise, and learning. *International Journal of Sports Science and Coaching*, 4(3), 451–463.

Fuelscher, I., Ball, K., & Macmahon, C. (2012). Perspectives on learning styles in motor and sport skills. *Frontiers in Psychology*, 3, 69. doi: 10.3389/fpsyg.2012.

Gibbons, T., Hill, R., McConnell, A., Forster, T., & Moore, J. (2002). *The path to excellence: A comprehensive view of development of U.S. Olympians who competed from 1984–1998*. United States Olympic Committee.

Gibson, J. J. (1977). The theory of affordances. In R. Shaw & J. Bransford (Eds.) *Perceiving, acting and knowing* (pp. 67–82). Hillsdale, NJ: Erlbaum.

Gilbert, W., Cote, J., & Mallett, C. (2006). Developmental paths and activities of successful sport coaches. *International Journal of Sports Science and Coaching*, 1(1), 69–76.

Gilbert, W., Lichtenwaldt, L., Gilbert, J., Zelezny, L., & Côté, J. (2009). Developmental profiles of successful high school coaches. *International Journal of Sports Science and Coaching*, 4(3), 415–431.

Greeno, J. G. (1994). Gibson's affordances. *Psychological Review*, 101(2), 336–342.

Gruzelier, J., Egner, T., & Vernon, D. (2006). Validating the efficacy of neurofeedback for optimising performance. *Progress in Brain Research*, 159, 421–431.

Guadagnoli, M., & Lee, T. (2004). Challenge point: A framework for conceptualizing the effects of various practice conditions in motor learning. *Journal of Motor Behavior*, 36(2), 212–224.

Hall, K., Domingues, D., & Cavazos, R. (1994). Contextual interference effects with skilled baseball players. *Perceptual and Motor Skills*, 78(3 Pt 1), 835–841.

Halvorsen, K., Eriksson, M., & Gullstrand, L. (2012). Acute effects of reducing vertical displacement and step frequency on running economy. *Journal of Strength and Conditioning Research*, 26(8), 2065–2070.

Hampson, D., St Clair Gibson, A., Lambert, M., Dugas, J., Lambert, E., & Noakes, T. (2004). Deception and perceived exertion during high-intensity running bouts. *Perceptual and Motor Skills*, 98(3 Pt 1), 1027–1038.

Handford, C. (2006). Serving up variability and stability. In K. Davids, S. Bennett, & K. M. Newell (Eds.) *Movement system variability* (pp. 73–84). Champaign, IL: Human Kinetics.

Handford, C., Davids, K., Bennett, S., & Button, C. (1997). Skill acquisition in sport: Some applications of an evolving practice ecology. *Journal of Sports Sciences*, 15(6), 621–640.

Helsen, W. F., Starkes, J. L., & Hodges, N. J. (1998). Team sports and the theory of deliberate practice. *Journal of Sport & Exercise Psychology*, 20(1), 12–34.

Hewett, T. E., Stroupe, A. L., Nance, T. A., & Noyes, F. R. (1996). Plyometric training in female athletes: Decreased impact forces and increased hamstring torques. *American Journal of Sports Medicine*, 24(6), 765–773.

Hodges, N. J., Chua, R. R., & Franks, I. M. (2003). The role of video in facilitating perception and action of a novel coordination movement. *Journal of Motor Behavior*, 35(3), 247–260.

Hodges, N., & Franks, I. (2002). Modelling coaching practice: The role of instruction and demonstration. *Journal of Sports Sciences*, 20(10), 793–811.

Hodges, N., Williams, A., Hayes, S., & Breslin, G. (2007). What is modelled during observational learning? *Journal of Sports Sciences*, 25(5), 531–545.

Holmes, P., & Calmels, C. (2008). A neuroscientific review of imagery and observation use in sport. *Journal of Motor Behavior*, 40(5), 433–445.

Hristovski, R., Davids, K., Araujo, D., & Passos, P. (2011). Constraints-induced emergence of functional novelty in complex neurobiological systems: A basis for creativity in sport. *Nonlinear Dynamics, Psychology, and Life Sciences*, 15(2), 175–206.

Ives, J., & Shelley, G. (2003). Psychophysics in functional strength and power training: Review and implementation framework. *Journal of Strength and Conditioning Research*, 17(1), 177–186.

Janelle, C. M., Barba, D. A., Frehlich, S. G., Tennant, L. K., & Cauraugh, J. H. (1997). Maximizing performance feedback effectiveness through videotape replay and a self-controlled learning environment. *Research Quarterly for Exercise and Sport*, 68(4), 269–279.

Janelle, C. M., Champenoy, J. D., Coombes, S. A., & Mousseau, M. B. (2003). Mechanisms of attentional cueing during observational learning to facilitate motor skill acquisition. *Journal of Sports Sciences*, 21(10), 825–838.

Jones, L., & French, K. (2007). Effects of contextual interference on acquisition and retention of three volleyball skills. *Perceptual and Motor Skills*, *105*(3 Pt 1), 883–890.

Magill, R. A. (2007). *Motor learning and control. Concepts and applications* (8th ed.). Boston, MA: McGraw Hill.

Magill, R. A., & Hall, K. G. (1990). A review of the contextual interference effect in motor skill acquisition. *Human Movement Science*, *9*(3–5), 241–289.

McEwen, S., Huijbregts, M., Ryan, J., & Polatajko, H. (2009). Cognitive strategy use to enhance motor skill acquisition post-stroke: A critical review. *Brain Injury*, *23*(4), 263–277.

Memmert, D., Baker, J., & Bertsch, C. (2010). Play and practice in the development of sport-specific creativity in team ball sports. *High Ability Studies*, *21*(1), 3–18.

Metsios, G. G., Flouris, A. A., Koutedakis, Y. Y., & Theodorakis, Y. Y. (2006). The effect of performance feedback on cardiorespiratory fitness field tests: Technical note. *Journal of Science and Medicine in Sport*, *9*(3), 263–266.

Nash, C. S., Sproule, J., Callan, M., McDonald, K., & Cassidy, T. (2009). Career development of expert coaches. *International Journal of Sports Science and Coaching*, *4*(1), 121–138.

Nash, C. S., Sproule, J., & Horton, P. (2011). Excellence in coaching: The art and skill of elite practitioners. *Research Quarterly For Exercise and Sport*, *82*(2), 229–238.

Newell, K. M. (2007). Kinesiology: Challenges of multiple agendas. *Quest*, *59*(1), 5–24.

Newell, K. M. (1986). Constraints on the development of coordination. In M. G. Wade & H. T. A. Whiting (Eds.) *Motor development in children. Aspects of coordination and control* (pp. 341–360). Dordrecht, Netherlands: Martinus Nijhoff.

Noehren, B., Scholz, J., & Davis, I. (2011). The effect of real-time gait retraining on hip kinematics, pain and function in subjects with patellofemoral pain syndrome. *British Journal of Sports Medicine*, *45*(9), 691–696.

Orrell, A. J., Eves, F. F., & Masters, R. W. (2006). Implicit motor learning of a balancing task. *Gait & Posture*, *23*(1), 9–16.

Parsons, J., & Alexander, M. (2012). Modifying spike jump landing biomechanics in female adolescent volleyball athletes using video and verbal feedback. *Journal of Strength and Conditioning Research*, *26*(4), 1076–1084.

Passmore, J. (2010). A grounded theory study of the coaching experience: The implications for training and practice in coaching psychology. *International Coaching Psychology Review*, *5*(1), 48–62.

Passos, P., Araújo, D., Davids, K., & Shuttleworth, R. (2008). Manipulating constraints to train decision making in rugby union. *International Journal of Sports Science and Coaching*, *3*(1), 125–140.

Peh, S., Chow, J., & Davids, K. (2011). Focus of attention and its impact on movement behaviour. *Journal of Science and Medicine in Sport*, *14*(1), 70–78.

Pinder, R., Davids, K., Renshaw, I., & Araújo, D. (2011a). Manipulating informational constraints shapes movement reorganization in interceptive actions. *Attention, Perception & Psychophysics*, *73*(4), 1242–1254.

Pinder, R. A., Renshaw, I., Davids, K., & Kerhervé, H. (2011b). Principles for the use of ball projection machines in elite and developmental sport programmes. *Sports Medicine*, *41*(10), 793–800.

Pinder, R., Renshaw, I., & Davids, K. (2009). Information-movement coupling in developing cricketers under changing ecological practice constraints. *Human Movement Science*, *28*(4), 468–479.

Post, P. G., Fairbrother, J. T., & Barros, J. C. (2011). Self-controlled amount of practice benefits learning of a motor skill. *Research Quarterly for Exercise and Sport*, *82*(3), 474–481.

Raab, M., Masters, R. W., Maxwell, J., Arnold, A., Schlapkohl, N., & Poolton, J. (2009). Discovery learning in sports: Implicit or explicit processes? *International Journal of Sport and Exercise Psychology*, *7*(4), 413–430.

Ranganathan, V., Siemionow, V., Liu, J., Sahgal, V., & Yue, G. (2004). From mental power to muscle power—gaining strength by using the mind. *Neuropsychologia*, *42*(7), 944–956.

Reid, M., Crespo, M., Lay, B., & Berry, J. (2007). Skill acquisition in tennis: Research and current practice. *Journal of Science and Medicine in Sport*, *10*(1), 1–10.

Renshaw, I., Davids, K., Shuttleworth, R., & Jia Yi, C. (2009). Insights from ecological psychology and dynamical systems. Theory can underpin a philosophy of coaching. *International Journal of Sport Psychology*, *40*(4), 580–602.

Renshaw, I., Oldham, T., Davids, K., & Golds, T. (2007). Changing ecological constraints of practice alters coordination of dynamic interceptive actions. *European Journal of Sports Sciences*, 7, 157–167.

Roberts, G. C. (2001). Understanding the dynamics of motivation in physical activity: The influence of achievement goals on motivational processes. In G.C. Roberts (Ed.) *Advances in motivation in sport and exercise* (pp. 1–50). Champaign, IL: Human Kinetics.

Roberts, G. C., Treasure, D. C., & Kavassanu, M. (1997). Motivation in physical activity contexts: An achievement goal perspective. In P. Pintrich & M. Maehr (Eds.) *Advances in motivation and achievement* (pp. 413–447). Stamford, CT: JAI Press.

Rucci, J., & Tomporowski, P. (2010). Three types of kinematic feedback and the execution of the hang power clean. *Journal of Strength and Conditioning Research*, 24(3), 771–778.

Salmoni, A., Schmidt, R., & Walter, C. (1984). Knowledge of results and motor learning: A review and critical reappraisal. *Psychological Bulletin*, 95(3), 355–386.

Segerståhl, K., & Oinas-Kukkonen, H. (2011). Designing personal exercise monitoring employing multiple modes of delivery: Implications from a qualitative study on heart rate monitoring. *International Journal of Medical Informatics*, 80(12), e203–e213.

Sheaves, E., Snodgrass, S., & Rivett, D. (2012). Learning lumbar spine mobilization: The effects of frequency and self-control of feedback. *Journal of Orthopaedic and Sports Physical Therapy*, 42(2), 114–124.

Sidaway, B., Bates, J., Occhiogrosso, B., Schlagenhaufer, J., & Wilkes, D. (2012). Interaction of feedback frequency and task difficulty in children's motor skill learning. *Physical Therapy*, 92(7), 948–957.

Skjesol, K., & Halvari, H. (2005). Motivational climate, achievement goals, perceived sport competence, and involvement in physical activity: Structural and mediator models. *Perceptual and Motor Skills*, 100(2), 497–523.

Smeeton, N., Williams, A., Hodges, N., & Ward, P. (2005). The relative effectiveness of various instructional approaches in developing anticipation skill. *Journal of Experimental Psychology. Applied*, 11(2), 98–110.

Smith, R. M., & Loschner, C. C. (2002). Biomechanics feedback for rowing. *Journal of Sports Sciences*, 20(10), 783–791.

Stoate, I., Wulf, G., & Lewthwaite, R. (2012). Enhanced expectancies improve efficiency in runners. *Journal of Sports Sciences*, 30, 815–823.

Travlos, A. K. (2010). Specificity and variability of practice, and contextual interference in acquisition and transfer of an underhand volleyball serve. *Perceptual and Motor Skills*, 110(1), 298–312.

Tremblay, L., & Proteau, L. (1998). Specificity of practice: The case of powerlifting. *Research Quarterly for Exercise and Sport*, 69(3), 284–289.

Valentini, N. C., & Rudisill, M. E. (2004). An inclusive mastery climate intervention and the motor skill development of children with and without disabilities. *Adapted Physical Activity Quarterly*, 21(4), 330–347.

Vereijken, B., & Whiting, H. (1990). In defence of discovery learning. *Canadian Journal of Sport Sciences*, 15(2), 99–106.

Vereijken, B., Whiting, H., & Beek, W. (1992). A dynamical systems approach to skill acquisition. *The Quarterly Journal of Experimental Psychology. A, Human Experimental Psychology*, 45(2), 323–344.

Vernon, D. (2005). Can neurofeedback training enhance performance? An evaluation of the evidence with implications for future research. *Applied Psychophysiology and Biofeedback*, 30(4), 347–364

Voigt, M., & Klausen, K. (1990). Changes in muscle strength and speed of an unloaded movement after various training programmes. *European Journal of Applied Physiology and Occupational Physiology*, 60(5), 370–376.

Wackerhage, H., Miah, A., Harris, R. C., Montgomery, H. E., & Williams, A. G. (2009). Genetic research and testing in sport and exercise science: A review of the issues. *Journal of Sports Sciences*, 27(11), 1109–1116.

Wall, M., & Côté, J. (2007). Developmental activities that lead to dropout and investment in sport. *Physical Education & Sport Pedagogy*, 12(1), 77–87.

Ward, P., Hodges, N. J., Starkes, J. L., & Williams, M. A. (2007). The road to excellence: Deliberate practice and the development of expertise. *High Ability Studies*, 18(2), 119–153.

Williams, A., & Ford, P. (2009). Promoting a skills-based agenda in Olympic sports: The role of skill-acquisition specialists. *Journal of Sports Sciences*, *27*(13), 1381–1392.

Wu, W. W., & Magill, R. A. (2011). Allowing learners to choose: Self-controlled practice schedules for learning multiple movement patterns. *Research Quarterly for Exercise and Sport*, *82*(3), 449–457.

Wulf, G. (2007). Self-controlled practice enhances motor learning: Implications for physiotherapy. *Physiotherapy*, *93*(2), 96–101.

Wulf, G., Shea, C., & Lewthwaite, R. (2010). Motor skill learning and performance: A review of influential factors. *Medical Education*, *44*(1), 75–84.

Yue, G., & Cole, K. (1992). Strength increases from the motor program: Comparison of training with maximal voluntary and imagined muscle contractions. *Journal of Neurophysiology*, *67*(5), 1114–1123.

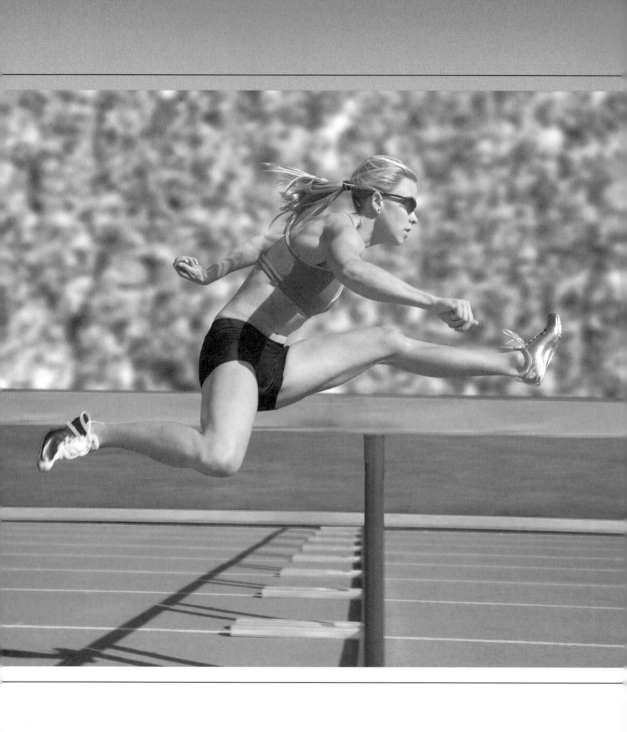

III

Training Mind, Body, and Brain

Throughout Units I and II we examined the fundamental physiological and psychological concepts behind the formation, execution, and learning of motor skills. In Unit III we explore these concepts as they relate to the underlying abilities contributing to motor skill production. Specifically, we emphasize postural control mechanisms and functional training.

10 | Postural Control Mechanisms

PURPOSE, IMPORTANCE, AND OBJECTIVES OF THIS CHAPTER

The purpose of this chapter is to examine postural control as a system that maintains body integrity and provides a foundational system supporting the execution of goal-directed movements. The nature and mechanisms of postural control exemplify psychological and physiological systems working in tandem and highlight the need to consider both systems when addressing postural control issues and motor skills in general.

After reading this chapter, you should be able to:

1. Define and describe muscle tone and its role in postural control and the relationships among tone, postural control, and skilled movement.
2. Explain the role of neural and biomechanical systems in regulating muscle tone and how each plays a role in the specific functions of tone.
3. Define and describe postural control, particularly in reference to the concepts of alignment and stability.
4. Discuss the contributions of sensory/reflexive systems, neuromuscular components, musculomechanical components, and CNS components in producing postural control.
5. Determine the reflexive, autonomic, voluntary levels of postural control during movements.
6. Define and explain reactive and proactive postural control, including anticipatory postural adjustments.
7. Compare and contrast posture and balance measurement tools.

The overt and observable execution of a motor skill hides the fact that much of the muscle actions and movements that underlie the skill go unnoticed. Like an iceberg with a massive support structure hidden under the water, the observable motor skill relies on muscles working behind the scenes to maintain postural control. **Postural control** is defined as the maintenance of body alignment and spatial orientation in order to put the body in a position to enable effective movement. The outcomes of postural control are stability and biomechanical alignment, which are necessary for effective motor skill execution as well as maintaining integrity of the musculoskeletal structures. The importance of training postural control has reached the popular fitness and sport settings but with little understanding and little scientific backing for training rationale. In this chapter, we look at the neuromuscular and psychological aspects of postural control and stability and alignment as outcomes of postural control. In Chapter 11, we examine postural control in health and performance. First it is necessary to define and examine muscle tone, as tone is essential to the maintenance of postural control.

MUSCLE TONE

Even when not contracting to make overt movements, muscle tissue has important roles in body functioning. Some of these roles are served by the maintenance of **muscle tone**. The definition of muscle tone is more straightforward than implied by fitness training centers that advertise "toning and sculpting." Muscle tone refers simply to the force with which the muscle resists lengthening, that is, its stiffness. High tone means the muscle is stiff and resistant to stretch; low tone means the muscle is compliant and stretches easily. Muscle stiffness is in a constant state of flux, and both high and low stiffness can be desirable at times.

Muscle tone serves to maintain a *base level of postural control*, to *regulate the storage and release of elastic energy* and to *regulate force dampening*. In maintaining postural control, stiffness of the relevant muscles are set to resist lengthening, thus limiting the sway amount or stiffening body segments and joints. This background level of activity, called *postural tone*, serves as a baseline level necessary for function during rest and activity. For example, along the length of the spine, the small paraspinal muscles like the intertransverse and interspinalis muscles are stiffened to maintain integrity of the vertebral column even during rest (Ebenbichler et al., 2001; see Fig. 10.1).

As we saw in previous chapters, the muscle elastic elements store and release force. This is notably evident in walking and running and serves to make movement more efficient. Altering tone is one way to regulate the amount of energy stored and released. For example, during running, the lower leg muscles stiffens to better and faster transmit force from the muscles to the ground and take advantage of the stretch–shorten cycle (Dumke et al., 2010; Sasaki & Neptune, 2006). In Figure 10.2 are landing sequence diagrams with the low and the high muscle tone in calf muscles. A compliant muscle is unable to prevent excessive ankle dorsiflexion, resulting in the heel crashing down with high-impact forces that are transmitted throughout the skeletal system. In contrast, calf muscles with high stiffness prevent the heel from hitting the ground and absorb the stretch forces for use in a plantar flexion recoil movement. Coinciding with the regulation of energy storage and release, the elastic elements help dampen rough movements to smooth them out and make them less jerky. Altering tone stiffens or slackens the elastic elements, thus regulating the amount of dampening.

Muscle tone is dependent on two factors, (1) the *viscoelasticity* of the muscle and tendon elastic elements and (2) the level of neural activation of the contractile elements. The first factor, which contributes to *passive tone*, is a result of the intrinsic properties of the muscle–tendon complex. Large muscles with rigid connective tissue are generally stiffer and have greater passive tone. The second factor contributes to *active tone* and is based on the fact that a contracted muscle is stiffer than a relaxed muscle. For example, a chronic baseline level of neural excitability, which often coincides with a sensitive muscle spindle, creates more tone by slightly contracting the muscle tissue, which in turn tugs on the elastic elements. This spindle gain can be regulated by both spinal and supraspinal centers.

There is no "right" amount of tone other than that which supports effective and skilled posture and movement. Poorly coordinated motor skills do not automatically imply faulty tone. On the other

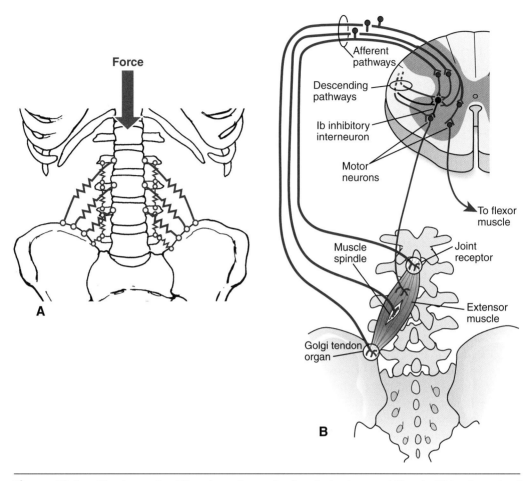

Figure 10.1 • Trunk muscle stiffness is used to maintain spinal column stability. **A.** This schematic of the vertebral column illustrates the inherent instability of the vertebral "tower," especially when subjected to forces. Moderate forces directly through the joint centers will minimally disrupt stability, but excessive and off-center forces may cause the spinal column to buckle. The surrounding connective tissue (ligaments, joint capsule) provide a measure of intrinsic support, but it is the musculature that enables dynamic stability under high loads. Here the muscles are shown to act as guy wires creating stability by maintaining levels of stiffness. Unbalanced stiffness may lead to spinal misalignment, but during dynamic situations, some unbalanced stiffness is necessary to enable movement. A base level of tone provides ongoing stability control and helps set reflex response characteristics. **B.** This schematic illustrates that reflex-based mechanisms are primarily responsible for maintaining stiffness and motion stability. Sensory signals arise from the paraspinal muscles, the disc, the vertebral joints (e.g., facet), and the capsule and ligaments. Reflex responses appear most strongly in the longissimus and multifidus muscles. (Reprinted from Holm, S. S., Indahl, A. A., & Solomonow, M. M. (2002). Sensorimotor control of the spine. *Journal of Electromyography & Kinesiology, 12*(3), 219–234, with permission from Elsevier.)

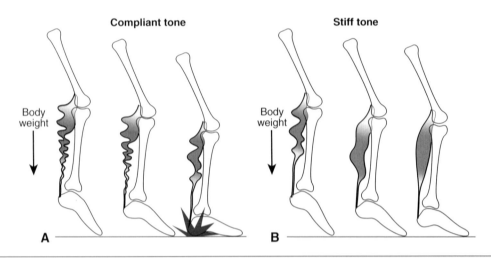

Figure 10.2 • Schematic of triceps surae muscle group with different levels of tone. **A.** The muscle complex is compliant, and thus, upon toe strike, the level of stiffness is too low to prevent a rapid ankle dorsiflexion and abrupt impact of the heel to the ground. **B.** There is a high level of tone present before toe strike, which prevents a rapid and long stretch of the triceps surae upon landing. Stretch force is absorbed, and heel impact is avoided.

hand, there are pathological conditions like upper motor neuron disease that may lead to conditions of excessive muscle tone (hypertonia) or too little tone (hypotonia). Other conditions, albeit not necessarily pathological, influence tone. Gender hormones, such as estrogen and progesterone, may lead to increased tissue elasticity in women (Burgess et al., 2010; Kubo et al., 2003). Decreased tendon stiffness may result from the biological aging process, but these changes are seen to be negative as a result of tissue degeneration (Magnusson et al., 2008). Increased temperature increases muscle elasticity; muscle damage from exercise or illness may stiffen the muscle–tendon mechanical properties or result in chronic neural activation. Disuse and atrophy and exercise history may further result in mechanical changes to the muscle–tendon complex (Magnusson et al., 2008).

■ Thinking It Through 10.1 Toning and Sculpting

Exercise programs are commonly advertised to "tone" and "sculpt." In this context, what do you think is meant by tone, or toning, and how do you think a toned body is obtained? Consider the role of flexibility training and strength training on muscle tone. After reading this section on muscle tone, what flaws do you see in the way that toning is advertised?

Postural Tone and Postural Control

The relationships among tone and posture and purposeful movement are like that of a human pyramid. As shown in Figure 10.3, the topmost person (Person 1) represents purposeful movement as he is preparing to jump and land. Person 1 is standing on the shoulders of Person 2, who represents postural control. Postural control must anticipate and dynamically change positions and alignment in order to provide a stable base from which Person 1 will jump. Moreover, Person 2 must provide reactive stability against the pushing forces of Person 1 as he jumps. Person 2, however, must be supported by Person 3, who represents postural tone. Purposeful movement will fail if either posture or tone is insufficient. Postural tone is set in advance, but it is not as dynamic or specific as postural control itself.

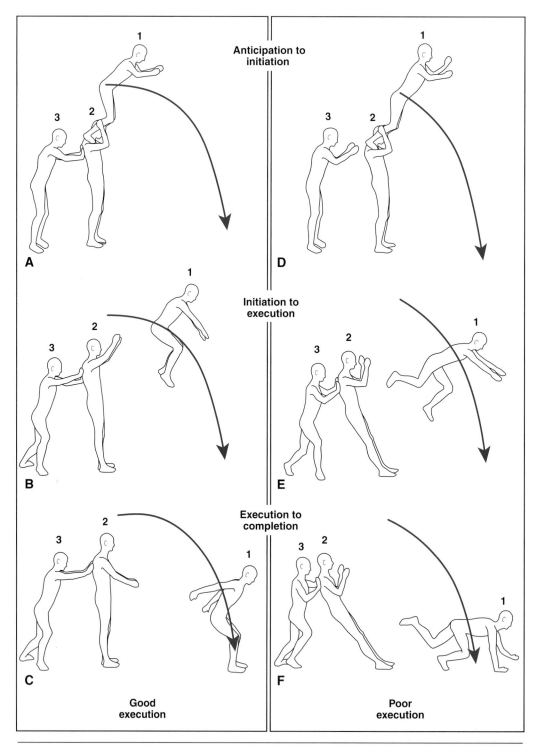

Figure 10.3 • The relationships among tone and posture and motor skills are illustrated here based on the original work of Walter Hess (see Stuart, 2005, for historical overview). In the left column, tone (3) and posture (2) work effectively, and the leap motor skill (1) can be executed effectively. Note in "**A**" that tone is set prior to the movement, and posture is also ready. In "**B**," tone is increased and posture helps in the movement, illustrating that the actions of posture can be very specific to the motor skill. In the second column, tone is unprepared (D,E,F), leading to poor postural control and, subsequently, a failed motor skill execution. See text for details.

POSTURAL CONTROL

As defined earlier, postural control maintains *body alignment* and *spatial orientation*. Alignment and orientation refer to positioning of our body segments and limbs to one another (alignment) and to the environment (orientation) at any given moment in time. It is an ongoing dynamic process aimed at creating stable positions that are ready for diverse actions regardless of the position or motion of the body. For example, good postural control allows one to maintain a stable position even during a disrupting external force, or enables an effective reach to a hand railing while falling. Spatial orientation has another purpose, and that is to maximize the available sensory information by placing our sensory systems into an effective configuration (Massion, 1998). In this regard, postural systems aim to keep the head upright to gather stable visual and vestibular information and to keep the feet on the ground to maximize body–ground referencing.

The common use of the term "posture" is often used synonymously with whole-body alignment, but this is misleading. Whole-body biomechanical alignment can be used synonymously with the term posture, but alignment also includes specific body segments, such as spinal alignment. Posture also includes a measure of spatial orientation, which is the positioning of the body to the environment. Thus, we may have slumped postures (alignment), prone and seated postures (orientation), and any number of combinations of alignment and orientation.

The primary outcome of alignment and orientation is stability. **Stability** is defined as a position that is resistant to disturbance or returns to its normal state after disruption (Pollock et al., 2000). For instance, each step in walking is a forward fall—a temporary state of instability leading back into a state of stability. Stability is a three-component interdependent system that includes whole-body stability, segmental stability, and joint stability. *Whole-body stability* orients the body to prevent or prepare for falls and is better known as *balance*. Equilibrium is a term used synonymously with balance and means that the forces acting on an object sum to zero. **Static balance** is defined as the ability to maintain the center of mass within the base of support during static or relatively steady body positions. Static balance circumstances include challenging body positions such as single leg stance and environmental challenges such as unstable support surfaces (Fig. 10.4). **Dynamic balance** is the ability to maintain the body in equilibrium during body movement, such as walking on slippery surfaces or controlled

---

| SIDE**NOTE** | **EVALUATING DIFFERENT POSTURES** |

The three basic posture orientations—standing, seated, and lying down—are often researched in different ways for different purposes. Standing posture is often the focus of motor control theory and computational biomechanics. Standing posture affords a rich exploration into the fundamental processes of whole-body coordination and interaction with the surrounding environment. Standing posture can be measured in numerous ways ranging from sophisticated to simple and qualitative to quantitative. Perhaps best of all, it is easy to manipulate standing posture to tease out motor control features and processes. Among these manipulations are biomechanical challenges (e.g., unstable support surfaces), physiological challenges (e.g., fatigue, single leg support), and psychological challenges (e.g., dual tasks, anxiety). On the other hand, seated and lying postures are most often viewed from rehabilitation and ergonomic standpoints. The reason for these approaches is that individuals in industrialized nations may spend the majority of their time in these postures that are now increasingly associated with musculoskeletal and psychosocial problems and associated health care costs and quality of life (Gallagher, 2005; O'Sullivan et al., 2011; Prins et al., 2008). The association between posture and health has some investigators and clinicians investigating non-Western postures, such as the squatting and kneeling postures used by many in the Arab countries that permit long duration use with minimal discomfort (Tetley, 2000).

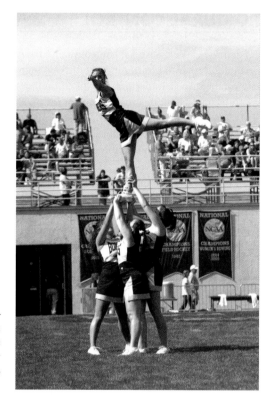

Figure 10.4 • Cheerleading routines are studies in postural control. The base positions and flyers require stabilization and orientation to the highest degree for aesthetics, safety, and motor skill execution. (Photo courtesy of Tim McKinney.)

landing from a jump. Because movement tends to destabilize the center of mass, dynamic balance may be termed controlled disequilibrium.

Segmental stability refers to the anchoring and stabilizing of body parts to provide a firm foundation upon which other body parts can move. Neutralizer, stabilizer, and fixator muscles play essential roles in segmental stability, such as the rhomboid muscles anchoring the scapula to prepare for arm movements. Segmental stability also prevents internal reactive forces from muscle actions to destabilize the rest of the body. *Joint stability* is dynamic process that maintains structural integrity of the joint while still permitting motion. Joint stability is not always considered an outcome of postural control because the joint has its own intrinsic mechanical stabilizers (e.g., ligaments, joint structure), but during dynamic and challenging situations, neuromuscular control plays an essential role in matching motion with stability.

Whole-body, segmental, and joint stability mechanisms are primarily distinguished by their primary purposes, but they do not work independently nor are their purposes singular. For instance, maintaining a balanced and stable upper body may serve to minimize destabilizing forces at the knee, thereby helping to maintain knee stability (McLean & Beaulieu, 2010). Similarly, segmental stabilization and positioning of the shoulder girdle may minimize damaging forces through the glenohumeral joint.

MECHANISMS OF POSTURAL CONTROL

Postural control actions involve many different systems with a fundamental goal to first provide stability against perturbations and, secondly, to minimize muscle activity (Kiemel et al., 2011). Figure 10.5 illustrates the contributions from sensory/reflexive systems, neuromuscular components,

Concepts in Action

From Research to Practice in Postural Control

Teasing out the mechanisms contributing to postural control takes a variety of different experimental paradigms and methodologies. Among the methods that continue to be used successfully is the introduction of a perturbation or destabilizing force to elicit a strong postural control action. Forces may be expected or unexpected and generated externally or internally. A. This experimental setup is designed to examine whole-body and segmental postural stability. The subject is blindfolded and headphoned to eliminate advance warning signals, EMG is gathered from trunk and leg muscles to assess whole-body postural actions, and EMG is gathered from the arms and shoulder girdle to assess segmental stability. A lightweight bucket is held out front while a weight above the bucket is held up by an electromagnet. The experimenter releases the weight without warning, causing an

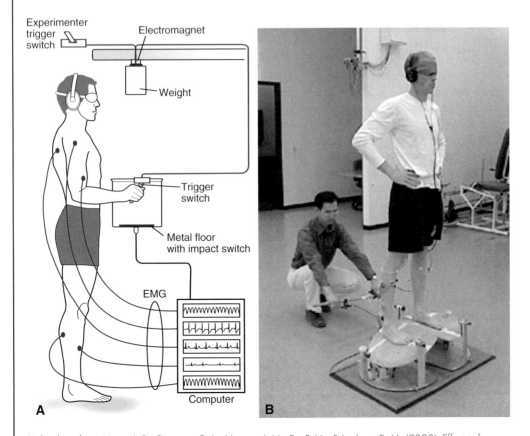

Right photo from Myers, J. B., Riemann, B. L., Hwang, J. H., Fu, F. H., & Lephart, S. M. (2003). Effects of peripheral afferent alteration of the lateral ankle ligaments on dynamic stability. *American Journal of Sports Medicine*, *31*(4), 498–506. Copyright 2003, American Orthopaedic Society for Sports Medicine. Reprinted by permission of SAGE Publications. (Bottom photo courtesy of Jeffrey C. Ives.)

continued on following page

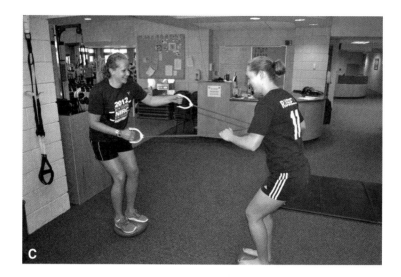

unexpected destabilizing force on the arms and whole body. Alternately, the subject may press a switch on the box to release the weight, thereby enabling preparation of the perturbation. Force plates and videography may be used to assess biomechanical outcomes. B. An experimental setup to look at joint stability by examining lower leg responses to ankle perturbations similar to the conditions causing an ankle inversion sprain. The subject's legs are instrumented with EMG to assess lower leg reflex responses while the platform is triggered by the experimenter to unexpectedly give way. C. Experimental results have led to innovations in clinical and applied settings. In this photo is an exercise with two sources of postural perturbation—asymmetric and variable upper body forces and an unstable support surface. Of course, more technologically sophisticated postural training systems exist, but the photo reveals that technology is secondary to knowledge and innovation.

musculomechanical components, and central nervous system (CNS) components. Sensory systems, namely, visual, somatosensory, and vestibular system, detect postural changes and provide rapid postural correction through reflexes. Of course, visual systems provide feedforward control mechanisms. Sensory systems provide ongoing monitoring of postural movements and from this provide continued low-level tonic corrective reflex actions and large postural corrections to gross perturbations.

Musculomechanical systems refer to those muscles with large postural control roles, such as paraspinal and abdominal muscles, working within biomechanical constraints. These components also include elastic element stiffness, muscle strength, muscle and joint health, and anthropometrics. For instance, some overweight individuals are biomechanically constrained by a low center of mass and exhibit less postural sway during normal standing (Błaszczyk et al., 2009). Neuromuscular components primarily comprise synergies that are both learned and innate (e.g., coordinative structures and CPGs) that provide postural control mechanisms. These synergies include specific patterns of spinal musculature activation in preparation for catching a heavy object, or a learned righting action during a fall.

The CNS oversees all postural control mechanisms subconsciously or consciously, but does not necessarily intervene. Multimodal sensory inputs are integrated in the CNS and evaluated to provide the CNS with the most relevant data regarding ongoing balance and orientation requirements. For

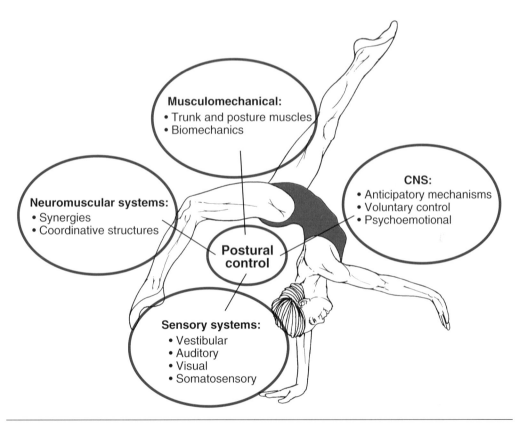

Figure 10.5 • System components of postural control.

instance, under conditions of poor vision, or challenging vestibular conditions, the CNS may rely more on proprioceptive inputs for postural control and downplay information from visual systems. This process is known as *multisensory* (or *sensory*) *reweighting* (see Chapter 4) and is defined as a decrease or increase in the influence of a particular sensory signal as conditions change. Changes in afferent information create situations in which information from one source may feature more prominently over another. Multisensory reweighting is suggested to be a critical feature of postural adaptability and poor reweighting is suggested to contribute to poor postural control that contributes to poor motor outcomes such as falling in the elderly (Jeka et al., 2010).

CNS systems may fine tune muscle tone and muscle mechanical properties depending on situational demands and make available some synergies versus others. The CNS provides most of what is known as *proactive* (or *predictive*) *postural control*. Proactive postural control prepares the body in advance of an anticipated postural disturbance, such as when visual systems provide advance warning of oncoming forces. In contrast, *reactive* (or *compensatory*) *postural control* includes all the adjustments that occur in response to postural disturbances. The nature of CNS-mediated reactive and proactive adjustments can be greatly influenced by learned behaviors and cognitive demands, including perception, psychoemotional state, and attention demands.

Levels of Postural Control

The four systems—sensory, neuromuscular, musculomechanical, and CNS—all contribute to three levels of postural control: (1) reflexive, (2) autonomic, and (3) voluntary. Each of these three levels of control is simultaneously active, but they do not work to the same extent under all conditions. For instance, spinal stability may be based more in reflexive actions than autonomic

---

SIDE**NOTE**	**ADAPTIVE POSTURAL MECHANISMS**

Figure 10.5 illustrates the four contributing systems to maintaining postural control. At different times, one system may dominate over the others, but what would happen if one or more systems were dysfunctional? Would postural control suffer greatly or would adaptations take place to enable the remaining systems to take over? Consider the case of blindness. Schmid et al. (2007) looked at acquired and congenitally blind subjects and compared them to normally sighted subjects on static balance tests and balance on a moving platform. Previous research has shown that both permanent and temporary blindness lead to a cross-modal reorganization of the visual cortex to take on somatosensory and auditory processing (Pascual-Leone & Hamilton, 2001), so the researchers hypothesized that blind individuals would have minimal or no postural deficits during normal situations. Their hypothesis was not confirmed, finding that blind individuals did not appear to make compensatory use of other enhanced sensory systems. Indeed, the researchers speculated that some of the larger sway characteristics of the blind subjects were to maximize somatosensory and vestibular sensory input. These findings led the authors to suggest that the postural visual pathways, unlike many other sensory pathways, are hardwired and little affected by cross-modal adaptation.

---

responses (Brown & McGill, 2009). Righting reflexes are a notable example of reflex mechanisms with minimal influence during normal balance challenges but under conditions of high postural disturbance (e.g., slip and fall) may play a prominent role.

Reflexive postural control is primarily a function of somatosensory, vestibular, and visual systems. The contributions of these sensory systems are evidenced during perturbed standing. As the upright body sways forward (due to gravity), the vestibular and visual systems detect movement and the dorsal side muscles may stretch (Gurfinkel' et al., 1974; Masani et al., 2003). In cases of disturbed posture, these mechanisms may produce a strong array of reflex actions (e.g., righting reflexes) to maintain and upright head and overall postural stability.

Autonomic postural control is a combination of innate and learned behaviors that provide subconscious postural corrections that are fast and task specific. Autonomic control may include a measure of reflex mechanisms, but in contrast to reflexes, autonomic postural control is more widespread and complex, is more adaptable to learning, and provides both reactive and proactive control. Examples of autonomic postural control include figure skaters not succumbing to dizziness following spins and, as shown in Figure 10.6, the trunk lean of a bicyclist that is necessary to stabilize and balance during raising the arm to signal a turn. Figure 10.6 also illustrates autonomic righting actions during an abrupt disruption. The flailing of the arms may appear to be vestibulospinal reflexes, but the specific patterning of the arms reveals them to be much more complex and coordinated and perhaps too rapid to be purely voluntary.

Voluntary postural control involves those postural adjustments made with conscious awareness. Voluntary control can be both reactionary and proactive. These may include whole-body stiffening before walking on ice or readying to catch a heavy object. Consider, for example, a novice exerciser playing catch with a heavy medicine ball. The first time the ball is caught, the person may be knocked over due to the unanticipated force of the ball. After this unpleasant experience, the novice begins to voluntarily stiffen the trunk and legs and take on a crouched and stable athletic posture in preparation to catch the ball. After considerable practice, the catching posture becomes less stiff, more efficient, and automatic. The exerciser no longer needs to think about postural stiffening as this becomes an ingrained component of the catching action.

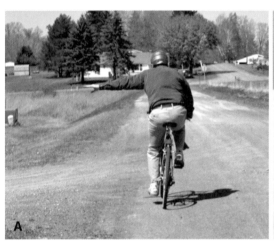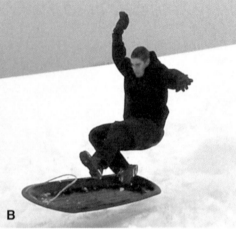

Figure 10.6 • Multiple systems work to maintain postural control under different conditions. **A.** To counteract the unbalanced forces created by the left turn signal, this bicyclist tilts the bike to the right and stabilizes the left side of the body by pressing down on the left pedal. This tilt, which may be unnoticed by the cyclist himself, is an autonomic postural adjustment to maintain balance and a straight line trajectory that has been set off course by the disruptive forces of raising the arm. (Photo courtesy of Whitman Ives.) **B.** This sledder has just hit a jump and has been destabilized at high speed. His right arm has shot up and his left arm out in order to maintain an upright trunk posture over the sled. These arm actions are a combination of autonomic postural synergies with vestibulospinal reflexes. (Photo courtesy of Jeffrey Ives.)

Control of Upright Stance and Fundamental Postural Control Strategies

Given that there are four basic mechanisms and three levels of postural control, how do these work together? Research on quiet versus perturbed upright stance have provided the most information on fundamental postural control strategies. During standing, the body acts like an *inverted pendulum* (Nashner, 1972), swaying fore and aft and side to side (Fig. 10.7). Gravity continually pulls the body into forward tilt that must be pulled back into vertical by dorsal side muscles. This sway cannot be eliminated even with training, suggesting that it is an intrinsic and necessary property of our motor control system (Bottaro et al., 2005). Sway helps keep somatosensory, vestibular, and visual systems active, but this does not mean that sway is corrected in an ongoing, feedback-based manner.

It has been long thought that forward sway stretches the calf muscles and causes a corrective stretch reflex (Gurfinkel' et al., 1974), but these data have now been challenged by ultrasound imaging evidence that during normal sway there are actually paradoxical, albeit very small, muscle length changes in the soleus and gastrocnemius (Loram et al., 2004). These changes, that is, the calf muscles shortening rather than lengthening during forward sway, make stretch reflex responses unlikely (Loram et al., 2004). That is, during forward sway, the calf muscles may actually shorten, which suggests that underlying postural tone and stretch reflex actions in these muscles are not sufficient to pull the body back to vertical. The control of "simple" sway may be a complex arrangement of force feedback from the Golgi tendon organs of the calf and cutaneous receptors in the feet coupling with anticipatory control mechanics and alpha–gamma linkage of the extrafusal and intrafusal fibers of the calf muscles and tibialis anterior (Loram et al., 2004, 2009). These automatic postural mechanisms may prompt "pulsed" intermittent ballistic contractions rather than continuous feedback-based muscle activation to set the body vertical, particularly if the amount of sensory feedback exceeds a threshold level (Bottaro et al., 2005; Milton et al., 2009). The normal subtle sway movements, sometimes considered

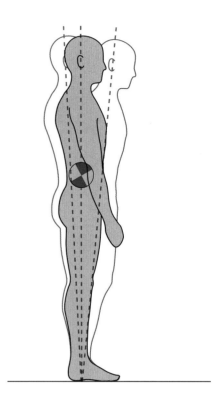

Figure 10.7 • Inverted pendulum model of postural control. Gravity topples the body forward; dorsal side muscles pull the body back to vertical. Rearward sway is minimal and cannot be corrected by pulsed muscle contractions to the same extent as forward sway.

to be "neural noise" or "chatter," are an outcome of neural processes but also enable the motor control system to monitor and prepare for a range of movements (Bottaro et al., 2005).

Ongoing CNS-mediated pulsed contractions do not eliminate the need to maintain base levels of postural muscle tone and reflex-mediated actions. The amount of tone and reflex sensitivity may serve to regulate the characteristics of the automatic pulsed contractions. In particular, a stiffer system may slow the sway and enable finer control of postural corrections (Bottaro et al., 2005). As conditions change, the contributions from sensory systems are reweighted and may play a more prominent role.

Under perturbed stance conditions, the involvement of reflex corrections increases. Regardless if the postural correction reflex is initiated with a stretch reflex, or vestibular, or visual input, the postural mechanisms generally begin at the point in contact with the support surface (e.g., foot/ankle). Then through a series of sequenced, coordinated, and minimized reflex and synergy activations and autonomic adjustments, the body is balanced. If this does not work to balance the body, such as when standing on slippery ice, then another strategy is adopted. For example, reflex activations may start at the knee or hip instead of the ankle. These various strategies are known as the ankle strategy, hip strategy, stepping strategy, and suspensory strategy.

Figure 10.8 illustrates these postural control strategies. Whole-body adjustments to maintain standing balance generally begin at the ankle. The **ankle strategy** provides the quickest way to maintain balance under normal circumstances. If the ankle strategy is not sufficient to maintain balance, the **hip strategy** may be used. The hip strategy enables a larger amount of correction and affords a different biomechanical profile than an ankle strategy. In particular, the hip strategy does not rely as much on foot friction with the support surface and thus may be more useful in cases of poor surface contact. Another strategy, the **suspensory strategy**, involves going into a crouching flexed behavior to lower the center of mass. This is most often done by those afraid to fall or those in an entirely unfamiliar environment. The elderly and very young are more likely to use this strategy. Hip, ankle, and suspensory

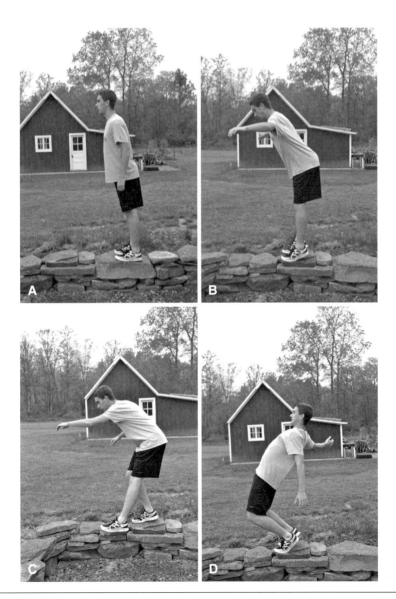

Figure 10.8 • There are four basic lower extremity postural strategies as illustrated by this walk along a stone wall. **A.** The ankle strategy is typically used on solid and stable surfaces, such as that afforded by the large rock. **B.** Upon stepping to the small and wobbly rock, the individual adopts a hip strategy with the ankle strategy. The hip strategy may use used without the ankle strategy. **C.** When the instability is too large, the person must take a step to avoid falling. **D.** A suspensory strategy is used when falling is imminent and the body collapses straight down to minimize fall consequences. (Photo courtesy of Jeffrey Ives.)

strategies are considered *fixed-point strategies* (Pollock et al., 2000). In more extreme balance challenges, a *change-in-support strategy* may be used. The two most common are taking a step (**stepping strategy**) and reaching for a support hold (Pollock et al., 2000).

At first glance, there seems to be a natural progression in strategy from ankle to hip and then to a change-in-support stance as more postural correction is needed. Yet, many physiological, biomechanical, psychological, or experiential factors can influence which strategy is employed. Physiological dysfunction, such as chronic ankle instability, and environmental and biomechanical circumstances, such as large external perturbation forces, may lead one to bypass an ankle strategy and use a hip or stepping strategy. Experiential and emotional factors also play a role in subconscious and conscious strategy selection. Dancers and gymnasts may avoid hip and stepping strategies as these are detrimental to performance. Fear of falling, pain, and other cognitive–emotional factors may lead one to favor a particular strategy over another.

■ Thinking It Through 10.2 Sway Strategies

Observe the posture strategy on a group of individuals by doing an eye-closed Romberg test and a self-initiated sway test. The Romberg test uses a gentle nudge to one's back between the shoulder blades to get the subject to sway in an anterior–posterior direction. Do gentle nudges and firmer nudges while standing on firm surfaces and on unstable surfaces (e.g., foam). The self-initiated sway test is simply having the subject sway forward and back to vertical repeatedly. Have them sway gently and then as far forward as they can without needing to take a step. Have them do this with eyes open and then with eyes closed. The point, where the body center of mass falls outside the base of support is considered the limit of stability. Be sure to spot your subjects should they stumble. Compare the postural control strategy between the gentle and firm nudges during the Romberg test and small and large sways during the self-initiated sway test. Did you notice any marked differences in the strategies among your subjects? For instance, did some people not adopt a different strategy during the firm nudge, unstable surfaces, or large sway? If so, can you identify why? Consider habitual activities (e.g., dancer, gymnast), injuries, or characteristics of the support surface.

Proactive Postural Control

Postural control actions are designed to react to disturbances that destabilize the body, as well as proactively prepare for anticipated disturbances. Reflexive postural mechanisms only participate in reactionary control, whereas autonomic and voluntary systems provide both reactive and proactive control. Proactive postural control comes in two basic forms. The first is based on upcoming or expected environmental circumstances or bodily actions. These postural adjustments are based largely on visual inputs and previous knowledge. For example, prior to stepping on ice the trunk may stiffen. The second form is referred to as **anticipatory postural adjustments**, or **APAs**. APAs are postural movements that accompany all or almost all planned movements and are designed to stabilize joints, body segments, or the whole body prior to the execution of the motor skill. They are, in fact, a subconscious component of the motor skill.

Figure 10.9 illustrates how APAs work. The subject in the figure pulls on the lever (biceps b. contraction) in reaction to an auditory stimulus. Reaction time of the elbow flexion is about 175 ms. Before the biceps b. contracts is an APA contraction of the gastrocnemius at a reaction time (110 ms) that is faster than voluntary reaction time. The gastrocnemius contracts to stabilize the body's center of mass to counteract the pulling force of the elbow flexion. This experiment reveals that the motor plan has two parts, the first is an anticipatory postural stabilization and the second is the goal-directed movement. According to Aimola et al. (2011) the CNS can predict only so far into the future when determining the consequences of a planned action and may tend to overcompensate with an overly strong APA when postural disturbances of a planned action are uncertain. In cases of unforeseen postural disruptions, such as from an external force or a slip, APAs may be nonexistent and postural adjustments made entirely by reactive mechanisms (Santos et al., 2010).

APAs are necessary components of even the most fundamental motor skills. During running, for example, leg stiffness is adjusted by APAs prior to striking the ground to accommodate different surface properties (Ferris et al., 1999). Among the most dramatic illustrations of anticipatory postural control is during falling or landing from a jump. While in flight and prior to ground contact, the

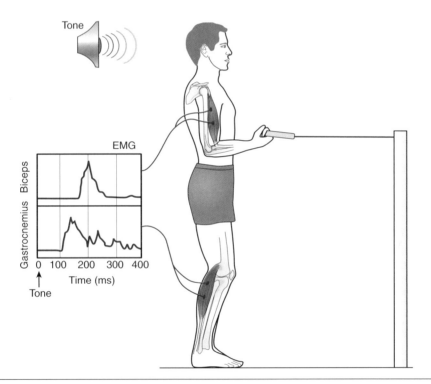

Figure 10.9 • Anticipatory postural control mechanisms. In this illustration, the subject reacts as fast as possible to an auditory stimuli by pulling on the handle. The premotor component of reaction time is a normal 175 ms. However, the gastrocnemius muscle activates long before this time, at about 110 ms following the stimulus and faster than voluntary reaction time allows. If the gastrocnemius muscle, along with other muscles not shown, did not activate, the individual would pull himself into the wall. Thus, the brain presets the gastrocnemius muscle to stabilize the body against the upcoming forward body motion anticipated by biceps flexion. (Figure based on Purves, D., Augustine, G. J., Fitzpatrick, D., et al. (Eds.) (2001). Motor control centers in the brainstem: Upper motor neurons that maintain balance and posture. In *Neuroscience* (2nd ed.). Sunderland, MA: Sinauer Associates.)

impact-absorbing limbs (legs or arms) contract to stiffen the muscles in order to prepare for impact forces. The precise coordination of this preactivation, such as the muscles involved and the timing and strength of contraction, is highly dependent on the task itself and is a preprogrammed phenomenon (Avela et al., 1996). In other words, the preactivation landing sequence is sent down from the CNS and appears to work with and be modified by inputs from visual, vestibular, and proprioceptive sensory systems. Moreover, this whole coordination mechanism appears to be alterable through practice.

APAs are highly sensitive to situations and circumstances. In the case of high postural instability, they can be turned off by the CNS, probably because the APAs might actually destabilize the body in such cases (Aruin et al., 1998). Stance width and direction of an oncoming perturbation also influence APA muscle activation in both trunk and leg muscles (Santos & Aruin, 2009). In a classic study, Zettel et al. (2002) found that APAs that accompany a stepping reaction could be modified to meet environmental challenges based simply on visual information and without practice. In this study, the researchers placed subjects on a moving platform that would jerk suddenly, making it necessary for the subjects to step forward to prevent falling. In some trials, an obstacle was placed in the normal step area, requiring the subjects to step higher and longer to get over the obstacle. The subjects were able to make this adjustment without falling. Even during the unpracticed trials the APAs were adjusted to counter the larger steps. Situations and circumstances differentially affect proximal and distal muscles and their roles in APAs: proximal and trunk muscles seem to be more patterned and active with normal and expected movements, and distal and limb muscle APAs may be more active during more unusual postural disruptions (Shiratori & Latash, 2000). Emotional states such as fear, anxiety, and deteriorated mood may slow or disorder APAs and make them less effective (Kitaoka et al., 2004; Uemura et al., 2012).

Leonard (1998) provided a useful summary of APAs that they have four characteristics: (1) they are modifiable through learning and experience, (2) they are adaptable to conditions and contexts of movement, (3) they are influenced by an individual's intention and emotional state, and (4) they can be either reactionary or anticipatory in order to minimize body displacement during the voluntary movements. It seems paradoxical that an anticipatory movement can be reactionary, but this may occur when a reactive movement done to stabilize the whole body (e.g., arm thrust to grab a hand rail) is preceded by an APA to stabilize the body part. The role of intention in postural adjustments was demonstrated in an elegant experiment by Earl and Frank (1992). These authors showed that leg and trunk postural control changed when subjects had to lift a tray with wine glasses versus tumblers. The fragile and unstable wine glasses required more precision, which modified the postural control. These authors also showed that postural control changed if the task was self-paced versus an externally timed pace.

Attention, Cognitive Involvement, and Postural Control

Postural control is understood to be background motor activity that typically works without a great deal of conscious awareness. Researchers have shown that when individuals consciously try to maintain standing postural stability, such as minimizing sway, they interfere with automatic processes that lead to more sway and less efficiency (Huxhold et al., 2006; Nafati & Vuillerme, 2011). When given a mild cognitive or motor challenge that diverts attention away from posture itself, the amount of static postural sway appears to lessen (Nafati & Vuillerme, 2011). Demanding cognitive challenges, however, may tax cognitive resources and postural control may become more variable and less controlled (Kuczyński et al., 2011). Under these circumstances, postural control may be maintained, but performance on the simultaneous cognitive task may suffer (Redfern et al., 2001; Resch et al., 2011). These results may be more pronounced in elders and less pronounced in subjects with task-related experiences (Berger & Bernard-Demanze, 2011; Kuczyński et al., 2011; Swanenburg et al., 2009).

During postural threats, uncertain environmental conditions, and stressful and emotionally taxing circumstances, voluntary postural control often takes over, and efficient postural control becomes compromised (Huffman et al., 2009). These negative situations are experimentally induced by removing vision, creating unstable surfaces, minimizing support surface size, elevating the support surface, or creating stressful and anxiety-producing cognitive dual tasks (see accompanying Sidenote box). For instance, Huffman et al. (2009) reported that a number of postural sway measures became larger in amplitude when a person was standing on a force platform at a 3.2-m height. Their data suggested that under threatening and stressful situations individuals "reinvest" conscious control into their posture. This may result in supraspinal mechanisms reducing reflex gains (Hoffman and Koceja, 1995; Llewellyn et al., 1990) and more muscle coactivation and stiffness (Stins et al., 2011). On the other hand, some investigators believe that the minimal and efficient postural sway observed under fully automatic conditions may also reveal increased muscle stiffness (see Stins et al., 2011, for commentary), but this may be a consequence of greater reflex sensitivity responding quicker to small sway movements and not conscious control causing cocontraction.

What these studies show is that with increasing complexity and uncertainty (no vision, unstable surfaces, balance beam), individuals tend to override automatic processes and take voluntary control of postural mechanisms. Voluntary control may result in a number of different outcomes depending on environmental and psychological factors. If the voluntary control is reactive, then sway may increase because these mechanisms are slower than reflex or automatic mechanisms. If on the other

SIDE**NOTE**	**POSTURAL CONTROL IN CONSTRUCTION WORKERS**

Falls in construction workers are a leading cause of severe workplace injuries. Working at heights on unstable platforms increases this risk by imposing physical constraints but also by increasing worker anxiety. Min et al. (2012) evaluated postural sway characteristics, heart rate responses, and subjective measures of balance difficulty in expert and novice construction workers on low and high scaffolds with and without handrails. Higher elevations equivalent to a second floor height (C, D) and the lack of handrails (A, C) increased postural instability, increased cardiovascular stress, and was perceived to make balance more difficult, all of which were more pronounced in novice workers. These results illustrate the vicious cycle of postural control, particularly in inexperienced individuals. Challenging conditions that demand excellent postural control also create psychophysiological stress that reduces control.

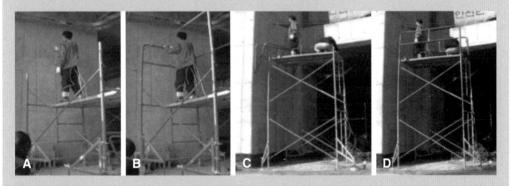

Reprinted from Min, S., Kim, J., & Parnianpour, M. (2012). The effects of safety handrails and the heights of scaffolds on the subjective and objective evaluation of postural stability and cardiovascular stress in novice and expert construction workers. *Applied Ergonomics, 43*(3), 574–581, with permission from Elsevier.

hand voluntary control is proactive, then the sway parameters may be reduced as an outcome of high levels of cocontraction stiffness.

A POSTURAL CONTROL MODEL

The complexity of different systems, different levels, and proactive versus reactive postural control can be further understood by modeling postural control. Figure 10.10 illustrates these control mechanisms. This schematic, an extension of our motor control schematic diagrams in Chapters 2 and 5 and based on the work of Massion et al. (Massion, 1998; Massion et al., 2004), shows postural control and motor skill mechanisms as separate systems working side by side and interacting. Essential to this model are internal "schemas" or body plans that provide reference points and requirements for stability and orientation based on gravity, biomechanics, anthropometrics, and environmental and situational needs. In this model, postural control has subsystems for alignment and orientation designed for stability ("stability") and orientation designed to optimize interaction with the environment and afferent flow ("orientation"). Automatic postural control arises out of these subcortical schemas and from spinal networks to provide basic balance and orientation control mechanisms. Here reflex gain and postural tone may be

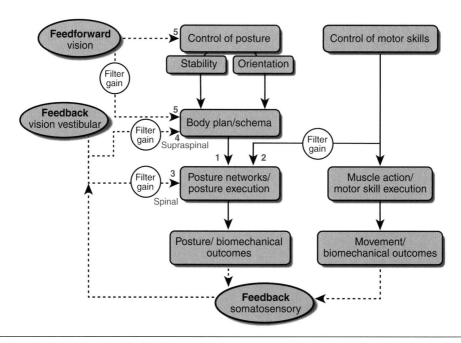

Figure 10.10 • Summary schematic of postural control mechanisms. *Dashed lines* represent sensory information and *solid lines* motor commands. (*1*) Automatic postural control provides basic stability and orientation control mechanisms arising out of schemas. (*2*) Voluntary postural commands and autonomic APAs arise directly alongside motor skill commands. (*3*) Reflexive postural control arises from feedback from somatosensory, vestibular, and visual sources. The reflexive system includes tonic and phasic postural reflexes and ongoing modulation of postural muscle tone. (*4*) Afferent flow is also used to update the internal body schema. (*5*) Feedforward control by visual systems provides the bulwark of most postural adjustments and ongoing control. The filter/gain circles represent points where feedforward and feedback commands may be adapted by filtering or by changing the gain setting. See text for more details. (Adapted from Massion, J. (1998). Postural control systems in developmental perspective. *Neuroscience and Biobehavioral Reviews*, *22*(4), 465–472.)

set as well as coordinated activation of postural muscles and postural pattern generators and synergies. Afferent signals are under constant filtering and regulation, that is, multisensory reweighting. The schematic also depicts that a component of motor skill commands are postural control commands. These components are voluntary and automatic proactive postural commands, such as APAs. APAs and other proactive commands are under filter and gain control as they integrate with ongoing postural control.

MEASURING POSTURAL ALIGNMENT, BALANCE, AND STABILITY

Direct measurement of postural control employs EMG to evaluate muscle activation patterns of postural support muscles during goal-directed movements, perturbed movements, or during quiet stance (Klous et al., 2011). Other clinical and research methods used to evaluate postural control are measures of postural control outcomes, that is, alignment, segmental stability, joint stability, and whole-body balance.

Postural Alignment

Standing static posture is commonly measured against a plumb line as shown in Figure 10.11. Digital photogrammetry and three-dimensional laser scanning aid in the quantification and precision of measurement. Both sagittal and frontal alignments are used to evaluate deviations from a theoretical ideal. This ideal, as shown in Figure 10.11, places the relevant joints in vertical alignment such

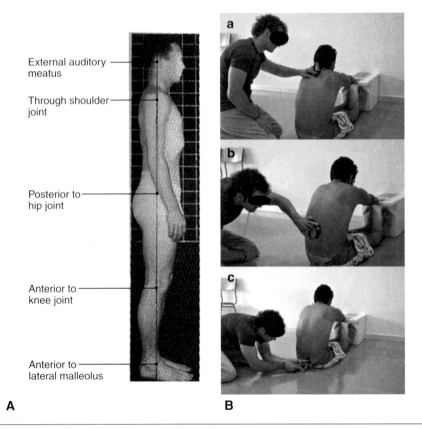

External auditory meatus

Through shoulder joint

Posterior to hip joint

Anterior to knee joint

Anterior to lateral malleolus

A

B

Figure 10.11 • Measurement of static posture. **A.** This classic photograph illustrates what is considered perfect posture, with all the relevant joints in biomechanical alignment. (From Kendall, F. P., McCreary, E. K., Provance, P. G. (1993). *Muscles: Testing and function* (4th ed.). Philadelphia, PA: Lippincott Williams & Wilkins.) **B.** Postural alignment, however, is more than whole-body alignment. Here is measurement of spinal curvatures in the sit-and-reach test. An inclinometer is placed at T_1 (a), T_{12} (b), and L_5 (c). (From López-Miñarro, P. A., Alacid, P., & Rodríguez-García, P. L. (2010). Comparison of sagittal spinal curvatures and hamstring muscle extensibility among young elite paddlers and non-athletes. *International SportMed Journal*, *11*(2), 301–312, Figure 2. Reproduced with permission from the *International SportMed Journal*.)

that forces and stresses through the musculoskeletal system are transferred directly through the joint centers (Kendall et al., 1993). It is thought that proper alignment places the body in a state of equilibrium and minimizes muscular activity necessary to maintain upright stance, which in turn decreases injury risk and the chance of developing chronic musculoskeletal pain (for review see Kritz & Cronin, 2008). Postural alignment is also evaluated in body segments, such as spinal alignment (e.g., kyphosis, scoliosis; see Fig. 10.11), leg alignment (e.g., bowlegs, knock-knees, femoral ante/retroversion), ankle/foot alignment (e.g., pes planus), and shoulder alignment (e.g., scapular winging).

Large deviations from the ideal posture are called *postural faults* and are suggested to be a result of muscle imbalances (stretch weakness or short and stiff muscles), structural defects from genetic causes, disease or injury, or habitual misuse. Misuse may be a result of emotional guarding, pain, chronically poor positioning during work or activities of daily living, or imbalanced exercise. Upon finding postural alignment problems, it is suggested that further assessment of muscle strength, muscle length, tone, and structural problems be evaluated (Kendall et al., 1993).

Interpreting postural alignment faults requires caution. Classifying "good" versus "poor" postural alignment is difficult because even gross misalignment is not always associated with poor health or performance outcomes. Indeed, many athlete groups, such as gymnasts, weight lifters, and cyclists, have

Concepts in Action

Using Digital Photogrammetry

Digital cameras and freely available digital photo editing software have made it relatively easy to make quantitative assessments of posture. To test the usefulness and precision of digital photography, take standard upright posture photos and workplace ergonomic photos. For the standard posture photos, take sagittal plane and frontal plane (from the back) posture photographs of subjects standing behind a plumb line (see Fig. 10.11 and below). Wear minimal and tight-fitting clothing, such as Lycra shorts and sport tops for women. Hair should be up to expose the ears and no shoes worn. The plumb line should be centered in the frontal view and aligned through the anterior aspect of the lateral malleolus in the sagittal view. Use a plumb line that has been carefully and visibly marked in 10-cm increments. These marks will serve as calibration marks in the software analyses. Alternately, use a long thin flexible measuring tape for the plumb line if it can be pulled straight and true. Set, plumb, and level the camera on a tripod such that the focus is centered on the midpoint the subject (near the pelvic girdle). Be sure the measurement marks on the plumb line

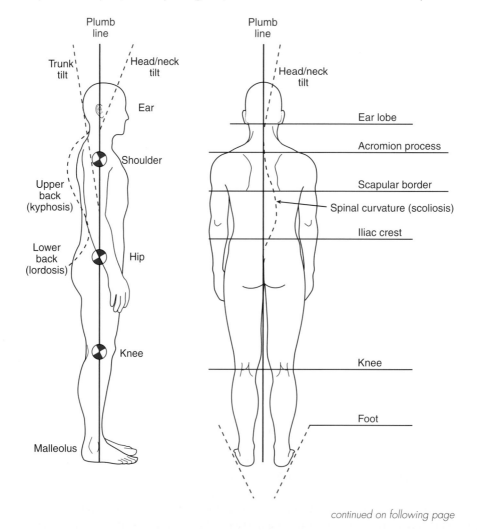

continued on following page

are visible, at least upon magnification. Take the frontal and sagittal pictures and load the pictures into ImageJ software. ImageJ is freely available from the National Institutes of Health Web site (http://rsbweb.nih.gov/ij/). Using the software, measure postural misalignment and asymmetries using the basic guidelines below or use your own scoring system. Measure angles of deviation and amount of deviation in centimeters from left side to right side and front to back. (It is not shown in the diagram, but note that deviations may be anterior, posterior, left, right, medial, and lateral. Also not shown is whole-body tilt.) Use the calibration on the plumb line to determine distances. Conduct the same tests but this time use both left and right single leg stance postures. Compare alignments among all three postures and identify what you consider to be postural misalignments. Discuss with the subject why these misalignments may exist. Consider injuries, habits, experiences, and psychological factors like stress.

Using the same photogrammetric system, evaluate work postures to evaluate job-related postural faults. Access the web pages below to evaluate trunk and arm postures (RULA: Rapid Upper Limb Assessment) and whole-body postures (REBA: Rapid Entire Body Assessment). With a partner, evaluate your normal postural position while in class and while studying.

http://ergo.human.cornell.edu/ahRULA.html
http://ergo.human.cornell.edu/ahREBA.html

been found to have poorer static alignment than nonathletes (Muyor et al., 2011; Tanchev et al., 2000; for review see Kritz & Cronin, 2008), which may reflect necessary and beneficial adaptations to sport participation (Kritz & Cronin, 2008; Uetake et al., 1998).

Dynamic posture is alignment or positioning during activities and is much more difficult to assess and interpret. For these reasons, dynamic assessments are often focused toward specific body segment

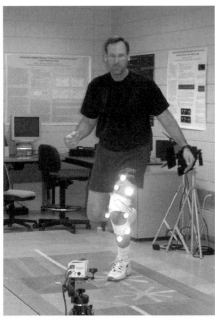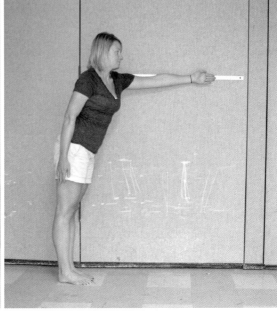

Figure 10.12 • Measuring stability and balance. On the left is a single-leg balance test done on a force platform. In this test, body center of mass sway parameters are measured by the force platform and specific knee stability measures measured by 3D cinematography. On the right is the functional reach test, which assesses functional balance performance. (Photos courtesy of Jeffrey Ives.)

Concepts in Action

Measuring Balance

Attempts have been made over the years to create balance tests that are objective, quantifiable, and useful across populations and levels of function and are able to both identify underlying problems in postural control mechanisms and predict future dysfunction. No such single test exists, but in its place are test batteries aimed at various populations. On the low end of technological sophistication is the Berg Balance Scale (BBS) designed for elders with impaired balance. Elders are evaluated on 14 different functional activities, ranging from picking up an object from the floor to standing on one leg. Each task is rated 0 to 4 based on criteria provided to the tester. An example question is shown below for the sit to stand movement.

SITTING TO STANDING INSTRUCTIONS: Please stand up. Try not to use your hand for support.

( ) 4 able to stand without using hands and stabilize independently
( ) 3 able to stand independently using hands
( ) 2 able to stand using hands after several tries
( ) 1 needs minimal aid to stand or stabilize
( ) 0 needs moderate or maximal assist to stand different activities

Among the first and most common computerized systems are those made by NeuroCom. Their most sophisticated system, the SMART EquiTest®, includes a rotating and translating force platform and a moveable visual surround. This system enables assessment in unstable and dynamic environments and provides normal reference values for a variety of populations. First used to evaluate elders and patients with a host of neurological conditions, computerized balance systems are now commonplace in athletic settings. Sway and center of pressure data are being used to evaluate the severity of injury and recovery outcomes in concussion injuries, back injuries, and lower extremity joint injuries.

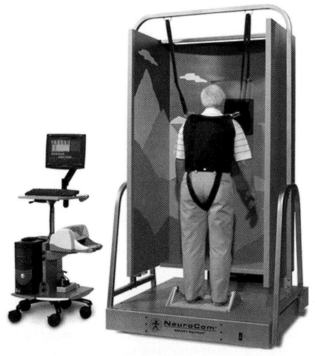

Image courtesy of Natus Medical Incorporated.

alignments, such as trunk alignment during a squat exercise and pelvic tilt during walking. Evaluating deviations or faults is often done subjectively in the field, but the widespread availability of digital still cameras and video has provided greater opportunity to quantify both dynamic and static posture.

Stability and Balance

Stability and balance measures vary widely in their nature and sophistication, ranging from timed "plank" tests to center of pressure measures on tilting computerized force platforms (Fig. 10.12). Body segment and joint stability assessments typically look at spinal stability, shoulder girdle stability, and knee and ankle stability. Whole-body stability (balance) measures are either timed measures of stance duration (e.g., single leg stance on an unstable platform) or sway characteristics. Sway characteristics include the direction, magnitude, and velocity of one's center of pressure objectively measured on computerized platforms and subjectively by visual observation. Large and jerky amounts of sway are considered to reflect poor postural control. Though standards and norms have been established for some balance measures (generally by equipment manufacturers) and some balance measures have been associated with injury and impairments, interpreting many balance tests for otherwise healthy individuals are often ambiguous (for reviews see Guskiewicz & Perrin, 1996; Shumway-Cook & Woollacott, 2005).

Less technologically sophisticated field-based tests for balance vary widely depending on the target population. Simple heel to toe walking and standing balance with eyes closed are among the common tests for frail elders, whereas challenging single leg stances with arm reaching movements are among those used for athletes. Recent field tests designed to assess postural control in athletes and relatively healthy adults include the Star Excursion Balance Test (Gribble & Hertel, 2003), the Balance Error Scoring System (Riemann et al., 1999), and the Functional Movement Screen test battery (Cook et al., 2006). Like other tests, they are often able to discriminate those with clear musculoskeletal injuries, but their ability to predict future injury and identify impaired postural mechanisms is inconsistent and unclear (Bressel et al., 2007). For example, O'Connor et al. (2011) determined that both low and high scores on the Functional Movement Screen were associated with higher injury rates in military personnel and that physical fitness scores were better predictors of injury than the Functional Movement Screen.

The inconsistent results shown by posture and balance tests are suggested to be a result of the tests being too general to assess specific postural control adaptations made by individuals in response to occupational or athletic demands (Bressel et al., 2007). Postural control tests are thus best used in conjunction with other tests and when aimed at a specific problem. For instance, Hicks et al. (2005) reported that prediction of successful treatment outcomes for low back pain sufferers included the patient's age and scores on tests for straight-leg raise, prone instability, aberrant motions, lumbar hypermobility, and fear-avoidance beliefs. These data confirm the use of stability and balance tests when they are specifically used to identify (1) limitations in functional capabilities, (2) adaptive motor or sensory strategies for movement, and (3) underlying sensory or motor or cognitive impairments. Stability tests are best suited in cases of dysfunction, for example, examining sway characteristics following a concussion, or comparing single leg stability of a noninjured leg to an injured leg. In some elderly and clinical populations, they may be used to predict the progression or risk of more dysfunction or disability.

■ Thinking It Through 10.3 The Clinical Test for Sensory Integration and Balance

The Clinical Test for Sensory Integration and Balance (CTSIB) is one of the most widespread test batteries to evaluate postural control. In its original form, the CTSIB test used subjective evaluations of standing sway during interacting conditions of support surface changes (hard surface, foam surface) and visual changes (eyes open, blindfolded, wearing a dome over the head). The dome, actually a modified Japanese lantern, is worn with eyes open and has horizontal reference marks inside that are visible. Now affectionately called the "foam-dome" test, the CTSIB is designed to reveal deficiencies in sensory

continued on following page

processing and sensory weighting. Given the six basic conditions below, can you determine the main postural problems that may occur at each condition? In particular, why does the dome condition differ from the blindfolded condition? Check your ideas with the originators of the test, Shumway-Cook and Horak (1986; see references for full citation).

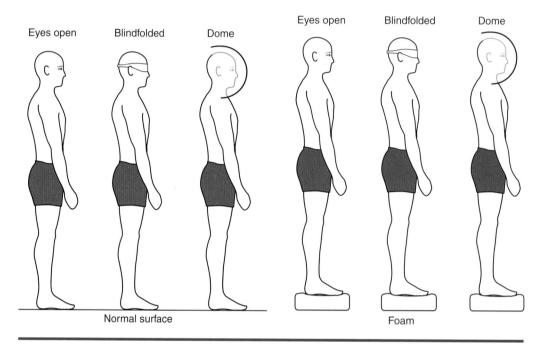

Eyes open   Blindfolded   Dome   Eyes open   Blindfolded   Dome

Normal surface   Foam

SUMMARY

Postural control is a foundational movement system designed to prepare the body for purposeful movement. The outcome of postural control mechanisms are biomechanical alignment and orientation in space. Together, these outcomes contribute to stability, and orientation further contributes to optimizing afferent information by proper orientation of the head and feet. Stability can be further broken down into whole-body stability (balance), segmental stability, and joint stability. Deviations in postural control contribute to instability and misalignment. Whole-body instability (poor balance) and misalignment (poor posture) are relatively simple to recognize, but uncovering their causes is more challenging. Further, measuring and uncovering the problems with segmental and joint stability are also challenging.

Postural control is controlled by three systems working in unison with one another. The "lowest" level is purely reflexive—largely by muscle spindles—that controls sway, joint stability, and overall muscle tone. Muscle tone provides a base from which specific postural control actions can be added and by itself serves to modulate force transmission throughout the body and the storage and release of elastic energy. The second level of postural control is autonomic. Autonomic control is based on both innate and learned behaviors that become automatic responses to both anticipated and unanticipated movements. The final level is purely voluntary. These are willful postural adjustments to maintain stability, generally in anticipation of an upcoming postural threat. These three levels of postural control mechanisms work through four systems: sensory, neuromuscular, musculomechanical, and the central nervous system.

Postural control is both reactive to disturbances and proactive to brace for anticipated perturbations. APAs are specific proactive postural mechanisms designed to stabilize body segments and enable whole-body balance in preparation for purposeful movements. APAs precede goal-directed movements and are highly modifiable and context specific. APAs and other proactive systems likely arise out of, or are triggered by, the motor control system as subcomponents of motor skill commands. Other postural mechanisms are controlled by a separate system and make use of internal body schemas that provide an internal model of the body's orientation and alignment based on multimodal sensory input.

Measurement of postural alignment and stability range from simple field tests to sophisticated computerized force platforms that can measure center of pressure and sway characteristics under a variety of perturbation conditions. Measures of alignment and balance for some populations may be used to help diagnose postural control problems and predict potential risks for falling or developing musculoskeletal problems. On the whole, however, the assessment of alignment and stability for relatively healthy persons to diagnose or predict problems remains inconclusive.

STUDY QUESTIONS

1. What is muscle tone and what regulates tone?
2. Muscle tone serves what purposes?
3. Define each of these terms: postural control, posture, segmental stability, joint stability, balance, and orientation.
4. Postural control is designed for alignment and orientation. Orientation has two functions: one to position the body to meet task and environmental constraints, and the second to position the body for better sensory feedback. Explain this latter concept.
5. What four systems contribute to postural control?
6. What are the three levels of postural control? Describe each in detail.
7. A person is standing in a closed room and the lights suddenly go out. Will the person begin to sway more or less? Explain your answer in detail.
8. An elderly person is standing at a curbside waiting to cross the road. The automobile traffic is heavy, there are many other pedestrians jostling about, and the pedestrian crossing lights are difficult to see. Explain in detail why this scenario creates a potential fall hazard for this person.
9. What is the difference between reactive and proactive postural control? Under what circumstances do we see these control mechanisms come into play? In your answer be sure to describe APAs.
10. Diagram the postural control model. Detail at which levels reflexive, automatic, and voluntary systems contribute.
11. How useful are postural alignment tests?
12. Describe two different field-based balance tests and two different measurements assessed by computerized balance testing. What can these tests reveal?

References

Aimola, E., Santello, M., La Grua, G., & Casabona, A. (2011). Anticipatory postural adjustments in reach-to-grasp: Effect of object mass predictability. *Neuroscience Letters*, *502*(2), 84–88.

Aruin, A., Forrest, W., & Latash, M. (1998). Anticipatory postural adjustments in conditions of postural instability. *Electroencephalography and Clinical Neurophysiology*, *109*(4), 350–359.

Avela, J. J., Santos, P. M., & Komi, P. V. (1996). Effects of differently induced stretch loads on neuromuscular control in drop jump exercise. *European Journal of Applied Physiology and Occupational Physiology*, *72*(5/6), 553–562.

Berger, L., & Bernard-Demanze, L. (2011). Age-related effects of a memorizing spatial task in the adults and elderly postural control. *Gait & Posture*, *33*(2), 300–302.

Błaszczyk, J., Cieślinska-Swider, J., Plewa, M., Zahorska-Markiewicz, B., & Markiewicz, A. (2009). Effects of excessive body weight on postural control. *Journal of Biomechanics*, *42*(9), 1295–1300.

Bottaro, A., Casadio, M., Morasso, P., & Sanguineti, V. (2005). Body sway during quiet standing: Is it the residual chattering of an intermittent stabilization process? *Human Movement Science, 24*(4), 588–615.

Bressel, E., Yonker, J., Kras, J., & Heath, E. (2007). Comparison of static and dynamic balance in female collegiate soccer, basketball, and gymnastics athletes. *Journal of Athletic Training*, *42*(1), 42–46.

Brown, S., & McGill, S. (2009). The intrinsic stiffness of the in vivo lumbar spine in response to quick releases: Implications for reflexive requirements. *Journal of Electromyography and Kinesiology*, *19*(5), 727–736.

Burgess, K., Pearson, S., & Onambélé, G. (2010). Patellar tendon properties with fluctuating menstrual cycle hormones. *Journal of Strength and Conditioning Research*, *24*(8), 2088–2095.

Cook, G., Burton, L., & Hoogenboom, B. (2006). Pre-participation screening: The use of fundamental movements as an assessment of function—Part 1. *North American Journal of Sports Physical Therapy*, *1*(2), 62–72.

Dumke, C. L., Pfaffenroth, C. M., McBride, J. M., & McCauley, G. O. (2010). Relationship between muscle strength, power and stiffness and running economy in trained male runners. *International Journal of Sports Physiology and Performance*, *5*(2), 249–261.

Earl, E. M., & Frank, J. S. (1992). The influence of task demands on the co-ordination of posture and movement. In M. Woollacott & F. Horak (Eds.) *Posture and gait: Control mechanisms, 1992* (Volume 1, pp. 135–138). XIth International Symposium of the Society for Postural and Gait Research, Portland, University of Oregon, United States.

Ebenbichler, G., Oddsson, L., Kollmitzer, J., & Erim, Z. (2001). Sensory-motor control of the lower back: Implications for rehabilitation. *Medicine and Science in Sports and Exercise*, *33*(11), 1889–1898.

Ferris, D., Liang, K., & Farley, C. (1999). Runners adjust leg stiffness for their first step on a new running surface. *Journal of Biomechanics*, *32*(8), 787–794.

Gallagher, S. (2005). Physical limitations and musculoskeletal complaints associated with work in unusual or restricted postures: A literature review. *Journal of Safety Research*, *36*(1), 51–61.

Gribble, P. A., & Hertel, J. (2003). Considerations for normalizing measures of the Star Excursion Balance Test. *Measurement in Physical Education and Exercise Science*, *7*(2), 89–100.

Gurfinkel', V., Lipshits, M., & Popov, K. (1974). Is the stretch reflex a basic mechanism in the system of regulation of human vertical posture? *Biofizika*, *19*(4), 744–748.

Guskiewicz, K. M., & Perrin, D. H. (1996). Research and clinical applications of assessing balance. *Journal of Sport Rehabilitation*, *5*(1), 45–63.

Hicks, G., Fritz, J., Delitto, A., & McGill, S. (2005). Preliminary development of a clinical prediction rule for determining which patients with low back pain will respond to a stabilization exercise program. *Archives of Physical Medicine and Rehabilitation*, *86*(9), 1753–1762.

Hoffman, M., & Koceja, D. (1995). The effects of vision and task complexity on Hoffmann reflex gain. *Brain Research*, *700*(1–2), 303–307.

Huffman, J., Horslen, B., Carpenter, M., & Adkin, A. (2009). Does increased postural threat lead to more conscious control of posture? *Gait & Posture*, *30*(4), 528–532.

Huxhold, O., Li, S., Schmiedek, F., & Lindenberger, U. (2006). Dual-tasking postural control: Aging and the effects of cognitive demand in conjunction with focus of attention. *Brain Research Bulletin*, *69*(3), 294–305.

Jeka, J., Allison, L., & Kiemel, T. (2010). The dynamics of visual reweighting in healthy and fall-prone older adults. *Journal of Motor Behavior*, *42*(4), 197–208.

Kendall, F. P., McCreary, E. K., & Provance, P. G. (1993). *Muscles: Testing and function* (4th ed.). Philadelphia, PA: Lippincott Williams & Wilkins.

Kiemel, T., Zhang, Y., & Jeka, J. (2011). Identification of neural feedback for upright stance in humans: Stabilization rather than sway minimization. *Journal of Neuroscience*, *31*(42), 15144–15153.

Kitaoka, K., Ito, R., Araki, H., Sei, H., & Morita, Y. (2004). Effect of mood state on anticipatory postural adjustments. *Neuroscience Letters*, *370*(1), 65–68.

Klous, M., Mikulic, P., & Latash, M. (2011). Two aspects of feedforward postural control: Anticipatory postural adjustments and anticipatory synergy adjustments. *Journal of Neurophysiology*, *105*(5), 2275–2288.

Kritz, M. F., & Cronin, J. (2008). Static posture assessment screen of athletes: Benefits and considerations. *Strength & Conditioning Journal*, *30*(5), 18–27.

Kubo, K., Kanehisa, H., & Fukunaga, T. (2003). Gender differences in the viscoelastic properties of tendon structures. *European Journal of Applied Physiology*, *88*(6), 520–526.

Kuczyński, M., Szymańska, M., & Bieć, E. (2011). Dual-task effect on postural control in high-level competitive dancers. *Journal of Sports Sciences*, *29*(5), 539–545.

Leonard, C. T. (1998). *The neuroscience of human movement*. St. Louis, MO: Mosby.

Llewellyn, M., Yang, J., & Prochazka, A. (1990). Human H-reflexes are smaller in difficult beam walking than in normal treadmill walking. *Experimental Brain Research*, *83*(1), 22–28.

Loram, I., Maganaris, C., & Lakie, M. (2004). Paradoxical muscle movement in human standing. *Journal of Physiology*, *556*(Pt 3), 683–689.

Loram, I., Maganaris, C., & Lakie, M. (2009). Paradoxical muscle movement during postural control. *Medicine and Science in Sports and Exercise*, *41*(1), 198–204.

Magnusson, S., Narici, M., Maganaris, C., & Kjaer, M. (2008). Human tendon behaviour and adaptation, in vivo. *Journal of Physiology*, *586*(1), 71–81.

Masani, K., Popovic, M., Nakazawa, K., Kouzaki, M., & Nozaki, D. (2003). Importance of body sway velocity information in controlling ankle extensor activities during quiet stance. *Journal of Neurophysiology*, *90*(6), 3774–3782.

Massion, J. (1998). Postural control systems in developmental perspective. *Neuroscience and Biobehavioral Reviews*, *22*(4), 465–472.

Massion, J., Alexandrov, A., & Frolov, A. (2004). Why and how are posture and movement coordinated? *Progress in Brain Research*, *143*, 13–27.

McLean, S. G., & Beaulieu, M. L. (2010). Complex integrative morphological and mechanical contributions to ACL injury risk. *Exercise and Sport Sciences Reviews*, *38*(4), 192–200.

Milton, J., Townsend, J., King, M., & Ohira, T. (2009). Balancing with positive feedback: The case for discontinuous control. *Philosophical Transactions. Series A, Mathematical, Physical, and Engineering Sciences*, *367*(1891), 1181–1193.

Min, S., Kim, J., & Parnianpour, M. (2012). The effects of safety handrails and the heights of scaffolds on the subjective and objective evaluation of postural stability and cardiovascular stress in novice and expert construction workers. *Applied Ergonomics*, *43*(3), 574–581.

Muyor, J. M., López-Miñarro, P. A., & Alacid, F. F. (2011). A comparison of the thoracic spine in the sagittal plane between elite cyclists and non-athlete subjects. *Journal of Back and Musculoskeletal Rehabilitation*, *24*(3), 129–135.

Nafati, G., & Vuillerme, N. (2011). Decreasing internal focus of attention improves postural control during quiet standing in young healthy adults. *Research Quarterly for Exercise and Sport*, *82*(4), 634–643.

Nashner, L. (1972). Vestibular postural control model. *Kybernetik*, *10*(2), 106–110.

O'Connor, F., Deuster, P., Davis, J., Pappas, C., & Knapik, J. (2011). Functional movement screening: Predicting injuries in officer candidates. *Medicine and Science in Sports and Exercise*, *43*(12), 2224–2230.

O'Sullivan, P., Smith, A., Beales, D., & Straker, L. (2011). Association of biopsychosocial factors with degree of slump in sitting posture and self-report of back pain in adolescents: A cross-sectional study. *Physical Therapy*, *91*(4), 470–483.

Pascual-Leone, A., & Hamilton, R. (2001). The metamodal organization of the brain. *Progress in Brain Research*, *134*, 427–445.

Pollock, A. S., Durward, B. R., Rowe, P. J., & Paul, J. P. (2000). What is balance? *Clinical Rehabilitation*, *14*(4), 402–406.

Prins, Y., Crous, L., & Louw, Q. (2008). A systematic review of posture and psychosocial factors as contributors to upper quadrant musculoskeletal pain in children and adolescents. *Physiotherapy Theory and Practice*, *24*(4), 221–242.

Purves, D., Augustine, G. J., Fitzpatrick, D., et al. (Eds.) (2001). Motor control centers in the brainstem: Upper motor neurons that maintain balance and posture. In *Neuroscience* (2nd ed.). Sunderland, MA: Sinauer Associates.

Redfern, M., Jennings, J., Martin, C., & Furman, J. (2001). Attention influences sensory integration for postural control in older adults. *Gait & Posture*, *14*(3), 211–216.

Resch, J., May, B., Tomporowski, P., & Ferrara, M. (2011). Balance performance with a cognitive task: A continuation of the dual-task testing paradigm. *Journal of Athletic Training*, *46*(2), 170–175.

Riemann, B. L., Guskiewicz, K., & Shields, E. W. (1999). Relationship between clinical and forceplate measures of postural stability. *Journal of Sport Rehabilitation*, *8*(2), 71–82.

Santos, M., & Aruin, A. (2009). Effects of lateral perturbations and changing stance conditions on anticipatory postural adjustment. *Journal of Electromyography and Kinesiology*, *19*(3), 532–541.

Santos, M., Kanekar, N., & Aruin, A. (2010). The role of anticipatory postural adjustments in compensatory control of posture: 1. Electromyographic analysis. *Journal of Electromyography and Kinesiology*, *20*(3), 388–397.

Sasaki, K., & Neptune, R. (2006). Muscle mechanical work and elastic energy utilization during walking and running near the preferred gait transition speed. *Gait & Posture*, *23*(3), 383–390.

Schmid, M., Nardone, A., De Nunzio, A., Schmid, M., & Schieppati, M. (2007). Equilibrium during static and dynamic tasks in blind subjects: No evidence of cross-modal plasticity. *Brain*, *130*(Pt 8), 2097–2107.

Shiratori, T., & Latash, M. (2000). The roles of proximal and distal muscles in anticipatory postural adjustments under asymmetrical perturbations and during standing on rollerskates. *Clinical Neurophysiology*, *111*(4), 613–623.

Shumway-Cook, A., & Horak, F. (1986). Assessing the influence of sensory interaction of balance. Suggestion from the field. *Physical Therapy*, *66*(10), 1548–1550.

Shumway-Cook, A., & Woollacott, M. H. (2005). *Motor control. Theory and practical applications* (2nd ed.). Philadelphia, PA: Lippincott Williams & Wilkins.

Stins, J., Roerdink, M., & Beek, P. (2011). To freeze or not to freeze? Affective and cognitive perturbations have markedly different effects on postural control. *Human Movement Science*, *30*(2), 190–202.

Stuart, D. (2005). Integration of posture and movement: Contributions of Sherrington, Hess, and Bernstein. *Human Movement Science*, *24*(5–6), 621–643.

Swanenburg, J., de Bruin, E., Uebelhart, D., & Mulder, T. (2009). Compromising postural balance in the elderly. *Gerontology*, *55*(3), 353–360.

Tanchev, P., Dzherov, A., Parushev, A., Dikov, D., & Todorov, M. (2000). Scoliosis in rhythmic gymnasts. *Spine*, *25*(11), 1367–1372.

Tetley, M. (2000). Instinctive sleeping and resting postures: An anthropological and zoological approach to treatment of low back and joint pain. *British Medical Journal*, *321*(7276), 1616–1618.

Uemura, K., Yamada, M., Nagai, K., Tanaka, B., Mori, S., & Ichihashi, N. (2012). Fear of falling is associated with prolonged anticipatory postural adjustment during gait initiation under dual-task conditions in older adults. *Gait & Posture*, *35*(2), 282–286.

Uetake, T. T., Ohtsuki, F. F., Tanaka, H. H., & Shindo, M. M. (1998). The vertebral curvature of sportsmen. *Journal of Sports Sciences*, *16*(7), 621–628.

Zettel, J., McIlroy, W., & Maki, B. (2002). Can stabilizing features of rapid triggered stepping reactions be modulated to meet environmental constraints? *Experimental Brain Research*, *145*(3), 297–308.

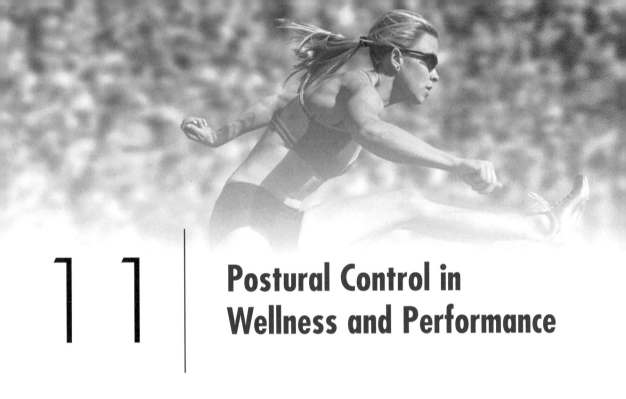

11 | Postural Control in Wellness and Performance

PURPOSE, IMPORTANCE, AND OBJECTIVES OF THIS CHAPTER

The purpose of this chapter is to examine the role that postural control plays in maintaining wellness, improving athletic performance, and prevention of sport-related injury. Postural control is seen as foundational to all of these, and breakdowns in postural control contribute to poorer health and poorer performance and increase the risk of injury. Specific strategies are provided to train postural control, and the evidence for their effectiveness is presented.

After reading this chapter, you should be able to:

1. Describe the relationship between wellness and postural control and potential reasons for poor postural control to develop.
2. Identify effective and noneffective postural control training methods for wellness and provide rationale for why some programs are effective.
3. Define core training and describe what it is most suited for.
4. Describe the relationship between sports performance and postural control and why postural control training for athletes is so perplexing.
5. Describe the relationship between sport injury and postural control, and give explicit guidelines for postural control training for injury prevention and rehabilitation.

In the previous chapter, postural control was seen to be a vital component of motor skill production and in maintaining musculoskeletal integrity. Specifically, the postural control outcomes of whole-body, segmental, and joint alignment and stability provide musculoskeletal integrity and a foundation upon which effective motor skills are enabled. It goes then that poor postural control may lead to a loss of integrity and a poor foundation, contributing to injury, dysfunction, and poor motor skill performance. The need to understand the role of postural control in wellness and performance and work with postural control problems in clients is an important area for exercise science practitioners. In this chapter, we look at these outcomes and the characteristics of effective postural control training programs for general populations and athletes.

WELLNESS AND POSTURAL CONTROL

Measurement difficulties aside, there is sufficient evidence and intuitive rationale to think that deviations in postural alignment or poor stability can be a result of underlying problems, may contribute to the development of future problems, or may hamper the development of high motor skill proficiency. Some postural control problems are clearly the result of pain, injury, disease, emotional guarding, or habitual misuse, but the extent to which postural dysfunction causes pain, injury, negative emotional affect, or movement problems has proven difficult to quantify in many areas. In this section, we examine postural control as a component in wellness and musculoskeletal health.

Maladaptive Postural Control

Poor postural control as evidenced by biomechanical misalignment or poor balance may result from a number of causes, including disease, injury, genetic deformities, and chronic adaptations to lifestyle factors. These lifestyle factors include chronic behaviors such as stress and chronic movement behaviors that arise from work and activities of daily living.

Behavioral states, such as joy and sadness, are reflected in physiological changes, overt movement actions, and subtle changes in tone and postural control (Horslen & Carpenter, 2011; Ma et al., 2006; Mondloch, 2012). Gross et al. (2010, 2012) have noted that specific emotions have specific movement qualities and that there are some generalities. Positive type behaviors are associated with stretching out and opening up type of movements and negative behaviors associated with withdrawing and bowing type movements, and all are rooted in tone and postural control. There is a growing body of evidence to suggest that chronic negative behaviors may lead to disordered muscle tone and associated postural changes. In particular, patients with depression and anxiety disorders have exaggerated fear responses and startle behaviors and disordered muscle tone (Lang & McTeague, 2009; Slósarska, 1986). Repeated physical

SIDE**NOTE**	**DIFFERENT POSTURE ORIENTATIONS AND HEALTH**

The three fundamental posture orientations are standing, seated, and lying down (prone or supine). Because prolonged standing is fatiguing, we often think that faulty standing postures produce the most dysfunction and discomfort. However, poor seated and lying postures can be just as injurious and contribute to medical costs. For instance, the constrained and prolonged seated postures of dental workers contribute to both low back and upper extremity musculoskeletal disorders (Morse et al., 2010; Valachi & Valachi, 2003), and even lying down in bed may contribute to some dysfunction (Normand et al., 2005; Zenian, 2010). Variations or extreme cases of these postures, such as stooping, squatting, kneeling, or constrained lying down, are serious problems in many occupations that contribute to poor performance and musculoskeletal breakdown. Further, they contribute to jobsite accidents, injuries, days lost, disability, and worker dropout (Gallagher, 2005). Accumulating evidence reveals relationships among nonstanding postures, psychosocial dysfunction, and musculoskeletal pain. In a review of musculoskeletal pain in children and adolescents, Prins et al. (2008) noted that children have high exposure to static seated postures while watching television, using a computer and during normal school activities. The duration of this exposure is a risk factor for developing upper body musculoskeletal problems. Moreover, psychosocial factors, including depression, mental stress (e.g., loneliness, anxiety), and psychosomatic complaints, were also related to musculoskeletal discomfort. The relationships among seated posture, psychosocial issues, and musculoskeletal problems have yet to be teased out, but it stands to reason that the reasons children sit for long hours may be related to negative psychosocial influences. Exercise science practitioners must continually address psychosocial issues influencing exercise programming and overall health and well-being.

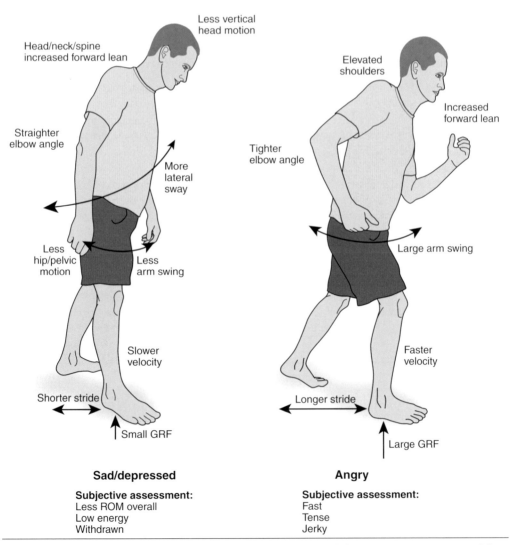

Figure 11.1 • Chronic behavioral states are reflected in these maladaptive movement patterns. These diagrams are based on clinical data from Michalak et al. (2009) and Sloman et al. (1987) comparing depressed mood patients versus nondepressed individuals. Additional experimental data on sad and depressed gait and data for angry gait, based on Roether et al. (2009) and Gross et al. (2012). GRF, ground reaction forces; indicative of how hard one strikes the ground with one's feet. All comparisons made to normal or contented gait. For more on the emotional content of movement, access the point light displays of Niko Troje's lab at *http://www.biomotionlab.ca/*.

and psychological trauma, fear, and associated stressors may result in conditioned and chronic muscular actions and excessively high or low muscle tone that may lead to maladapted postures like tightened shoulders or slumping and in some cases disordered gait (Michalak et al., 2009) (Fig. 11.1). Slumped postures, particularly among male children while seated, are associated with low back pain and psychosocial problems like negative self-worth and anxiety (O'Sullivan et al., 2011; see also accompanying SideNote).

Physiological and biomechanical causes of poor postural control are numerous. Diseases, injuries, and aging that contribute to deficits in musculoskeletal strength and integrity, peripheral (motor and sensory) and central nervous system (CNS) decline, and poorly functioning physiological systems all contribute to postural dysfunction. Poor vision and hearing, medications, and inadequate nutrition

Concepts in Action

Mind and Body Wellness through Postural Control Training

If muscle tone and postural dysfunction are outcomes of negative behaviors or mental states, it stands to reason that improving mental states could improve tone and posture. Furthermore, it could be that improving tone and posture could improve mental states. Numerous physical and psychophysical training methods are based on these ideas and use a variety of techniques to implement the "mind–body" approach. Various techniques may educate clients to relax tightened muscles, increase awareness of their bodies, move in free and unconstrained ways, and think (or image) positive thoughts (Bakal, 1999). The most widespread of these methods are Eastern martial arts (e.g., Tai Chi, yoga) and the Western movement reeducation techniques of the Feldenkrais method and the Alexander technique. These Western methods are purported to address movement dysfunction arising from excess muscle tone caused by storing negative emotions in the muscles in a form of "muscular armor." Both methods were developed by individuals (Moshe Feldenkrais, F.M. Alexander) based on their own posture and movement problems. Proponents of these methods maintain that by engaging in patterned and self-aware movements that emotional stress carried in the muscles as high tone can be released, thereby freeing up mind and body. Though there is some evidence of alternations in postural control (Cacciatore et al., 2011) and countless anecdotes to support the idea of wellness through a freed mind and body, solid experimental and clinical evidence is scarce (see Ives, 2003; Jain et al., 2004; and Woodman & Moore, 2012, for reviews).

may be especially powerful disruptors of postural control in the elderly. In relatively healthy populations, maladaptive postural control may be a result of sustained workplace postures, such as hours of seated work and repetitive assembly-line movements that are strongly linked to musculoskeletal disorders (Gallagher, 2005; Punnett & Wegman, 2004). Recent work has shown that a combination of obesity and low fitness contributes to poor postural control characteristics in adolescents and adults (Błaszczyk et al., 2009; King et al., 2012) and weight loss may contribute to postural stability (Hue et al., 2007). Caution must be urged in interpreting balance and sway laboratory data to real-world circumstances, for there are conflicting data based on age, level of fitness and health, occupational experiences, and more. For instance, overweight has been shown to lessen sway characteristics by providing a more solid base of support, but may lessen balance recovery (Błaszczyk et al., 2009).

Training for Postural Control

Recent years have seen an explosion of exercise programs aimed at "core," stability, and balance, including martial arts like yoga and Tai Chi. Designed to improve overall wellness or specific functional abilities like reducing the incidence of falls in the elders, these programs have been called "sensorimotor training," "neuromuscular training," and "proprioceptive training." Researchers have maintained that these descriptors are inappropriate and this type of training should instead refer to the intended outcome, such as balance training, joint and core stability training, or simply postural control training (Ashton-Miller et al., 2001; Taube et al., 2008). In this section, we examine in brief these programs in healthy and unhealthy adults.

Postural Control Training Methods

In their extensive review on healthy athletes and nonathletes, Zech et al. (2010) noted that most postural control interventions consisted of whole-body balance exercises on unstable platforms like wobble boards and foam surfaces with or without destabilizing forces. These exercises can include single leg stances, jumping and landing, rigorous strength and plyometric exercises, and unilateral strength training (see Behm et al., 2010). Postural control programs for less healthy populations and elders may be general strength training, martial arts, and systematically increasing the challenges of activities of daily living (Cress et al., 2005; Granacher et al., 2011). Though strength training may be of postural benefit to elderly and less healthy populations (Anderson & Behm, 2005), there seems to be no strong association between laboratory measures of strength and measures of postural control in young healthy populations, leading researchers to assert that these should be evaluated separately (Granacher & Gollhofer, 2011). Recent additions to postural control training techniques use computerized force platforms that provide instantaneous feedback on center of pressure movements (Behm et al., 2010). These techniques have emerged from the clinic and laboratory to be part of popular at-home video games, such as the Wii Fit. On the other end of the technology spectrum is the growing use of imagery techniques used by elders with postural control impairments (Pichierri et al., 2011).

Training for body segment stability is often synonymous with **core training**. The core is operationally defined as the axial skeleton, including shoulder and pelvic girdles, and all the soft tissue (ligaments, tendons, fascia, muscles) that attach to it (Behm et al., 2010). Muscles of the core specifically refer to the intrinsic muscles of the trunk but in practical usage must include the musculoskeletal system that attaches the trunk to the extremities and function more to stabilize and orient rather than move limbs. Trunk flexors, extensors, rotators, and lateral flexors (abdominal muscles, erector spinae, small paraspinal muscles, quadratus lumborum) are considered the main core muscles, but hip movers like the small rotators, iliacus and psoas, gluteals, and scapular stabilizers may also be considered core muscles. Addressing core stabilization is more than simply identifying muscles, as the core musculature may activate differently based on movement intentions and outcomes. For instance, differences in abdominal muscle activation are seen if the thorax moves on a stable pelvis or if the pelvis moves on a stable thorax (Vera-Garcia et al., 2011).

Among the core-specific training techniques are directed attempts to contract the abdominal and other core muscles in very specific manners. These techniques include specific exercises for the pelvic floor (Kegel exercises) and abdominal exercises to isolate the transverse abdominis muscle and then coactivate it with internal oblique muscles in a "hollowing" manner. The abdominal hollowing maneuver has been suggested to increase spine stability and decrease pain and dysfunction in patients with disordered motor control (O'Sullivan et al., 1998). Recent research, however, has shown that more global activation of the back and abdominal muscles produces a stronger bracing action and provides stronger stability against both expected and unexpected perturbations and poses a more robust stabilization technique for most people to learn (Grenier & McGill, 2007; Vera-Garcia et al., 2007) (Fig. 11.2). However, further research has suggested that consciously focusing on trunk bracing maneuvers, as opposed to taking on a "natural" stability technique, may lead to asymmetric muscle activation and less spinal stability (Brown et al., 2006). Brown et al. (2006), in accord with discovery learning tenets, noted that eventually individuals must find their own motor strategies for trunk and spinal stability.

■ Thinking It Through 11.1 Breathing and Posture Combined

Many of the same muscles controlling trunk stabilization are also responsible for breathing. These muscles contract and relax cyclically with every breath, which seemingly creates a problem when isometric trunk stabilization is necessary and high contraction effort is required, such as when lifting weights. Researchers have looked at this issue in a variety of ways by assessing EMG patterns and trunk stability measurements during a variety of breathing challenges (Shirley et al., 2003; Wang & McGill, 2008). Among the findings of these studies is that during high exertion physical activity requiring heavy breathing, the back and trunk musculature have a global increase in activity to maintain spinal stabilization. At the end of inspiration when the lungs are at full capacity, trunk stability is increased even more. During inspiration the back extensors are activated, which may be a response to increase spine stiffness. During expiration there may be a relaxing of the abdominal muscles and a reduction in stability. With these findings in mind, evaluate the role of breathing during weight-lifting exercises, in particular, how should one breathe while lifting? Does it matter if the lifting is done while standing, sitting, or lying down? Read the articles by Shirley et al. (2003) and Wang and McGill (2008) and see what these authors have to say.

Core training aims first to stabilize the spine and pelvis to prevent low back injury and pain, and second, to provide a stable center base from which limb movements and associated motor skills can be effectively carried out. Core training almost always includes trunk flexion, extension, and rotation movements, but only recently have isometric exercises, like lateral planks, become popular. Research from Stuart McGill and his colleagues have identified a series of exercises useful to stabilize the spine and prevent low back injury (Hicks et al., 2005; McGill, 2002). More important than the exercises themselves is how they are done: biomechanical form and a strong measure of isometric actions with the purpose to build core muscle endurance and neuromuscular control more so than strength.

Trunk-specific exercises like lateral planks are *primary core training* because the core is emphasized. Other exercises for the core, called *secondary core training*, emphasize noncore movements that require extensive core stabilization. Many different exercise programs fall into this category, ranging from unilateral weight lifting to standing on unstable surfaces (Anderson & Behm, 2005; Behm et al., 2010). Core stabilization training in these situations is a result of overcoming extreme stabilization challenges caused by the primary task (Fig. 11.3). When unstable surfaces are used during weight lifting, the lifting intensity is reduced, but core muscle activation is increased. And though the level of trunk activation may not be maximal, it is more important to train muscle timing, stiffness control, and endurance over training for strength (Behm et al., 2010). Further, researchers have concluded that no core muscle could be singled out as the most important, in part because patterns of postural muscle activation are task and situation dependent (Anderson & Behm, 2005; Behm et al., 2010).

Outcomes of Postural Control Training

For hundreds of years, exercise has been prescribed to fix misaligned posture, including severe abnormalities like scoliosis. Because posture abnormalities may be associated with muscle tightness and

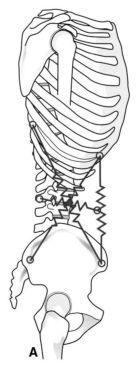
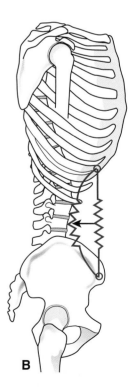

Figure 11.2 • A comparison of abdominal bracing (**A**) versus abdominal hollowing (**B**). During hollowing, the isolated contractions of the transverse abdominis and internal obliques pull the rectus abdominis muscle inward (see *arrow*), reducing its effective moment arm and ability to produce stabilizing torques. On the left, the bracing maneuver maintains the positioning of the rectus abdominis and activates additional stabilizing muscles. (Adapted from Grenier, S., & McGill, S. (2007). Quantification of lumbar stability by using 2 different abdominal activation strategies. *Archives of Physical Medicine and Rehabilitation, 88*(1), 54–62.)

A   B

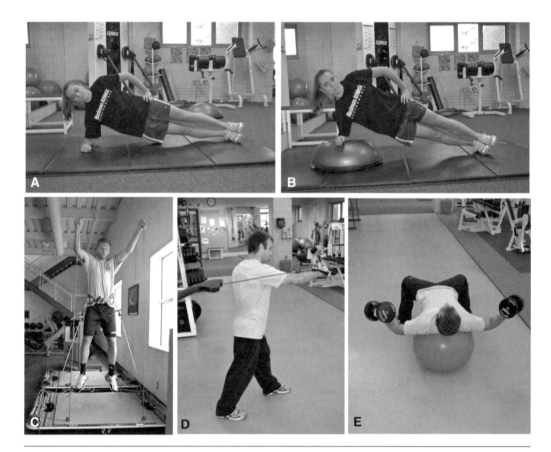

Figure 11.3 • Primary **(A,B)** versus secondary **(C–E)** core training methods. **A.** Standard side plank exercises. **B.** Side plank exercises made more challenging by the addition of an unstable support surface. **C.** Using handheld elastic bands during vertical jumping creates midair trunk loading that must be stabilized in the absence of any ground support surface. **D.** High levels of core stabilization are necessary to support the primary task of a standing unilateral cable press. The asymmetric loading, coupled with no trunk support surface, creates the need for high core muscle activation. **E.** The primary lifting task under the unstable stability ball requires high levels of core stabilization for support. (Photos courtesy of Jeffrey C. Ives.)

weakness and asymmetries, it has been suggested that exercise training, in the form of stretching, calisthenics, and resistance training, may be an effective treatment. On the whole, however, there is little evidence showing demonstrable effects of exercise leading to either better or worse static posture in relatively healthy persons (Hrysomallis & Goodman, 2001). Even exercise programs touted to improve posture and carriage, like Pilates-based exercise, have only been shown to be minimally effective at best (Kloubec, 2010; Kuo et al., 2009).

Targeting specific body segment stability or alignment has shown to be more effective than targeting whole-body postural alignment, particularly in clinical populations. There is consistent evidence showing some improvement in scoliosis and other spinal deformities when treated with targeted exercises in young children and adolescents (Fusco et al., 2011; Hawes, 2003), and adults with hyper- and hypolordosis (Scannell & McGill, 2003). Among the successful treatments for scoliosis include those that fall directly in line with discovery learning, that is, patient control over the training program, psychophysical considerations, and other factors consistent with constraint-based approaches (see Weiss & Turnbull, 2011). Findings of improvements to spinal segment stability and an associated reduction in trunk musculoskeletal disorders and low back pain has also been discussed by McGill (2002, 2004). McGill has noted that specifically targeted mechanisms of trunk stability and neuromuscular control are the key elements of a trunk stability program.

Whole-body balance training is now suggested to be a component of any fitness program aimed at improving functional health, including improvement of activities of daily living and preventing falls. Yet understanding what makes for an effective balance training program that transfers to improved real-life activities is still being uncovered. It is well established that balance training in healthy and unhealthy persons improve clinical measures of static and dynamic sway and balance, and these results can be found across a vast array of balance training methods (DiStefano et al., 2009; Zech et al., 2010). These results should not be interpreted, however, that all balance programs have equal effects on improving functional balance outside the laboratory.

Granacher et al. (2011) have recently reviewed evidence on balance and fall prevention exercise programs for the elderly and noted that traditional programs are effective in reducing fall incidence but not necessarily for fall recovery and reducing fall severity. Traditional approaches to fall prevention in elders are multifaceted strategies aimed at improving patient-related factors and environmental factors. Patient factors include muscle strength, poor vision, medications, self-efficacy, and postural control. Environmental factors include obstructed walkways, poor lighting, and so forth. Effective fall reduction programs vary in scope, but typically include strength training, increasing balance challenges by minimizing the base of support by using single leg or tandem stances, changing sensory input such as closing eyes, and increasing instability by unstable support surfaces and movements of one's center of mass (Fig. 11.4). It is imperative that any training for elders address self-efficacy issues regarding beliefs and symptoms that influence how one performs the tasks for these beliefs may pose more restrictions than actual physical limitations (Liu-Ambrose et al., 2004; Rejeski & Brawley, 2006; Wolf et al., 1997). For example, in a large study of elders undergoing computerized balance training versus Tai Chi training, it was found that the Tai Chi group did not improve on computerized balance scores but did reduce the incidence of falls (Wolf et al., 1997). The authors ascribed the fall prevention success, in part, to confidence gained by the elderly participants.

Recent evidence suggests that adding more task-specific functionality to these programs could be even more effective and, in addition, provide mechanisms to better recover during a fall. Task-specific functionality include the addition of perturbation training and multitask balance training to mimic the causes of falls in real-world activities and high-velocity strength training that trains neuromuscular mechanisms necessary to recover from falls (Granacher et al., 2011). These suggestions are directly in line with research showing that proactive postural control to activate bracing muscles faster and with better coordination dramatically reduce impact forces on the arm when arresting a fall (Lo & Ashton-Miller, 2008). In sum, postural control training to reduce fall injury risk should follow a systems approach in which multiple task demands are meshed with environmental and individual-specific constraints.

Common balance exercises, such as wobble board exercises and movements on foam-cushioned mats, have been shown to improve various laboratory measures of balance, and have been shown to improve some functional performance like walking speed in impaired individuals. Balance exercises have even been shown to improve reflex responses to perturbations in elderly subjects. Generic balance exercise may improve some aspects of motor performance in otherwise healthy persons, for example, single leg balance training may improve leg strength, but specifically focused balance training can have a much larger impact on skills and abilities like vertical jump height, hopping stability, strength, and injury prevention. Taube et al.'s (2008) review noted that balance training for postural stability has direct consequences to sensory systems, motor systems, spinal sensorimotor integration, and cortical and other supraspinal adaptations (Fig. 11.5). These authors also noted a high degree of specificity of training in that both spinal and corticospinal changes were task specific.

■ Thinking It Through 11.2 Balance in the Workplace

Balance and falls are serious concerns in many workplace settings. Slips, trips, and falls account for a large number of injuries in occupations ranging from hospital workers to construction workers. Construction workers, in particular, face the real risk of disabling injury or death in falls from high platforms. Hsiao and Simeonov (2001) summarized that the conditions workers face come down to challenges in proactive and reactive balance control within a dynamic systems model. As shown below, the interaction of the environment, the individual, and task constraints must be considered. Environmental physical constraints include unstable surfaces due to loose and slippery materials on roofs, steeply pitched roofs, confined spaces, and unstable ladders and scaffolds. Being on roofs and other high elevations, especially when sloped, creates visual ambiguity and perception problems. For example, think about the visual confusion that may occur if the worker in the photo below were to look up from the task and look around from

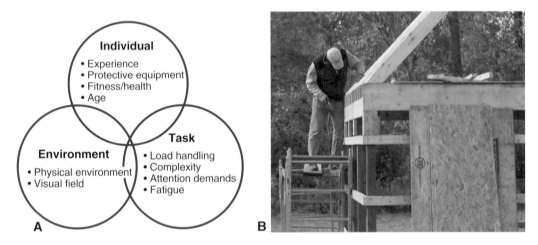

Construction, farm, and other manual labor jobs provide ample opportunities for injury due to disordered postural control and the need for balance. **A.** The three component dynamic systems model of constraints related to construction worker falls based on Hsiao and Simeonov (2001). **B.** This photo demonstrates many of the constraints noted by Hsiao and Simeonov. The worker is standing on an unstable platform (scaffolding planks) and checking his balance by leaning against the building. Leaning may further indicate fatigue is setting in. The multitask challenge (scaffold balance, holding the lumber, swinging the hammer) has a high attention demand. It is likely that the postural stiffness throughout the trunk and legs is large and postural fatigue a likely outcome that may increase the risk of falling or musculoskeletal injury. (Photo courtesy of Jeffrey Ives.)

his high perch. Task-related factors include heavy load handling, fatiguing situations, and complex and dual-task situations requiring considerable attention demands. Individual factors include age, fitness and health, experience, and use of safety equipment. Among the recommendations to prevent falls, these authors suggested a better understanding of individual capabilities (e.g., fatigue and balance control) and balance training with high attentional demands while doing tasks.

With this in mind, ponder the exercise prescription needs for a typical construction worker. What would be of most benefit: an aerobic exercise program, a strength training program, or a form of occupation-specific functional training for fall prevention? Given the realistic scenario that an individual will not engage all three types over the course of a typical week, prioritize an exercise program for these needs.

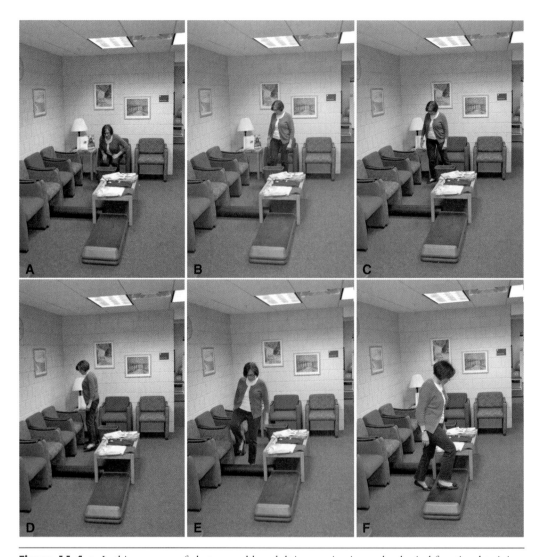

Figure 11.4 • In this sequence of photos, an older adult is engaging in psychophysical functional training. Constraints, in the form of obstacles and decision making, make the simple sit to stand to walk task more challenging. Physical obstacles of steps and narrow pathways require side steps, high steps, and fall awareness. Cognitive constraints include having the client read the headlines from the magazines and newspapers on the table and engage in conversations. (Photo courtesy of Jeffrey Ives.)

In summary, exercises for body segment stability and balance can have positive effects on health and performance, particularly for populations with declining function. Balance exercises in particular should follow a dynamic systems constraint-based approach by maximizing real-world environmental challenges and necessary task requirements and target the physiological and psychological declines in the individuals being served. This may mean that some populations require more strength training, some might need muscle endurance training, and others may need dual-task challenges. It is particularly important to address behavioral issues in populations struggling with movement apprehension and cognitive and emotional dysfunction.

SIDE**NOTE**	**INVESTIGATING FALL PREVENTION AND OBSTACLE AVOIDANCE**

Weerdesteyn et al. (2008) conducted one of the more elegant studies looking at how older individuals respond to obstacles to prevents falls and how training may influence their fall prevention performance. Using a special treadmill that could drop an obstacle onto the treadmill belt (see below), participants were filmed with high-speed video to assess their obstacle-avoiding stepping patterns. Some of the subjects underwent a training program for 10 sessions over 5 weeks that included walking in crowded rooms, stepping over obstacles and walking on unstable or irregular surfaces like stepping stones, and various sit to stand and reaching movements. Many of these tasks were done with visual challenges, dual-task motor challenges (e.g., carrying a grocery bag), and dual-task cognitive challenges (e.g., repeating a story). The participants also engaged in fall recovery motor skill training based on martial arts. In contrast to a control group that did not engage in training, the trained subjects had more successful obstacle avoidance on the treadmill, generally by having longer strides over the obstacle. These authors noted that other researchers have used generic strength training interventions and had found similar results. This led the authors to suggest that the self-efficacy benefits of exercise are at least partly responsible for improved obstacle avoidance.

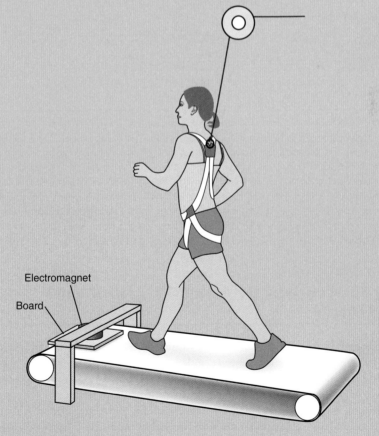

The experimental treadmill setup like that used by Weerdesteyn et al. (2008). The bridge over the front of the treadmill housed an electromagnet that held up a metal and wood board. The magnet could be controlled by a computer to drop the board onto the treadmill at random times during the gait cycle. The person was instructed to step over, not on or around, the object.

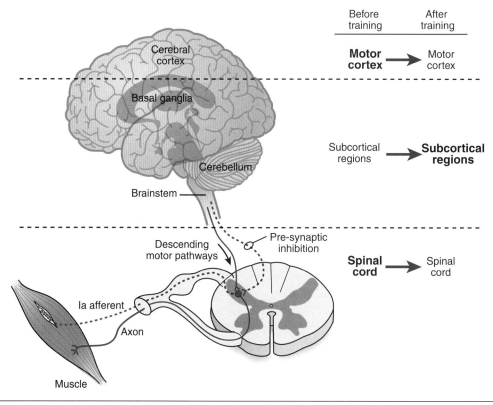

Figure 11.5 • CNS changes resultant from postural control training. On the left are the primary structures and regions thought to be involved in postural control learning, ranging from cortical and higher-level brain structures to subcortical regions to the spinal cord. On the right are the areas of change following training. Cortical regions decrease in activity, subcortical regions are thought to increase in activity and overall importance, and the spinal cord lessens activity. The reduced spinal activity and decreased reflex excitability is likely from presynaptic inhibition from supraspinal centers. (Adapted from Taube, W., Gruber, M., & Gollhofer, A. (2008). Spinal and supraspinal adaptations associated with balance training and their functional relevance. *Acta Physiologica*, *193*, 101–116. With permission from Wiley-Blackwell, Copyright 2008 Scandinavian Physiological Society, doi: 10.1111/j.1748–1716.2008.01850.x.)

POSTURAL CONTROL IN ATHLETES AND SPORT PERFORMANCE

The very nature of most sporting activities requires athletes to perform forceful and precise movements while in off-balance positions or be subjected to large amounts of destabilizing forces. Figure 11.6 depicts the postural control needs during a coordinated sporting action and the potential outcomes during an uncoordinated action. Outstanding postural control is thus imperative for athletes, yet identifying the postural control characteristics associated with high-level performers is more ambiguous than assessing postural control faults in injured and unhealthy individuals. As seen previously, sporting activities may contribute to postural misalignment in athletes, and exercises to correct this misalignment are largely unsuccessful (Hrysomallis & Goodman, 2001). In regard to stability and balance, the balance performance of "balance athletes" (e.g., gymnasts, dancers, surfers) may or may not be better than other athletes or nonathletes. Balance performance appears to be specific to the conditions and situations imposed by the sport-specific activities (Hrysomallis, 2011). Furthermore, there are data

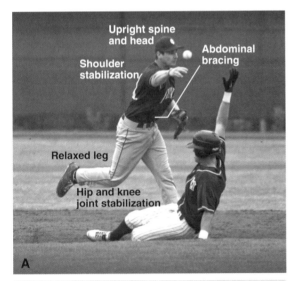

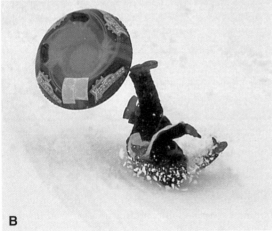

Figure 11.6 • Postural control needs during athletic performance and preparing for destabilizing forces. **A.** The player making the double play throw must have considerable support from postural control mechanisms to enable a strong and accurate throw, all while avoiding the runner and preparing for impact should avoidance fail. In this case, the player's preparation for impact forces will minimize the chance of injury. (Photo courtesy of Greg Schneider.) **B.** Unpredictability and suddenness of a perturbation leaves the body unprepared for stability changes and reliant on reactive mechanisms. A lack of practice at "wiping out" and disorientation have left this sledder in a vulnerable headfirst position going down the hill. (Photo courtesy of Jeffrey Ives.)

showing that higher-level athletes may perform better or worse than their lower-level counterparts on standard force platform stability tests or that balance and sport performance may be correlated in low- but not high-level performers (see Behm et al., 2010, and Hrysomallis, 2011, for reviews). There is a large amount of research on athletes of many different sports using many different postural control measures and many different performance measures, and the only firm summary that can be made is that relationship between postural control measures and athletic performance are more complex that can be elucidated by current measures of posture and performance (Zech et al., 2010).

Training Postural Control for Sport Performance

With such ambiguity in the relationship between measures of postural control and athletic performance, does it make sense to specifically train postural control? Researchers and clinicians generally agree the answer is yes for two reasons. The first is that the standard postural tests may simply not be sufficient to tease out the true relationship between postural control and performance, and despite this, there is some evidence to pursue training programs for performance improvement in some classes of athletes. Second, there is strong evidence that postural control training may reduce the risk of musculoskeletal injury, and this is a sufficient reason by itself.

■ Thinking It Through 11-3 Interpreting Balance Scores in Athletes

Computerized force plate balance assessments measure the amount of sway by changes in foot pressure on the force plate. From these data, measurements like sway velocity and sway distance are gathered. It is well recognized that persons with pathologies and the elderly sway more than young healthy persons and challenging situations (e.g., eyes closed) cause more sway. But does more sway always mean poorer postural control or balance? Consider research on expert surfers compared to recreational surfers and swimmers (control subjects) by Chapman et al. (2008). All subjects were evaluated for postural sway under eyes open and eyes closed conditions, under conditions with the head tilted back, and conditions in which they had a concurrent mental task. Under normal condition of eyes open, the expert surfers swayed more than the swimmers. Under the challenging conditions of no vision and with the head tilted back, all subjects swayed more as expected. During the dual-task cognitive challenges, sway was only minimally affected (tended to be less), but the expert surfers still swayed more than the recreational surfers and control subjects. In an assessment of balance in ballet dancers, Hugel et al. (1999) found that the dancers' performance was more negatively affected (more sway velocity) by eyes closed than a control group of nondancers. Perrin et al. (2002) compared static and dynamic balance in expert judoists, ballet dancers, and controls. On most measures of sway with eyes open and closed and on a moving platform, the judoists swayed less than the controls and less than the dancers. In fact, on a couple of measurements, the dancers swayed more than the controls. Altogether these data reveal that expert balancers (surfers, judoists, dancers) may sway more or may sway less than controls and they may be more affected by challenging balance situations than controls. Overall, how would you interpret these data? Consider differences in these activities (and training) that could lead to these balance differences (e.g., Gentile's classification scheme). Also consider if increased sway is really a negative outcome or a positive outcome of training.

One purpose of postural control training is to improve trunk stability in order to improve motor skill execution. Unfortunately, there is little evidence in athletes and relatively healthy persons that demonstrate that trunk or core training actually improves performance. This lack of data, however, should not necessarily be interpreted that core training does not work. Rather it reflects an overall lack of data, measurement difficulties in determining core muscle function, and a general difficulty in determining the contribution of abilities into specific motor skill performance (Behm et al., 2010).

Balance training in recreational athletes and fit and active persons has been shown in some cases to improve vertical jump height, rate of muscle tension development, and some sport performance and agility tests (Zech et al., 2010). Balance training has been shown to improve laboratory measures of balance in active and athletic populations, but to date, no balance training program has been shown to be superior to resistance training for improving the performance or underlying abilities (e.g., sprint speed, jump height) of accomplished athletes. This does not necessarily rule out that aspects of postural control training may induce neural changes in athletes that could eventually manifest itself in better on field performance (for reviews, see Hrysomallis, 2011; Taube et al., 2008; Zech et al., 2010).

Given these findings, a number of researchers have provided recommendations for postural control training to improve athletic performance. These recommendations are first that postural control training should not replace other conditioning programs and younger and nonelite athletes are more likely to gain benefits than elite athletes. Next, postural control training must be multifaceted, comprehensive, rigorous, and sport specific. Programs can be incorporated into other conditioning exercises, such as sport-specific strength training programs done under both stable and unstable conditions (Anderson & Behm, 2005). Finally, programs should emphasize proactive postural mechanisms by creating uncertainty and the need for rapid decision making, which may force postural control systems to "expect the unexpected."

Additional recommendations can be found for trunk stability (e.g., core) training programs for athletes who are merging strength and stability training. McGill (2002, 2004; see also Behm et al., 2010) emphasized that no single core muscle should be singled out because the intensity and control of trunk musculature is task and situation dependent. Athletes should be coached to use abdominal bracing techniques during lifting, particularly during instability conditions. Athletes may utilize unstable surfaces (e.g., wobble boards) or unstable weights during lifting to force the need for increased core activation and stabilization. Unstable weights are most often the use of unilateral lifts to create an asymmetric load on the body segments. Regardless of the instability technique used, there is a decrease in the amount of weight that can be lifted, which may hamper the development of maximum strength if overused.

REHABILITATION AND PREVENTION OF SPORT JOINT INJURY

Unlike the previous section in which postural control training provides an uncertain benefit to athletic performance, such training has resulted in demonstrable reductions in sport-related musculoskeletal injuries. These injuries include ankle and knee sprains and, to a lesser extent, shoulder injuries. To better understand how postural control training may help prevent injury or reinjury, it is helpful to take a brief look at the control of joint stability and the etiology of a traumatic joint injury.

Control of Joint Stability

We have seen that one outcome of postural control is joint stability. Also contributing to joint stability is a static mechanical support system based on joint structure and musculotendinous and ligamentous

SIDE**NOTE**	**RESEARCHING ATHLETE POSTURAL CONTROL**

Measuring postural control in athletes, in particular during real-life sporting actions, requires creativity to produce valid and reproducible results. Consider, for example, jumping into the air and reaching to catch an off-target object. Such a movement causes the body to land in a skewed fashion, which has been hypothesized to be a prime cause of musculoskeletal injury. Measuring this type of body action using typical laboratory equipment would limit the freedom and spontaneity of the movement and call into question the validity of the results. Dempsey et al. (2012) addressed some of these validity issues by using the set up shown in the figure on the next page. Experimental subjects leaped to catch a ball that was airborne using a pendulum and gantry system in a huge open room that provided realistic visual perception of an overhead pass in Australian football. The gantry system enabled the balls to arrive in various directions in a reproducible manner, but the direction was not known in advance by the subjects. The subjects were outfitted with reflective markers for 3-D biomechanical video analysis and the only instructions given were to land on a specific leg. A force platform gathered ground reaction force data and was large enough to minimally influence the subjects' attention on trying to land on a small target. These authors found that the ball direction (toward or away from the subject) and the reach distance had a large influence on knee stability during landing. In particular, when the subject needed to reach out for the ball while it was coming toward him top photos knee valgus forces were highest. These valgus forces have been suggested to increase injury risk. The authors found other results regarding trunk and knee movements that are contrary to popular knee stability training guidelines, such as "knees over toes." Based on their findings, these authors suggested that knee stability training should avoid torso flexed postures, avoid external rotation of the foot and knee, and avoid internal rotation of the hip. Instead, the trunk should be upright and the feet and knees pointed in the direction of travel. Of course, learning to do this in the flow of the game remains a challenge, and reproducing these findings is necessary to consider them trustworthy.

continued on following page

| SIDE**NOTE** | **RESEARCHING ATHLETE POSTURAL CONTROL** (Continued) |

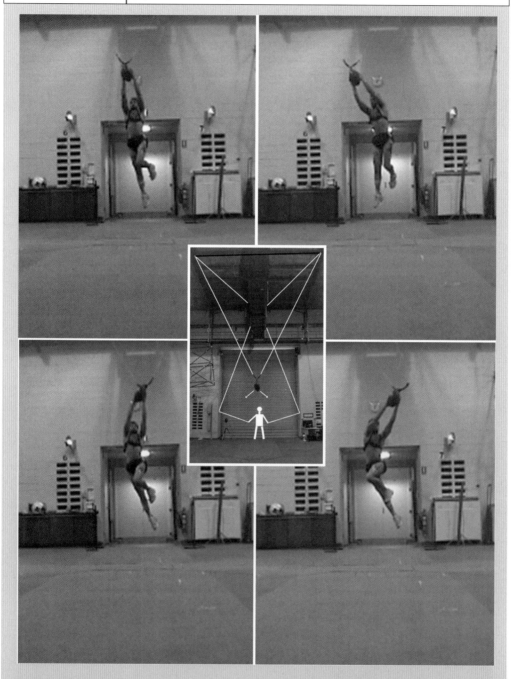

Reprinted and adapted from Dempsey, A., Elliott, B., Munro, B., Steele, J., & Lloyd, D. (2012). Whole body kinematics and knee moments that occur during an overhead catch and landing task in sport. *Clinical Biomechanics, 27*(5), 466–474, with permission from Elsevier.

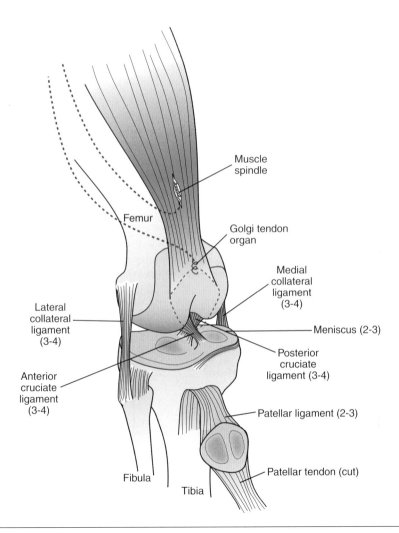

Figure 11.7 • Knee joint stability mechanisms. This diagram illustrates the key features of the knee joint (and similar highly mobile joints) responsible for static and dynamic stabilization. The meniscus, capsule and capsular ligaments (collateral), intracapsular ligaments (cruciate), and surrounding muscle–tendon complexes provide mechanical stabilization. Shown with each tissue is the number of different types of sensory endings found within that tissue. Varying tissue mechanical properties, coupled with the response characteristics of different sensory endings, enable feedback regarding joint stress and strain, compressive forces, positions, and movement.

tissues. Tissues in and around a joint have specific roles to maintain joint function, from providing mechanical stabilization to producing nutrients or lubrication. Figure 11.7 illustrates that for the knee many tissues in the joint are likely to have at least one type of sensory ending and often three to four different receptor types. Other than Golgi tendon organs and muscle spindles, each of these tissues may contain pacinian corpuscles, Meissner's corpuscles (skin), Ruffini endings, Golgi tendon–like endings, and free dendritic endings (Hogervorst & Brand, 1998; Solomonow & Krogsgaard, 2001).

These receptors may participate directly in reflex arcs, act as modifiers to muscle spindle activity in both local and distal muscles, help maintain and monitor tissue homeostasis like inflammation, provide pain signals, and provide feedback to the CNS regarding joint integrity and joint action (Beckman & Buchanan, 1995; Hogervorst & Brand, 1998). The variety of receptors in some tissues marks these tissues as highly important stimulus receivers and underscores the role that sensory detection plays in maintaining joint stability.

At rest, the mechanical support structures are important for stability, but during dynamic actions, joint stability relies on postural control mechanisms, both reactive and proactive (Riemann & Lephart, 2002a,b; Solomonow & Krogsgaard, 2001). Figure 11.8 illustrates a model of joint stability based on Riemann and Lephart's (2002a) functional joint stability model and coinciding with our previous model of postural control. This model depicts joint stability arising primarily from postural control and mechanical systems and, to a lesser extent, motor skill proficiency. It can be speculated that more coordinated motor skill execution may lead to fewer off-balance forces and, thus, lower injury risk (Gabbett et al., 2012). The figure also depicts reflex responses as separate from other reactive postural mechanisms to set apart their contributions as joint stabilizers. The knee anterior cruciate ligament (ACL), for example, has a direct reflex arc to activate the hamstrings musculature, helping to pull the tibia back into place following anterior displacement forces (Solomonow et al., 1987). Shoulder capsule and ligamentous sensory systems appear to have similar functions in maintaining glenohumeral positioning and stiffness (Hundza & Zehr, 2007; Myers et al., 2004; Nyland et al., 1998; Riemann & Lephart, 2002b).

Despite the presence of these reflex arcs, Figure 11.8 shows the contribution from these reflexes to be uncertain. They have been shown to be variable across joints or type of perturbation, or too weak

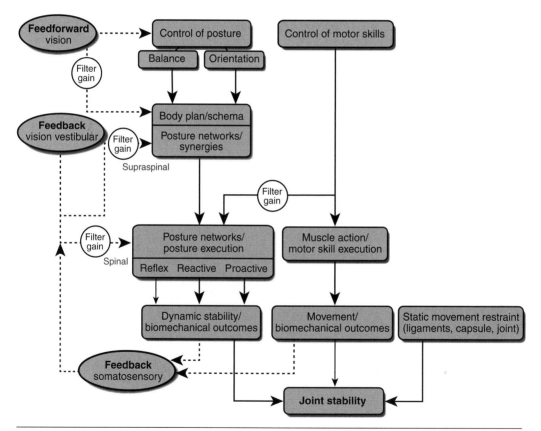

Figure 11.8 • Schematic of joint stability mechanisms. Dynamic postural mechanisms and static mechanical restraints are seen as direct controllers of stability. Reflex control is shown separate from other reactive mechanisms to illustrate a separate and less understood contribution. A *thin arrow* connects motor skill outcomes with stability as well, for smoother, and more coordinated movements likely reduce destabilizing joint forces and avoid environmental hazards. Dashed lines are sensory information, dark lines are motor commands.

to sufficiently stabilize a perturbed joint. Numerous research reports on knee and ankle joint stability and mechanisms have been unable to conclusively document the strength of reflex control in joint stability, particularly under large perturbation forces (see discussions in Friemert et al., 2010; Solomonow & Krogsgaard, 2001). Muscle spindle stretch reflex responses have been shown at times to be capable of stabilizing a perturbed joint, but less is known about the joint mechanoreceptors (Friemert et al., 2010). Nevertheless, even if spindle and joint receptor reflexes are insufficient to create joint stability by themselves, they have far-reaching effects that may be even more important. For instance, the most important role of knee ligament receptors may be to modulate the muscle spindle stretch reflex than directly activate skeletal muscle. Furthermore, distal joints and muscles can be affected, for example, ankle problems have been shown to affect gluteal muscles and hip motion (Beckman & Buchanan, 1995) and hip motion affects soleus reflex excitability (Kawashima et al., 2006).

It is increasingly understood that feedforward and anticipatory postural control are required to maintain and ready the joint for large disturbances (Palmieri-Smith et al., 2008). Preactivation of knee and ankle musculature, for example, not only controls dampening and force transmission but braces the joints against destabilizing forces. Furthermore, in highly trained individuals, proactive postural control not only prepares the joints for expected stresses but also for unexpected stresses and perturbations. Uncertainty in task requirements creates changes in proactive postural control such that it is more flexible and adaptable (Leukel et al., 2012). Movement training to prepare for the unexpected, as described below, is a key element in successful injury prevention programs.

Etiology of Sport-Related Joint Injury

In a typical sport-related joint injury, the joint is subjected to rapid and excessive forces. These forces may be from external contacts, such as collision with another player, or noncontact forces due to abrupt changes in body position or unexpected environmental conditions (e.g., hole in the ground or slippery surfaces). The vast majority of lower extremity joint injuries are noncontact, meaning that the body's own forces and movements have led to injury. This further means that controlling the body's forces and movements may decrease the potential for injury. Ligaments are a likely injured tissue, but cartilage, joint capsule, tendons, bursae, tendon sheaths, the surrounding skin, and other tissue in the area may be damaged.

Following a joint injury, the stability of the joint may be compromised for several reasons. The most noticeable is a reduction in mechanical stability due to weakened and damaged connective tissues. Changes in tissue mechanical properties also change the nature of the stimulus–response characteristics of the receptors within the tissue and, subsequently, the nature of the information sent to the CNS. Receptors may respond differently to changes in force, velocity, or acceleration or may no longer be directionally tuned after tissue damage. Joint stabilizing reflexes initiated from ligaments or meniscus receptors may no longer work satisfactorily (Al-Dadah et al., 2011; Krogsgaard et al., 2011). When the ACL or other ligaments are damaged, the sensory signals often result in aberrant reflexes or poor kinesthesia (Krogsgaard et al., 2011; Solomonow et al., 1987). Pain can also affect muscle activation. For example, low back pain may alter the subconscious and automatic activation of gluteal muscles during gait and change gait biomechanics (Himmelreich et al., 2008). In all of these cases, the poor motor control can be considered to be a result of inappropriate sensory functioning or inappropriate perception combined with maladaptive voluntary motor control strategies.

This change in sensory signaling after injury must be reinterpreted by the CNS in regard to joint movement, joint health, and joint stability. That is, the brain must relearn the meaning of the altered sensory signaling, and if it does not, joint stability may remain compromised. For example, arthrogenic muscle inhibition may continue long after injury, weakening the surrounding joint musculature. Finally, sensory endings and neurons themselves may be damaged, leading to a loss in sensory function.

Joint surgery itself causes extensive joint damage, such as tendon or ligament grafting to replace damaged tissue. Newly grafted tissue does not have sensory innervation, which raises the question if the new tissue gets restored proprioceptive function. Recent evidence shows that these tissues may reinnervate and provide sensory signaling after months of healing. Grafts can (but not always) regenerate new mechanoreceptor afferent pathway and reflex arcs (Tsuda et al., 2003). It is thought that existing mechanoreceptors may grow new afferent neurons, and it is unknown if new receptors can also be grown. Why some persons have strongly restored sensory pathways and others do not is unclear, but there is some evidence that the level of regeneration is tied to the amount or quality of rehabilitation exercises. Whereas reinnervation may occur in cases of injury repair, there is no evidence of other sensory morphological changes as a result of training. For instance, neither intrafusal fiber hypertrophy nor morphological adaptations to tendon organ pathways have been found. These findings highlight that training for injury rehabilitation should focus on relearning postural stabilization and not tissue healing *per se*.

Mechanical insufficiency by the supporting connective and muscle tissue can most likely be overcome by traditional rehabilitation training, but it is just a part of the overall mechanisms that control the joint's stability. The nervous system must be trained to provide postural control, particularly proactive control.

Risk Factors for Joint Injury

Given the complex and multifaceted nature of joint stability, it is no surprise that risk factors for injury are also complex and multifaceted. Because female athletes compared to their male counterparts have been shown to have a two to four times the risk for serious knee and ankle injury, those looking at risk factors have emphasized gender differences. Risk factors for ankle and knee (primarily ACL) injuries have been identified as modifiable and nonmodifiable, with most attention placed on those that appear modifiable through training or other interventions (Hewett et al., 2010; McLean & Beaulieu, 2010). Among the nonmodifiable risk factors thought to put females at more risk are shallower and less robust joint structures, increased joint laxity, smaller ligament size and less robust ligament morphology, greater body fat, and less favorable structural alignment such as increased femoral anteversion and larger Q-angle (for reviews, see Donaldson, 2012; Hewett et al., 2010; McLean & Beaulieu, 2010; Myer et al., 2008). Among the modifiable risk factors are poor leg muscle coordination leading to poor jumping control, excessive knee wobble, and unstable landing mechanics; altogether these are called the "high-risk" biomechanical profile (Hewett et al., 2010; McLean & Beaulieu, 2010). This high-risk biomechanical profile has been the target of most intervention programs. There is a growing consensus that poor trunk and hip control of female athletes may also pose as a risk factor (McLean & Beaulieu, 2010; Mendiguchia et al., 2011) and attention has begun to turn there as a target for intervention.

Among other risk factors for sport injury is fatigue. Epidemiological and circumstantial evidence associates fatigue with an increased risk of musculoskeletal injury (Gabbett, 2004; Rahnama et al., 2002). These data are supported by experimental studies showing fatigue lowers tissue strength, changes muscle activation patterns, and alters sensory and reflex function (Gehring et al., 2009; see Alentorn-Geli, 2009a, for review). A disturbance in postural control is theorized to have a large influence on injury risk. Paillard (2012) noted that both local muscular fatigue and general fatigue lead to a cascade of physiological and neurological breakdowns that contribute to disordered postural control (see Fig. 11.9). In his review, Paillard noted that decreased physiological performance, such as muscle weakness, leads to compensatory motor strategies and a reweighting of sensory information. A loss of energy substrates, a buildup of metabolic byproducts, dehydration, altered tissue mechanics, altered contractile characteristics, and changing movement biomechanics lead to altered proprioceptive, visual, and vestibular sensitivity and a reweighting toward visual information. This change contributes to an altered postural body schema that may inaccurately reflect actual body mechanics and geometry. Together with CNS fatigue, these postural mechanisms become insufficient to proactively or reactively adjust to postural disturbances.

Training Programs

Since the mid-1990s, there has been an ongoing shift in the rehabilitation and prevention strategies for joint injuries in sports involving running, cutting, jumping, and other potential noncontact injury mechanisms. This shift has been accompanied by a large number of research studies, culminating in

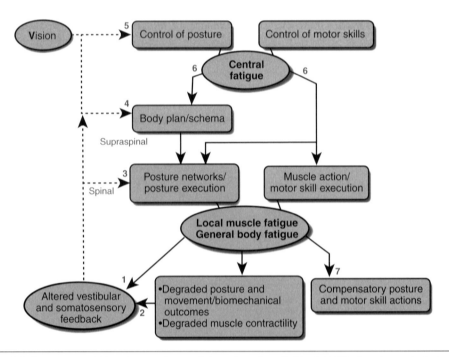

Figure 11.9 • Postural disturbances due to fatigue, based on Paillard (2012). Local muscle fatigue and general fatigue lead to degraded muscle function, posture, and motor skill performance. This degradation may be sufficient to increase injury risk by itself, but additional mechanisms also add to the risk. The fatigue itself leads to proprioceptive dysfunction (*1*) and the degraded posture and motor skills also lead to faulty proprioception (*2*). Disordered proprioception is fed back to the spinal networks (*3*) and leads to modified reflexes and possibly modified pattern generators. Disordered proprioception is also responsible for erroneous information to the CNS leading to an aberrant body schema (*4*) and faulty information upon which to base posture and motor skill commands (*5*). An increased reliance on vision may be a compensatory adaption. Central fatigue may contribute to the aberrant body schema and disordered motor commands (*6*) that further constrain posture and motor skill control. Eventually compensatory strategies (*7*) will be adopted, including altered neural recruitment, changes in coordination and anticipatory postural adjustments, altered stiffness control, increased or decreased reflex excitability, increased spindle gain, increased use of proximal muscles and proximal postural control strategies (e.g., hip strategy), increased reliance on nonfatigued sensory sources, and increased filtering of sensation from fatigued sources.

recent years with several comprehensive scientific and evidence-based reviews of what works and what does not. As might be expected based on lower extremity joint injury prevalence, much of this work has focused on young female athletes. Some interventions have further focused on modifying risk factors; some have targeted specific injuries (e.g., recovery from ACL surgery), while others have looked solely at injury prevalence following training.

The most notable finding from the extensive reviews is that training programs, when done correctly, can positively impact the modifiable risk factors and can reduce joint injury rates in male and female athletes by improving postural control mechanisms. Some of these programs may also improve physical abilities like vertical jump height and sport-specific function (for review, see Noyes & Barber Westin, 2012). These results are not without negative findings, but the methodologically sound and reliable studies show positive benefits (see reviews by Alentorn-Geli et al., 2009b; Hübscher et al., 2010; Lerch et al., 2011; Noyes & Barber Westin, 2012). Another consensus is that mediocre adherence by younger and nonelite athletes is a problem and limits the effectiveness of prevention and rehabilitation programs (Lerch et al., 2011).

Preventative balance training alone can help reduce the incidence of ankle sprains, particularly in those with a history of injury, but this training has little influence on knee or upper extremity injury rates or severity (Hübscher et al., 2010). Multi-intervention programs (balance, strength, agility), however, not only reduce ankle injuries even more but can reduce knee injury rates, reduce the overall risk of lower extremity injuries, and may reduce some cases of upper extremity injuries (see also Alentorn-Geli et al., 2009b). Given sufficient rigor, adherence, and duration of training for injuries treated conservatively without an operation, researchers have found a reduced incidence of recurrent lower limb joint sprains and "giving-way" episodes and better dynamic balance but inconsistent results for other measures like edema, muscle reflex times, and knee function scores (Zech et al., 2009).

There is a growing consensus on what works and what does not. Hewett et al. (2006) summarized several key features of effective programs for knee and ankle injury prevention based on an extensive meta-analysis of the literature. The most successful programs are multifaceted, are of longer duration (e.g., 60 minutes per session), and last at least 6 weeks. They involve various forms of jumping, leaping, or hopping, generally in the form of plyometric training. Most programs incorporate running, cutting, and strength training. The successful programs emphasize movement quality and postural control over fitness development, and teaching movement quality is the foremost responsibility of instructors.

Concepts in Action

Evaluating Knee Injury Risk

Excessive knee valgus (knee inward buckling) upon landing is suggested to be indicative of poor knee stability control and a risk factor for knee injury, particularly in females. In the photos below are three females landing from a depth jump. **A.** This 8-year-old girl displays unilateral valgus of her left knee. **B.** A young adult female athlete displays similarly poor valgus movements. **C.** In contrast, this 10-year-old girl shows what looks to be good knee control during landing, suggesting that females are not automatically at risk.

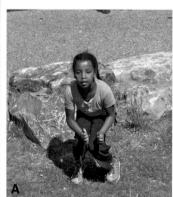 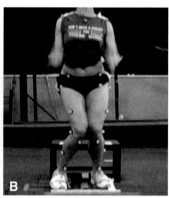 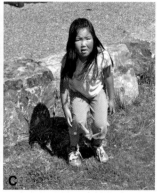

A,B. Photos courtesy of Jeffrey Ives. **C.** Reproduced from Myer, G., Ford, K., & Hewett, T. (2011). New method to identify athletes at high risk of ACL injury using clinic-based measurements and freeware computer analysis. *British Journal of Sports Medicine, 45*(4), 238–244, with permission from BMJ Publishing Group Ltd.

continued on following page

Exactly what constitutes poor knee control and how to measure it with simplicity and validity was investigated by Myer et al. (2011) using standard video cameras and ImageJ software. These authors used digital cameras set up for sagittal and frontal views and used screen snapshots to capture individual images upon which to make measurements. These images were loaded into ImageJ available from the National Institutes of Health (www.nih.gov), and knee angles were measured. These angles, along with anthropometric and strength data, were input into a knee injury risk nomogram that provides an injury risk profile. A sample of the nomogram is shown below. See if you can use the Myer et al. (2011) techniques to evaluate the injury risk of several of your classmates. Access the article (see references for complete citation) and follow their instructions for photography and analysis. Use the nomogram to determine injury risk.

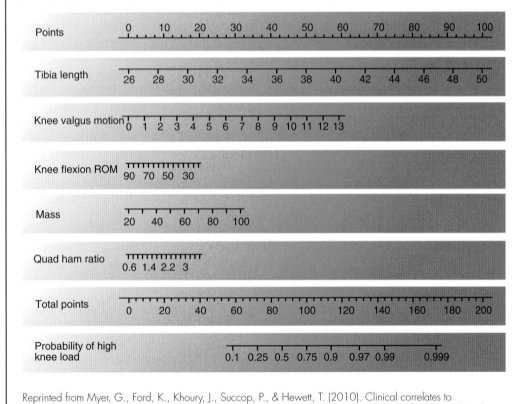

Reprinted from Myer, G., Ford, K., Khoury, J., Succop, P., & Hewett, T. (2010). Clinical correlates to laboratory measures for use in non-contact anterior cruciate ligament injury risk prediction algorithm. *Clinical Biomechanics, 25*(7), 693–699, with permission from Elsevier.

The successful programs have similarities in how movement quality is taught. The first is the use of critical analysis of movement technique and the use of feedback by instructors. Sport-specific injury prevention strategies, such as landing techniques, must be identified. Next, athletes are encouraged to use imagery alongside instructor verbal and visual cues in order to formulate movement solutions, rather than simply follow prescriptions. Finally, athletes are encouraged to evaluate movements, for example, using video, and devise their own prevention strategies. Other authors have noted that successful programs include core and trunk control (Alentorn-Geli et al., 2009b) and sport-specific perception–action situations, such as fatigue, decision making, external focus of attention, and randomness (McLean & Beaulieu, 2010).

Recent summative findings have emphasized the need for individual-specific programs regardless of gender, but with the caveat that training programs for women should account for the nonmodifiable gender differences in joint structure and skeletal alignment (McLean & Beaulieu, 2010). In particular, specific postural alignment at landing impact for females should differ from males because of the hip and knee structural differences, and these landing strategies should emphasize more hip and trunk control (McLean & Beaulieu, 2010; Mendiguchia et al., 2011).

The programs shown to be effective follow deliberate practice and exploratory learning strategies. They are designed to overcome weaknesses (poor biomechanics and poor movement patterns), and movements are repeated in different contexts to solidify the basic movement patterns and to make them adaptable to changing environments. Though instructors must identify specific areas for improvement (e.g., reducing valgus knee motion), it is up to the athlete to figure out the best way to reach that goal. From what we have learned in previous chapters, this type of training targets the psychophysiological systems as much as musculoskeletal systems.

SUMMARY

Postural control mechanisms are essential to maintain joint integrity and balance and produce efficient and effective movement. Poor postural control may develop from genetic factors, poor physical and mental health, and chronic motor behaviors. Occupational demands are among the leading causes of poor postural adaptations leading to poor health outcomes, and mental stress is being increasingly recognized to play a role in the relationship between posture and health. Specific postural alignment and balance control in athletes may develop consequent to long-term exposure to sport-specific training and may not reflect ideal values suggested for healthy persons.

Postural control training as a component of multifaceted training regimens in nonathletes can have a marked effect on overcoming some musculoskeletal problems, improve some aspects of functional performance, and prevent falls in those persons with dysfunction and poor health. Training programs, however, are rather ineffective in improving static posture except in severe cases like scoliosis. Successful training programs for wellness and injury prevention fall directly in line with dynamic systems constraint-led approaches, emphasizing activity-specific tasks, specific and highly challenging environmental constraints, and psychophysical challenges. Under these guidelines, programs combining strength, power, and balance exercises appear the most successful. Training programs targeting the core musculature and spinal stability should focus on endurance and control and should enable the exerciser to develop their own best strategies for stabilization. Core training programs can directly target core muscles (primary core training) or require high core stability during another primary task (secondary core training).

Postural control training to improve athletic performance has yet to be conclusively shown. In contrast, training to decrease athletic musculoskeletal injuries has substantial support. Most athletic joint injuries are noncontact, and addressing risk factors for injury, including poor trunk and leg neuromuscular coordination, has shown to be successful. Targeted programs underscoring postural control in challenging situations, particularly when these programs emphasize movement coordination, proactive postural control, and sport-specific challenges, are successful in reducing the risk of knee and ankle injuries and some shoulder injuries.

STUDY QUESTIONS

1. What chronic behaviors may lead to poor postural control, particularly alignment?
2. What factors other than behaviors may lead to poor postural alignment and poor balance?
3. Let's say a person has a "permanent" slumping, cowering posture that can be traced to years of psychological trauma and stress. What reason best explains the mechanisms of neuromuscular adaptations that could have taken place?

4. What are the risk factors for sport-related joint injury?
5. Postural control training has been shown to be effective for some things and not effective for other things. Discuss these differences in detail.
6. What should be the focus of core training?
7. Joint stability is dependent on what factors? What causes instability?
8. Discuss the key elements to postural control training for wellness purposes. Include in your answer the concepts of constraints and discovery learning. Also include an explanation for the need for psychological training.
9. Discuss the key elements to postural control training for athletes. Include in your answer the concepts of constraints and discovery learning. Discuss gender differences and how training programs address risk factors for joint injury.
10. Explain why the terms "sensorimotor training," "neuromuscular training," and "proprioceptive training" may be considered inappropriate.
11. A person has healed from torn knee ligaments and has no overt pain, but the knee is still unstable. It often "gives way" and causes the person to collapse at unpredictable times. What do you think is the matter?
12. Describe the role of fatigue in postural control.

References

Al-Dadah, O. O., Shepstone, L. L., & Donell, S. T. (2011). Proprioception following partial meniscectomy in stable knees. *Knee Surgery, Sports Traumatology, Arthroscopy*, *19*(2), 207–213.

Alentorn-Geli, E., Myer, G., Silvers, H., Samitier, G., Romero, D., Lázaro-Haro, C., et al. (2009a). Prevention of non-contact anterior cruciate ligament injuries in soccer players. Part 1: Mechanisms of injury and underlying risk factors. *Knee Surgery, Sports Traumatology, Arthroscopy*, *17*(7), 705–729.

Alentorn-Geli, E., Myer, G. D., Silvers, H. J., Samitier, G., Romero, D., Lázaro-Haro, C., et al. (2009b). Prevention of non-contact anterior cruciate ligament injuries in soccer players. Part 2: A review of prevention programs aimed to modify risk factors and to reduce injury rates. *Knee Surgery, Sports Traumatology, Arthroscopy*, *17*(8), 859–879.

Anderson, K., & Behm, D. G. (2005). The impact of instability resistance training on balance and stability. *Sports Medicine*, *35*(1), 43–53.

Ashton-Miller, J. A., Wojtys, E. M., Huston, L. J., & Fry-Welch, D. D. (2001). Can proprioception really be improved by exercises? *Knee Surgery, Sports Traumatology, Arthroscopy*, *9*(3), 128–136.

Bakal, D. A. (1999). *Minding the body: Clinical uses of somatic awareness*. New York: The Guilford Press.

Beckman, S. M., & Buchanan, T. S. (1995). Ankle inversion injury and hypermobility: Effect on hip and ankle muscle electromyography onset latency. *Archives of Physical Medicine and Rehabilitation*, *76*(12), 1138–1143.

Behm, D., Drinkwater, E., Willardson, J., & Cowley, P. (2010). The use of instability to train the core musculature. *Applied Physiology, Nutrition, and Metabolism*, *35*(1), 91–108.

Błaszczyk, J., Cieślinska-Swider, J., Plewa, M., Zahorska-Markiewicz, B., & Markiewicz, A. (2009). Effects of excessive body weight on postural control. *Journal of Biomechanics*, *42*(9), 1295–1300.

Brown, S., Vera-Garcia, F., & McGill, S. (2006). Effects of abdominal muscle coactivation on the externally preloaded trunk: Variations in motor control and its effect on spine stability. *Spine*, *31*(13), E387–E393.

Cacciatore, T., Gurfinkel, V., Horak, F., Cordo, P., & Ames, K. (2011). Increased dynamic regulation of postural tone through Alexander Technique training. *Human Movement Science*, *30*(1), 74–89.

Chapman, D. W., Needham, K. J., Allison, G. T., Lay, B. B., & Edwards, D. J. (2008). Effects of experience in a dynamic environment on postural control. *British Journal of Sports Medicine*, *42*(1), 16–21.

Cress, M., Buchner, D. M., Prohaska, T., Rimmer, J., Brown, M., Macera, C., et al. (2005). Best practices for physical activity programs and behavior counseling in older adult populations. *Journal of Aging and Physical Activity*, *13*(1), 61–74.

DiStefano, L. J., Clark, M. A., & Padua, D. A. (2009). Evidence supporting balance training in healthy individuals: A systematic review. *Journal of Strength and Conditioning Research*, *23*(9), 2718–2731.

Donaldson, P. (2012). Does generalized joint hypermobility predict joint injury in sport? A review. *Clinical Journal of Sport Medicine*, *22*(1), 77–78.

Friemert, B., Franke, S., Gollhofer, A., Claes, L., & Faist, M. (2010). Group I afferent pathway contributes to functional knee stability. *Journal of Neurophysiology*, *103*(2), 616–622.

Fusco, C., Zaina, F., Atanasio, S., Romano, M., Negrini, A., & Negrini, S. (2011). Physical exercises in the treatment of adolescent idiopathic scoliosis: An updated systematic review. *Physiotherapy Theory and Practice*, *27*(1), 80–114.

Gabbett, T. (2004). Incidence of injury in junior and senior rugby league players. *Sports Medicine*, *34*(12), 849–859.

Gabbett, T., Ullah, S., Jenkins, D., & Abernethy, B. (2012). Skill qualities as risk factors for contact injury in professional rugby league players. *Journal of Sports Sciences, 30*(13), 1421–1427.

Gallagher, S. (2005). Physical limitations and musculoskeletal complaints associated with work in unusual or restricted postures: A literature review. *Journal of Safety Research*, *36*(1), 51–61.

Gehring, D., Melnyk, M., & Gollhofer, A. (2009). Gender and fatigue have influence on knee joint control strategies during landing. *Clinical Biomechanics*, *24*(1), 82–87.

Granacher, U., & Gollhofer, A. (2011). Is there an association between variables of postural control and strength in adolescents? *Journal of Strength and Conditioning Research*, *25*(6), 1718–1725.

Granacher, U., Muehlbauer, T., Zahner, L., Gollhofer, A., & Kressig, R. (2011). Comparison of traditional and recent approaches in the promotion of balance and strength in older adults. *Sports Medicine*, *41*(5), 377–400.

Grenier, S., & McGill, S. (2007). Quantification of lumbar stability by using 2 different abdominal activation strategies. *Archives of Physical Medicine and Rehabilitation*, *88*(1), 54–62.

Gross, M., Crane, E. A., & Fredrickson, B. L. (2010). Methodology for assessing bodily expression of emotion. *Journal of Nonverbal Behavior*, *34*(4), 223–248.

Gross, M. M., Crane, E. A., & Fredrickson, B. L. (2012). Effort-shape and kinematic assessment of bodily expression of emotion during gait. *Human Movement Science*, *31*, 202–221.

Hawes, M. C. (2003). The use of exercises in the treatment of scoliosis: An evidence-based critical review of the literature. *Pediatric Rehabilitation*, *6*(3–4), 171–182.

Hewett, T. E., Ford, K. R., Hoogenboom, B. J., & Myer, G. D. (2010). Understanding and preventing ACL injuries: Current biomechanical and epidemiologic considerations—Update 2010. *North American Journal of Sports Physical Therapy*, *5*(4), 234–251.

Hewett, T., Ford, K., & Myer, G. (2006). Anterior cruciate ligament injuries in female athletes: Part 2, a meta-analysis of neuromuscular interventions aimed at injury prevention. *American Journal of Sports Medicine*, *34*(3), 490–498.

Hicks, G., Fritz, J., Delitto, A., & McGill, S. (2005). Preliminary development of a clinical prediction rule for determining which patients with low back pain will respond to a stabilization exercise program. *Archives of Physical Medicine and Rehabilitation*, *86*(9), 1753–1762.

Himmelreich, H. H., Vogt, L. L., & Banzer, W. W. (2008). Gluteal muscle recruitment during level, incline and stair ambulation in healthy subjects and chronic low back pain patients. *Journal of Back and Musculoskeletal Rehabilitation*, *21*(3), 193–199.

Hogervorst, T., & Brand, R. (1998). Mechanoreceptors in joint function. *Journal of Bone and Joint Surgery*, *80*(9), 1365–1378.

Horslen, B. C., & Carpenter, M. G. (2011). Arousal, valence and their relative effects on postural control. *Experimental Brain Research*, *215*(1), 27–34.

Hrysomallis, C. (2011). Balance ability and athletic performance. *Sports Medicine*, *41*(3), 221–232.

Hrysomallis, C. C., & Goodman, C. C. (2001). A review of resistance exercise and posture realignment. *Journal of Strength and Conditioning Research*, *15*(3), 385–390.

Hsiao, H., & Simeonov, P. (2001). Preventing falls from roofs: A critical review. *Ergonomics*, *44*(5), 537–561.

Hübscher, M., Zech, A., Pfeifer, K., Hänsel, F., Vogt, L., & Banzer, W. (2010). Neuromuscular training for sports injury prevention: A systematic review. *Medicine and Science in Sports and Exercise*, *42*(3), 413–421.

Hue, O., Simoneau, M., Marcotte, J., Berrigan, F., Doré, J., Marceau, P., et al. (2007). Body weight is a strong predictor of postural stability. *Gait & Posture*, *26*(1), 32–38.

Hugel, F. F., Cadopi, M. M., Kohler, F. F., & Perrin, P. P. (1999). Postural control of ballet dancers: A specific use of visual input for artistic purposes. *International Journal of Sports Medicine, 20*(2), 86–92.

Hundza, S., & Zehr, E. (2007). Muscle activation and cutaneous reflex modulation during rhythmic and discrete arm tasks in orthopaedic shoulder instability. *Experimental Brain Research*, *179*(3), 339–351.

Ives, J. (2003). Comments on "the Feldenkrais Method: A dynamic approach to changing motor behavior." *Research Quarterly for Exercise and Sport*, *74*(2), 116–123.

Jain, S., Janssen, K., & DeCelle, S. (2004). Alexander technique and Feldenkrais method: A critical overview. *Physical Medicine and Rehabilitation Clinics of North America*, *15*(4), 811–825.

Kawashima, N., Yano, H., Ohta, Y., & Nakazawa, K. (2006). Stretch reflex modulation during imposed static and dynamic hip movements in standing humans. *Experimental Brain Research*, *174*(2), 342–350.

King, A., Challis, J., Bartok, C., Costigan, F., & Newell, K. (2012). Obesity, mechanical and strength relationships to postural control in adolescence. *Gait & Posture*, *35*(2), 261–265.

Kloubec, J. A. (2010). Pilates for improvements of muscle endurance, flexibility, balance, and posture. *Journal of Strength and Conditioning Research*, *24*(3), 661–667.

Krogsgaard, M. R., Fischer-Rasmussen, T., & Dyhre-Poulsen, P. (2011). Absence of sensory function in the reconstructed anterior cruciate ligament. *Journal of Electromyography and Kinesiology*, *21*(1), 82–86.

Kuo, Y. L., Tully, E. A., & Galea, M. P. (2009). Sagittal spinal posture after Pilates-based exercise in healthy older adults. *Spine*, *34*, 1046–1051.

Lang, P., & McTeague, L. (2009). The anxiety disorder spectrum: Fear imagery, physiological reactivity, and differential diagnosis. *Anxiety, Stress, and Coping*, *22*(1), 5–25.

Lerch, C., Cordes, M., & Baumeister, J. (2011). Effectiveness of injury prevention programs in female youth soccer: A systematic review. *British Journal of Sports Medicine*, *45*(4), 359.

Leukel, C., Taube, W., Lorch, M., & Gollhofer, A. (2012). Changes in predictive motor control in drop-jumps based on uncertainties in task execution. *Human Movement Science*, *31*(1), 152–160.

Liu-Ambrose, T. T., Khan, K. M., Eng, J. J., Lord, S. R., & McKay, H. A. (2004). Balance confidence improves with resistance or agility training. *Gerontology*, *50*(6), 373–382.

Lo, J. J., & Ashton-Miller, J. A. (2008). Effect of pre-impact movement strategies on the impact forces resulting from a lateral fall. *Journal of Biomechanics*, *41*(9), 1969–1977.

Ma, Y., Paterson, H., & Pollick, F. (2006). A motion capture library for the study of identity, gender, and emotion perception from biological motion. *Behavior Research Methods*, *38*(1), 134–141.

McGill, S. (2002). LBD risk assessment. In S. McGill (Ed.) *Low back disorders: Evidence-based prevention and rehabilitation* (pp. 149–159). Champaign, IL: Human Kinetics.

McGill, S. (2004). Linking latest knowledge of injury mechanisms and spine function to the prevention of low back disorders. *Journal of Electromyography and Kinesiology*, *14*(1), 43–47.

McLean, S. G., & Beaulieu, M. L. (2010). Complex integrative morphological and mechanical contributions to ACL injury risk. *Exercise and Sport Sciences Reviews*, *38*(4), 192–200.

Mendiguchia, J., Ford, K. R., Quatman, C. E., Alentorn-Geli, E., & Hewett, T. E. (2011). Sex differences in proximal control of the knee joint. *Sports Medicine*, *41*(7), 541–557.

Michalak, J., Troje, N., Fischer, J., Vollmar, P., Heidenreich, T., & Schulte, D. (2009). Embodiment of sadness and depression—Gait patterns associated with dysphoric mood. *Psychosomatic Medicine*, *71*(5), 580–587.

Mondloch, C. (2012). Sad or fearful? The influence of body posture on adults' and children's perception of facial displays of emotion. *Journal of Experimental Child Psychology*, *111*(2), 180–196.

Morse, T., Bruneau, H., & Dussetschleger, J. (2010). Musculoskeletal disorders of the neck and shoulder in the dental professions. *Work*, *35*(4), 419–429.

Myer, G., Ford, K., & Hewett, T. (2011). New method to identify athletes at high risk of ACL injury using clinic-based measurements and freeware computer analysis. *British Journal of Sports Medicine*, *45*(4), 238–244.

Myer, G. D., Ford, K. R., Paterno, M. V., Nick, T. G., & Hewett, T. E. (2008). The effects of generalized joint laxity on risk of anterior cruciate ligament injury in young female athletes. *American Journal of Sports Medicine*, *36*(6), 1073–1080.

Myers, J., Ju, Y., Hwang, J., McMahon, P., Rodosky, M., & Lephart, S. (2004). Reflexive muscle activation alterations in shoulders with anterior glenohumeral instability. *American Journal of Sports Medicine*, *32*(4), 1013–1021.

Normand, M., Descarreaux, M., Poulin, C., Richer, N., Mailhot, D., Black, P., et al. (2005). Biomechanical effects of a lumbar support in a mattress. *Journal of the Canadian Chiropractic Association*, *49*(2), 96–101.

Noyes, F. R., & Barber Westin, S. D. (2012). Anterior cruciate ligament injury prevention training in female athletes: A systematic review of injury reduction and results of athletic performance tests. *Sports Health: A Multidisciplinary Approach*, *4*(1), 36–46.

Nyland, J., Caborn, D., & Johnson, D. (1998). The human glenohumeral joint. A proprioceptive and stability alliance. *Knee Surgery, Sports Traumatology, Arthroscopy*, 6(1), 50–61.

O'Sullivan, P., Smith, A., Beales, D., & Straker, L. (2011). Association of biopsychosocial factors with degree of slump in sitting posture and self-report of back pain in adolescents: A cross-sectional study. *Physical Therapy*, 91(4), 470–483.

O'Sullivan, P., Twomey, L., & Allison, G. (1998). Altered abdominal muscle recruitment in patients with chronic back pain following a specific exercise intervention. *Journal of Orthopaedic and Sports Physical Therapy*, 27(2), 114–124.

Paillard, T. (2012). Effects of general and local fatigue on postural control: A review. *Neuroscience and Biobehavioral Reviews*, 36(1), 162–176.

Palmieri-Smith, R., Wojtys, E., & Ashton-Miller, J. (2008). Association between preparatory muscle activation and peak valgus knee angle. *Journal of Electromyography and Kinesiology*, 18(6), 973–979.

Perrin, P., Deviterne, D., Hugel, F., & Perrot, C. (2002). Judo, better than dance, develops sensorimotor adaptabilities involved in balance control. *Gait & Posture*, 15(2), 187–193.

Pichierri, G., Wolf, P., Murer, K., & de Bruin, E. (2011). Cognitive and cognitive-motor interventions affecting physical functioning: A systematic review. *BMC Geriatrics*, 11, 29. doi:10.1186/1471–2318–11–29.

Prins, Y., Crous, L., & Louw, Q. (2008). A systematic review of posture and psychosocial factors as contributors to upper quadrant musculoskeletal pain in children and adolescents. *Physiotherapy Theory and Practice*, 24(4), 221–242.

Punnett, L., & Wegman, D. H. (2004). Work-related musculoskeletal disorders: The epidemiologic evidence and the debate. *Journal of Electromyography and Kinesiology*, 14(1), 13–23.

Rahnama, N., Reilly, T., & Lees, A. (2002). Injury risk associated with playing actions during competitive soccer. *British Journal of Sports Medicine*, 36(5), 354–359.

Rejeski, W., & Brawley, L. (2006). Functional health: Innovations in research on physical activity with older adults. *Medicine and Science in Sports and Exercise*, 38(1), 93–99.

Riemann, B., & Lephart, S. (2002a). The sensorimotor system, part I: The physiologic basis of functional joint stability. *Journal of Athletic Training*, 37(1), 71–79.

Riemann, B., & Lephart, S. (2002b). The sensorimotor system, part II: The role of proprioception in motor control and functional joint stability. *Journal of Athletic Training*, 37(1), 80–84.

Roether, C., Omlor, L., Christensen, A., & Giese, M. (2009). Critical features for the perception of emotion from gait. *Journal of Vision*, 9(6), 15.1–32.

Scannell, J. P., & McGill, S. M. (2003). Lumbar posture—Should it, and can it, be modified? A study of passive tissue stiffness and lumbar position during activities of daily living. *Physical Therapy*, 83, 907–917.

Shirley, D., Hodges, P. W., Eriksson, A. E. M., & Gandevia, S. C. (2003). Spinal stiffness changes throughout the respiratory cycle. *Journal of Applied Physiology*, 95, 1467–1475.

Sloman, L., Pierrynowski, M., Berridge, M., Tupling, S., & Flowers, J. (1987). Mood, depressive illness and gait patterns. *Canadian Journal of Psychiatry*, 32(3), 190–193.

Slósarska, M. M. (1986). Non-specific physiological changes of depressed patients as manifested by reactions to simple stimuli. *International Journal of Psychosomatics*, 33(3), 17–20.

Solomonow, M. M., Baratta, R. R., Zhou, B. H., Shoji, H. H., Bose, W. W., Beck, C. C., et al. (1987). The synergistic action of the anterior cruciate ligament and thigh muscles in maintaining joint stability. *American Journal of Sports Medicine*, 15(3), 207–213.

Solomonow, M., & Krogsgaard, M. (2001). Sensorimotor control of knee stability. A review. *Scandinavian Journal of Medicine & Science in Sports*, 11(2), 64–80.

Taube, W., Gruber, M., & Gollhofer, A. (2008). Spinal and supraspinal adaptations associated with balance training and their functional relevance. *Acta Physiologica*, 193, 101–116.

Tsuda, E., Ishibashi, Y., Okamura, Y., & Toh, S. (2003). Restoration of anterior cruciate ligament-hamstring reflex arc after anterior cruciate ligament reconstruction. *Knee Surgery, Sports Traumatology, Arthroscopy*, 11(2), 63–67.

Valachi, B., & Valachi, K. (2003). Mechanisms leading to musculoskeletal disorders in dentistry. *Journal of the American Dental Association*, 134(10), 1344–1350.

Vera-Garcia, F., Elvira, J., Brown, S., & McGill, S. (2007). Effects of abdominal stabilization maneuvers on the control of spine motion and stability against sudden trunk perturbations. *Journal of Electromyography and Kinesiology*, 17(5), 556–567.

Vera-Garcia, F., Moreside, J., & McGill, S. (2011). Abdominal muscle activation changes if the purpose is to control pelvis motion or thorax motion. *Journal of Electromyography and Kinesiology*, *21*(6), 893–903.

Wang, S., & McGill, S. (2008). Links between the mechanics of ventilation and spine stability. *Journal of Applied Biomechanics*, *24*(2), 166–174.

Weerdesteyn, V., Nienhuis, B., & Duysens, J. (2008). Exercise training can improve spatial characteristics of time-critical obstacle avoidance in elderly people. *Human Movement Science*, *27*(5), 738–748.

Weiss, H. R., & Turnbull, D. (2011). The Integrated Scoliosis Rehabilitation/ISR Scoliologic best practice program: A synthesis of four approaches of physiotherapy for the treatment of scoliosis (pp. 94–101). In Fusco, C., Zaina, F., Atanasio, S., Romano, M., Negrini, A., & Negrini, S. (Eds.). Physical exercises in the treatment of adolescent idiopathic scoliosis: An updated systematic review. *Physiotherapy Theory and Practice*, *27*(1), 80–114.

Wolf, S., Barnhart, H., Ellison, G., & Coogler, C. (1997). The effect of Tai Chi Quan and computerized balance training on postural stability in older subjects. Atlanta FICSIT Group. Frailty and Injuries: Cooperative Studies on Intervention Techniques. *Physical Therapy*, *77*(4), 371–381.

Woodman, J., & Moore, N. (2012). Evidence for the effectiveness of Alexander Technique lessons in medical and health-related conditions: A systematic review. *International Journal of Clinical Practice*, *66*(1), 98–112.

Zech, A., Hübscher, M., Vogt, L., Banzer, W., Hänsel, F., & Pfeifer, K. (2009). Neuromuscular training for rehabilitation of sports injuries: A systematic review. *Medicine and Science in Sports and Exercise*, *41*(10), 1831–1841.

Zech, A., Hübscher, M., Vogt, L., Banzer, W., Hänsel, F., & Pfeifer, K. (2010). Balance training for neuromuscular control and performance enhancement: A systematic review. *Journal of Athletic Training*, *45*(4), 392–403.

Zenian, J. (2010). Sleep position and shoulder pain. *Medical Hypotheses*, *74*(4), 639–643.

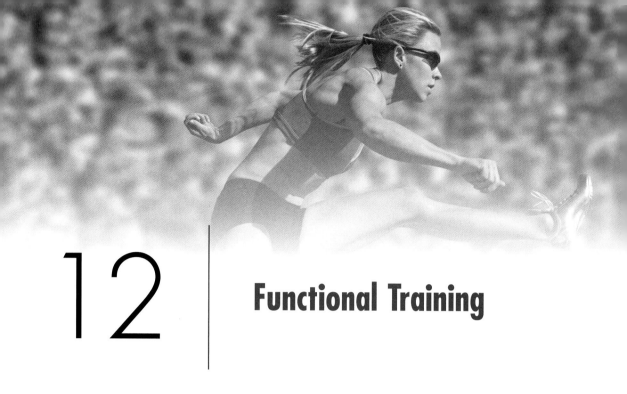

12 | **Functional Training**

PURPOSE, IMPORTANCE, AND OBJECTIVES OF THIS CHAPTER

Improving physiological abilities such as strength and power through traditional training programs does not necessarily lead to better performance on the field, at home, or at work. The purpose of this chapter is to examine the concepts and guidelines for functional training designed to maximize the transfer of physiological gains made during training to real-world performance. Understanding the essential elements of functional training, which are rooted directly in the concepts of discovery learning, constraints-based practice, and deliberate practice, provides a basis for creating programs that maximize transfer and, therefore, maximize performance.

After reading this chapter, you should be able to:

1. Define and describe the key elements of functional training and how functional training differs from practice and conventional physical training.
2. List and describe the physical and psychological contributors to the production of strength and power and the difficulties and controversies in strength and power testing and training.
3. Explain the key components to transfer strength and power gains from the weight room to the athletic playing field.
4. Define functional psychophysical training and explain the steps to creating a psychophysical training program in athlete populations and nonathlete populations.
5. Explain the benefits and shortcomings of using virtual reality as a functional training mode.

Throughout this text, we have examined the properties of learning and practice as they contribute to the development of skilled motor performance. Motor skill performance also relies on underlying abilities, and enhancing abilities are common targets for improving performance. Yet improved abilities only increase capability for skilled performance and do not always transfer to improved performance on the field. Maximizing transfer is the goal of **functional training**, which has been defined as bringing real-life situational needs and constraints to the training environment (Ives & Shelley, 2003). Functional training differs from conventional training in that the goal is to maximize transfer of abilities rather

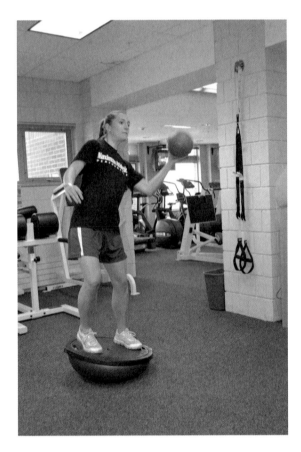

Figure 12.1 • Maximal forces cannot be developed during medicine ball throwing because muscle actions are constrained by the need to balance. (Photo courtesy of Jeffrey Ives.)

than maximize the abilities themselves. Indeed, functional training often does not permit full muscle activation, even at maximal effort, because segmental stability and balance may be upset (McGill et al., 2009) (see Fig. 12.1). Functional training differs from practice in that the goal is to develop physiological abilities rather than technical, motor, and mental skills. According to Tomljanović et al. (2011), traditional strength training is designed to improve the muscle quality and energetic potential, whereas functional training serves to improve control and coordination of these qualities. Functional training is not a substitute for training or practice but serves as a bridge between the two.

Functional training programs are as diverse as the number of different sports and occupations. Devising a functional training program that truly maximizes transfer can be difficult and requires considerable thought on the part of trainers, athletes, and coaches. In this chapter, we examine the keys to maximizing transfer of abilities to improve performance on the athletic field, at the workplace, and in activities of daily living. In particular, we look at strength and power training as they are the most common training programs for most athletes and are becoming commonplace for nonathletes as well. We highlight the role of psychological factors and motor behavior in functional training and look at virtual reality as one method of manipulating psychological constraints in functional training.

DEFINITIONS AND CONCEPTS IN STRENGTH AND POWER

Strength and power training are considered so essential to the development of athletic performance that numerous lay and scholarly journals are singularly devoted to just this type of training. The importance of strength and power training as a component of wellness and health in nonathlete populations

| SIDE**NOTE** | A RECENT HISTORY OF STRENGTH AND POWER TRAINING RECOMMENDATIONS |

The role of strength training as an important part of an exercise program has changed dramatically in recent years. Nowhere is this more evident than in the position stands on the quality and quantity of physical activity to develop and maintain fitness for adults put out by the American College of Sports Medicine (ACSM). Over time the ACSM policy has fundamentally changed in regard to resistance training. It was not until 1990 that the position stand included resistance training as a part of well-rounded fitness program for adults (American College of Sports Medicine, 1990). Training recommendations were very simple: One set of 8 to 12 repetitions of moderate intensity, 8 to 10 different exercises, and conducted at least 2 days per week. In 1998, the recommendations changed to state that multiple-set regimens may provide greater benefits, that programs should be progressive and individualized, and added that older and frail individuals could also benefit from strength training (American College of Sports Medicine, 1998). In 2011, the position stand again made fundamental changes with greater elaboration on resistance training exercise prescriptions and population-specific recommendations (Garber et al., 2011). Among the notable changes was the inclusion of high-intensity training to over 80% of one-repetition maximum (1-RM), a recommendation of 2 to 4 sets, and redefining the training as strength and power training, including for elders. Newly added in the 2011 statement was the recommendation for "neuromotor" exercise training for the purpose of maintaining functional performance. These exercises include motor skill training with balance, agility, coordination and gait components, and "multifaceted" exercises like martial arts. Despite the appropriateness of these recommendations, the continuing additions to the position stand have resulted in unrealistic expectations for exercisers. The number of hours and days for cardiovascular (>4 days), resistance (>2–3 days), neuromotor (>2–3 days), and flexibility (>2–3 days) training exceeds any practical schedule for the vast majority of people and calls attention to the need for exercise programming that targets multiple systems and outcomes. Well-planned functional exercise programs can do just that.

is increasingly recognized, resulting in major sport and exercise science organizations working with national governments to craft detailed position papers on the topic (Garber et al., 2011; Stratton et al., 2004). Yet despite documentation of strength and power training methods back to the ancient Greeks, debate still continues about the best ways to train, particularly in producing gains that transfer to better performance on the playing field, at work, and at home.

Strength is defined as the maximum force or torque one can exert under specific task constraints. That means that strength can be determined by a one-repetition maximum (1-RM) bench press, a maximal voluntary isometric (MVIC) squat lift, a knee extension on an isokinetic dynamometer, or the number of bricks a mason can lift on one pallet. The task constraints may include movement speed (e.g., fast vs. isometric), movement or contraction type (e.g., concentric vs. eccentric; isoinertial vs. isokinetic), postures, and muscle involvement. Power as used in the context of strength training and conditioning is defined as the rate in which strength or force is exerted, or force times velocity. Maximum power is the point at which force multiplied by the speed of movement is maximal. On the typical force–velocity curve, the point of peak power is normally at the center of the curve (Fig. 12.2).

Numerous subcategories of strength and power have been identified. Among these are high-speed strength, low-speed (or high-load) strength, reaction strength, explosive strength, and skill strength (Newton & Dugan, 2002). Table 12.1 details the differences among these measures, and Figure 12.2 illustrates the relationships among low-speed, high-speed, and peak power areas on the force–velocity curve. Note that skill strength is context specific and cannot be categorized according to load or speed (Fig. 12.3).

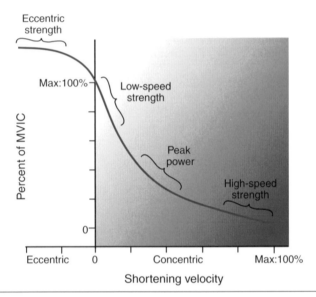

Figure 12.2 • Force–velocity curve and training zones. Low-speed strength training makes use of heavy loads. Using very heavy loads is considered neural training. High-speed strength training includes ballistic training some plyometric training. Peak power training is typically at about 30% of MVIC, but this number can vary greatly. The eccentric training range shown is with supramaximal loads and stands apart from eccentric work that accompanies high speed stretch-shorten cycle movements.

Strength and power are defined in different ways because tasks require different variations of strength and power, and strength and power are not necessarily generalizable across the strength and power spectrum (Bishop et al., 2011; Roig et al., 2009). Though there is some measure of a general strength component (Hortobagyi et al., 1989), strength and power gains made during training are mostly specific to the training variables used. Gains made in training are specific to movement velocity (Behm & Sale, 1993), mode of contraction (Folland & Williams, 2007; Roig et al., 2009), metabolic demands (Harris et al., 2007), and task demands (Roig et al., 2009). The basis for specificity of strength and power training are seen in metabolic adaptations, hypertrophy adaptations, and neural adaptations. Of these, the specificity of neural adaptations to specific training variables appears to be the most prominent and perhaps the most important because neural changes have the most variability and thus must be targeted most precisely (Folland & Williams, 2007; Roig et al., 2009).

The Physiology of Muscular Force Production and Training

The physiological mechanisms of force production are well known and are described in basic kinesiology and exercise physiology textbooks and review articles (e.g., Aagaard, 2010). Briefly, force and power production are dependent on muscle mass, muscle morphology (motor unit type and fascicle arrangement), fatigue and metabolic properties, stretch–shorten cycle and other elastic element factors, biomechanical and anthropometric characteristics, and the neural control of motor unit behavior, including intramuscular and intermuscular coordination (Cormie et al., 2011a). Experience, motivation, and other psychological factors are necessary to put forth the maximal effort required of strength tasks. For example, inexperienced individuals may simply not know how to energize themselves to put forth a full strength contraction (Aagaard, 2010).

The fundamental characteristics of training include overload, specificity, fatigue, variation, intention, and effort (Cormie et al., 2011b). These characteristics are manipulated, along with

TABLE 12.1	Different Strength Qualities	
Measure	**Conditions**	**Comments/Examples**
High-speed strength	<30% MVC with maximal velocity	Light loads lifted with maximal velocity, "speed strength." Normally a ballistic action. Peak power measures may fall in this category. Normally assessed by jump squats.
High-load (low-speed) strength	>70% MVC with maximal velocity	Maximal strength (1-RM loads) to typical 8-RM loads. Includes both neural and hypertrophy training.
Reaction strength	Stretch–shorten movements	Ability to reverse direction from high-load eccentric contraction to concentric contraction (e.g., from a drop jump to vertical jump plyometric exercise). Minimal reversal time indicates strong reaction strength; plays a role in agility and activities requiring repetitive jumps (e.g., basketball).
Explosive strength	Varied loads Rate of force development	Measured by fastest rate of force/tension development or time to reach a specific force level. Really a measure of power. Generally requires computerized dynamometry to measure, such as force–time curve during isometric contractions.
Skill strength	Task specific	Skill strength involves functional performance measures of skills and abilities that are task specific. For example, box lifting for workers in material handling jobs and blocking sled pushing for football players.

other training variables such as sets, repetitions, volume, and simple versus complex movements. Training variables are cycled in and out over time to create specific times of stress and recovery to different systems. This cycling, called *periodization*, may occur over days (*microcycles*) or weeks (*mesocycles*). For instance, cycling between upper and lower body exercises over the course of a week (microcycle) and cycling between high-load training and high-repetition training over the course of weeks (mesocycle) may result in less overall training volume and better strength gains (Bloomer & Ives, 2000).

The physiological and neurophysiological adaptations that arise from strength and power training have been well investigated with strong evidence of changes in muscle and tendon hypertrophy and fascicle arrangement, changes in metabolic and endocrine factors, and widespread changes in neural factors (Aagaard & Andersen, 2010; Andersen & Aagaard, 2010; Carroll et al., 2011; Cormie et al., 2010, 2011b; Folland & Williams, 2007). Coinciding with these adaptations are changes in function, such as improved jump height, easier occupational lifting, faster walking speed in the elders, and faster sprint performance (Bishop et al., 2011; Cormie et al., 2010; Protas & Tissier, 2009). Despite all of what is known about strength and power, there are considerable gaps in knowledge and controversies over even the most basic tenets of training (Carpinelli, 2009). The greatest gaps exist in determining training methods that will improve actual day-to-day motor skill performance, whether that is on the athletic field, jobsite, or activities of daily living. These problems are further highlighted in the measurement of strength and power, which suffers from the conflict between reliability and ecologic validity (Reilly et al., 2009). That is, the most reliable and repeatable testing methods are not necessarily valid in terms

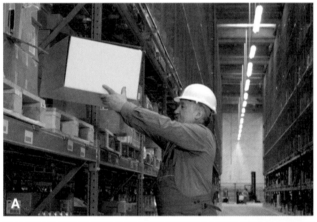

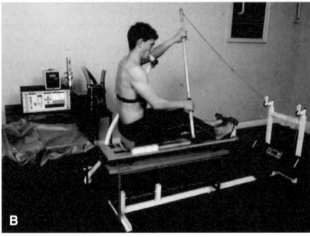

Figure 12.3 • Skill-based measures are useful in occupational settings and in evaluating aerobic fitness. **A.** Box lifting is used to evaluate lifting capacity workers engaged in manual material handling. Box size, weight, and placement height are all manipulated to evaluate job-specific capabilities. **B.** Assessing aerobic power is also functional and dependent on specific motor skill proficiencies. This kayak ergometer provides better measures aerobic performance in kayakers than do generic tests. (Image from Reilly, T., Morris, T., & Whyte, G. (2009). The specificity of training prescription and physiological assessment: A review. *Journal of Sports Sciences*, 27(6), 575–589. Reprinted by permission of Taylor & Francis Ltd (http://www.tandf.co.uk/journals).)

of identifying the important strength components of athletes (Abernethy et al., 1995; Cronin & Sleivert, 2005) or workers in vocational settings (Lee et al., 2001). (See the Thinking It Through box for more insight to this problem.)

■ Thinking It Through 12.1 Functional Strength and Fitness Testing

Evaluating functional strength and power in athletics and occupations has long been a challenge due to reliability, validity, and logistical issues. Taking measurements in the field during actual tasks, for example, is beset by problems of reliability and logistics. Simplifying complex skill–strength tasks so that they may be reliably performed in the laboratory raises questions of validity, that is, does the test accurately reflect the demands of real-life performance? Bridging the gap between reliability and validity is the goal of

continued on following page

functional testing using simulated or real-life strength devices. Functional tests often come in the form of test batteries, sometimes called "combines" in athletes and job-related fitness tests in occupational settings. In the figures below are three examples of functional strength testing related to push–pull tasks. On the right is squat–push test ("jammer") used by football players to assess blocking ability. In the middle is an 80-kg dummy used by firefighters to test and train for personnel rescue, and on the right is a push–pull machine used by some European police forces to assess the ability to restrain or push away a suspect. Which expression of strength do you think best reflects the strength and power demands required of the activity? Why?

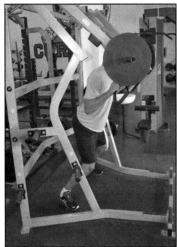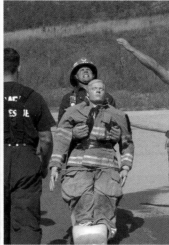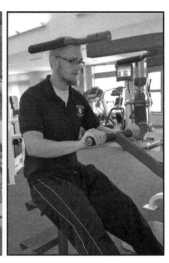

Left and **right** photos courtesy of Jeffrey C. Ives and **middle** photo courtesy of U.S. Air Force and 2nd Lt. John Ross.

STRENGTH AND POWER AND PERFORMANCE IN ATHLETES

Athleticism is almost synonymous with strength and power, even including athletic feats in aerobic type activities such as swimming and cycling. Strength and power are often thought to be associated with speed and agility, but this association is generally weak (Marcovic, 2007). Speed is defined as linear velocity and is measured by sprint times, typically 100, 40, or 10 m. Agility is defined as the capability to stop and start and change directions and typically implies the ability to move laterally in a nonstandard gait, such as slide steps or carioca. Quickness refers to acceleration or how fast speed can be developed, particularly from a stationary start. All four of these abilities—strength, power, speed, and agility—are considered essential components of athletic success in many sports.

Transfer of Training Gains to the Playing Field

Athletes engage in a vast array of training programs to improve strength and power abilities and overall sport performance. Despite the apparent sophistication of athlete training programs, there exists much uncertainty if gains made in the weight room equal gains made on the playing field. Perhaps even more confusing is the apparent paradox that a variety of strength and power training methods may improve laboratory performance measures like vertical jump height and sprint speed, but identifying better on-field performance has proved difficult to tease out, especially in highly trained athletes (Abernethy et al., 1995; Cronin & Sleivert, 2005; Harris et al., 2007; Young, 2006). Ziv and Lidor (2010) summarized from their review on vertical jumping in volleyball players that "there are not enough data to support the argument that the higher the players jump, the more wins the team is able to accumulate." Moreover, there is evidence to suggest that strength and power training may actually reduce functional performance, such as sprint acceleration (Moir et al., 2007). These findings are also supported by numerous authors who have pointed out that strength and power assessments do not necessarily discriminate successful from less successful athletes (for reviews see Abernethy et al., 1995; Cronin & Sleivert, 2005), though these results are dependent on the sport and level of performance (e.g., Lawton et al., 2011). Reilly et al. (2009) urged caution in interpreting data showing correlations between measures of strength and performance because causality remains undetermined.

Overall, it is difficult to generalize that elite performers are more powerful, stronger, or faster than their subelite counterparts. In a similar manner, it is difficult to state that strength and power training will improve on-field performance of high-level athletes, or even many aspects of performance of subelite performers. The inability to consistently correlate strength and power with high-level sports performance has led researchers to further investigate missing elements of strength and power production in sport. There is growing recognition that maximal transfer of performance is dependent on intramuscular and intermuscular coordination factors (Young, 2006). Eminent sport scientist Per Aagaard and his colleagues (Aagaard & Andersen, 2010) noted in their extensive review that improved neural function, including improved coordination, were among the adaptations enabling even aerobic athletes to benefit from heavy resistance training (see Concepts in Action box). The high-intensity and explosive strength training found to be successful can be considered functional to running, cycling, and skiing because it addressed the rapid cyclic nature of the activities and developed necessary stretch–shorten cycle mechanisms and contract–relax coordination.

Concepts in Action

Strength and Power Training for Aerobic Athletes

Up until recently, endurance athletes rarely engaged in strength and power training. It was thought that aerobic metabolic systems would suffer and hypertrophied muscle mass would cause extraneous weight, decreased capillary density, and less efficient movement. These perceptions were reinforced by studies on concurrent or combined strength and aerobic training on recreational and subelite athletes that showed that aerobic performance did not improve or decline (e.g., Dudley & Djamil, 1985). These findings have been countered by other researchers, and differences in results ascribed, in part, to key differences in training regimens (Andersen & Aagaard, 2010). In their review, Andersen and Aagaard (2010) concluded that high-level aerobic athletes (runners, skiers, cyclists) may gain performance benefits with the right kind of high-intensity strength training. These authors noted three fundamental benefits of strength training for aerobic athletes: (1) an increase in type IIA fiber area with a concurrent decrease in type IIX fiber area, (2) changes in neural function, and (3) increased musculotendinous stiffness. As shown in the diagram on the next page, these changes lead to increases in force and power without hypertrophy or a loss in endurance, improved movement efficiency, and improved capillary blood flow—all of which lead to better endurance performance. Other authors have suggested that better coordination leading to improved running mechanics and force sharing among muscles may also contribute (Bonacci et al., 2009) and have directly noted these factors as contributing to the elite performance of aerobic athletes (Jones, 2006).

An important conclusion from this body of research is that not all training is effective. Endurance performance gains have best, or only, been demonstrated with high-intensity (>85% of 1-RM) loading and/or explosive exercises conducted over long time periods (>8 weeks). Lower-intensity loadings of few sets for shorter time periods are unsuccessful. The take-home point here is that researchers and coaches of elite endurance athletes recommend that a portion of the endurance training be replaced by high-intensity strength and power training (Jones, 2006; Yamamoto et al., 2010).

continued on following page

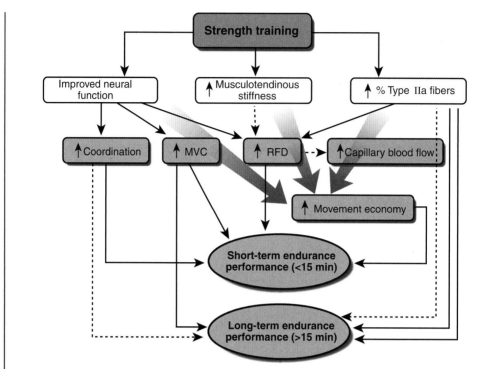

This schematic is based on data from Andersen and Aagaard (2010) and Bonacci et al. (2009). *Solid arrows* represent experimentally confirmed connections, whereas *dashed lines* are hypothesized and require experimental verification. The *thick gray line* illustrates that neural function, stiffness, and type IIA fibers are likely have an influence on movement economy, but the exact nature of those effects are yet unknown. MVC, maximal voluntary contraction; RFD, rate of force development.

Improving transfer is the purpose of functional strength and power training regimens. Maximizing transfer requires maximizing specificity to create coordination mechanisms tuned to sport skills (Young, 2006). Functional training programs range from concurrent but separate skill and strength training, to complex and cross training, to overloaded skill-based tasks (see Reilly et al., 2009, for review). In the latter category are pulling of weighted sleds, wearing of weighted vests, and restraining harnesses, all designed to enable development of specific strength and power coordination mechanisms. A shortcoming in these techniques is that they often overlook that functional coordination in sport depends a great deal on cognitive factors like rapid decision making, overcoming time constraints, and uncertainty of motor actions (Handford et al., 1997; Young & Farrow, 2006). For instance, Gabbett and Benton (2009) found that an agility test involving rapid decision making in response to an external stimulus was a better predictor of on-field performance when compared to standard agility tests in rugby players. This type of *reactive agility* testing, as illustrated in Figure 12.4, uses real people to provide sport-specific stimuli and perceptual cues and results in more effective testing (Young et al., 2011).

These missing factors have prompted researchers to investigate more closely the specific forms of strength and power production and how they fit within a systems approach and deliberate practice models to better transfer to on-field performance. According to Newton and Dugan (2002), the key biomechanical features of the movements must be identified through direct testing, discussions with experts, or scientific literature searches. Contraction type, range of motion, and speed of movement are just a few of the movement characteristics that need to be clarified. Analysis of high-level performers may reveal certain qualities these athletes possess and provide starting points for training. Others maintain that the perceptual challenges of the sport or task also need to be considered,

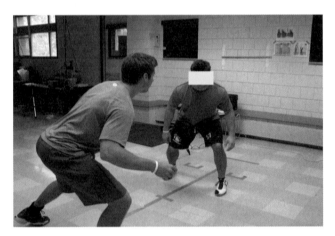

Figure 12.4 • Reactive agility testing. This photo shows a reactive agility test based on Gabbett and Benton (2009). The athlete (*front*) charges toward the tester (*back*) who then cuts to the left or right. The athlete reacts and cuts with the tester and then finishes the run through a photo timing gate (not shown). (Photo courtesy of Irik Johnson.)

including reaction time, decision making, environmental stability, time pressures, psychological stress, and other psychological constraints (Handford et al., 1997; Ives & Shelley, 2003; Passos et al., 2008). Psychophysical challenges introduced into the training environment create task-specific coordination changes and better the transfer of strength and power to the athletic field. This has led to the development of functional psychophysical training.

Athletic Performance and Functional Psychophysical Training

A football lineman exploding from a crouched position is a precisely crafted motor skill taking into account a multitude of environmental, task-, and individual-specific constraints. Footing, timing, characteristics of the opponent, game circumstances, tendencies of teammates, fatigue, injuries, and desire are just a few of the factors that play a role in the formation of the explosive motor commands. Consider also the "warrior athlete" who must calm his heart rate and his mind to aim and fire his weapon after sprinting to the top of a hill amid exploding shells. Taking such information into account in designing and implementing **functional psychophysical training** (or simply psychophysical training) programs was described by Passos et al. (2008) and more specifically by Ives and Shelley (2003) in their framework to manipulate these constraints into effective strength and power training programs. The four steps in functional psychophysical training are identified below.

1. Determine the physiological, perceptual, and psychomotor factors and skills required for successful performance. This information can come from the scientific literature as well as coaches and athletes themselves. It may be necessary to draw upon data from similar sports if that is the only data available. It is imperative that sport-specific characteristics be identified, because the psychological skills for one sport, or generic skills, may not work for another sport (Birrer & Morgan, 2010). In workplace settings, this is called a *task and demand analysis*, in which the requirements of the task (e.g., loading boxes onto a conveyor belt) and demands on the body (e.g., spinal compressive forces, strength, cognitive processing) are evaluated both subjectively and objectively (Sell et al., 2010). A task and demand analysis requires assessment of psychological factors like decision making, time pressures, and apprehension to fully understand the nature of the job.

2. Using the data from # 1 above, determine the specific constraints that influence movement and performance outcomes and the obstacles that need to be overcome for performance to improve. Define these obstacles and constraints as problems to be solved. Compare and contrast this list to the specific characteristics and abilities of the individual athlete or worker. For instance, the volleyball net is a constraint that needs to be overcome by the player. A volleyball player may

have difficulty with the net because of an insufficient reach due to a short stature, poor jump height, poor reaching technique during jumping, or may have poor timing that prevents her from reaching her maximal jump height at the right moment. Of course, stature cannot be changed, but constraints that influence the other factors may be movement of teammates or defenders that create jump timing problems, the net that forces biomechanical alterations, fear of injury from landing on someone's foot, or unfavorable muscle strength or body mass index that limits jump height.

3. Create a training environment that addresses strength or power as well as the psychomotor and mental factors necessary for performance. As a starting point, address mental effort, attention, and intention to determine the mental factors necessary for training. Training need not address all of these factors at once and can progress from simple to more complex. These psychological constraints should not overshadow the need for rigorous physiological challenges necessary to stress metabolic, morphologic, and neuromuscular systems. Yet, these constraints should pose sufficient a challenge to create psychophysical instability that requires adaption to take place.

4. Carefully present constraints, obstacles, and cues in a fashion that allows the athlete to discover on their own the best way to accomplish goals. Monitor progress and present new constraints and obstacles when learning plateaus.

A number of functional training techniques incorporate some of the features above. For instance, "small games" practice (Bishop et al., 2011) aims at improving agility and repeated sprint performance within the context of game-like decision making. Even simple jumping drills up against a wall or while reaching for an object incorporate environmental and cognitive constraints seen in basketball or volleyball. Using unstable landing surfaces such as a foam pad and teaching effective injury prevention landing strategies may then free up the athlete to maximize jump height during chaotic game situations. In their example on functional psychophysical training for volleyball players, Ives and Shelley (2003) reported data from a variety of sources that many psychophysical factors influenced the quality and effectiveness of vertical jumping for hitting. Among these factors were technical skills, "tight sets," proximity to the net, attention on defensive players and their movements, ball timing and other factors influencing optical flow and action–perception coupling, and movement variability. Using these data to formulate a psychophysical functional training program, these authors recommended a progression of constraints, including tight space constrained plyometric drills and the addition of a ball and defensive player(s) during jump and landing drills.

FUNCTIONAL PSYCHOPHYSICAL TRAINING FOR NONATHLETES

It has been well documented that general exercise in all forms—aerobic, anaerobic, flexibility, and strength—can have dramatic effects on health and wellness across the age span and across the health continuum (Garber et al., 2011). Nevertheless, functional exercise prescriptions are quickly finding their place alongside or in place of general exercise programs for the added benefits they can provide. For instance, functional training is recommended for healthy persons in physically and psychologically demanding activities, particularly the military, police, fire, and rescue work (Sell et al., 2010). Functional training for these professionals, sometimes referred to as **tactical training**, is often aimed at high-stress environments, interpersonal engagement (e.g., personnel carries and body drags), and equipment use. In their review of load carriage performance for soldiers, Knapik et al. (2012) reported that the largest gains in performance were a result of training that included progressive and overloaded load-carrying activities (i.e., functional activities) in addition to other exercise programming, particularly upper body strength exercises.

■ Thinking It Through 12.2 Firefighter Tactical Training

Firefighters, police, military, and other public safety and rescue personnel are the focus of tactical strength and conditioning. These individuals perform under conditions of uncertain and severe environmental challenges, high psychological stress and urgency, and danger. Physiological needs change from moment to moment, ranging from cardiovascular endurance to running speed, extreme balance, and high muscular strength. In the left photo below, a firefighter holds a high-powered hose with a fatiguing and awkward posture. The heavy turnout gear, smoke, perilous fire, and urgency make the task more physically and psychologically stressful. On the right, the danger of ladder climbing is evident. With this in mind, can you conduct a basic task and demand analysis for these firefighting conditions? As part of your analysis, describe the relationships among the task demands, physiological requirements, and psychological requirements. You may need to consult the current literature to aid you in your analysis.

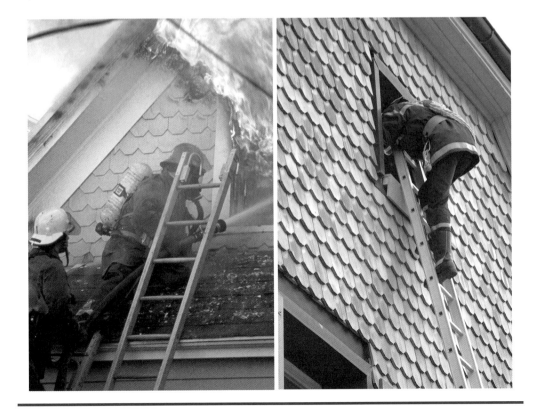

A host of evidence arising from studies on the elderly, from the rehabilitation literature, and on general wellness suggests that persons not engaged in sports or rigorous occupations also benefit from functional training to improve *functional health*. According to Ives and Keller (2008), functional health is the "capacity to participate in a wide range of activities of daily living, regardless of any underlying pathology or physical or mental illness" (p. 74). Functional health is characterized by a highly adaptable motor system that accomplishes movement goals while taking into account individual deficits and environmental and task challenges.

SIDE**NOTE**	**MAINTAINING FUNCTIONAL CAPABILITY AFTER EXTREME INACTIVITY**

Extended periods of extreme inactivity, such as long-term bed rest or the microgravity environment of space, result in serious degradation of physiological performance. Recovery from these negative effects—most notably a loss in muscle mass and function—normally takes weeks or months. Some occupations like special military forces, however, require high levels of muscle function immediately following extended periods of extreme inactivity. Extreme inactivity may be necessary during covert surveillance that may have soldiers in quiet horizontal positions for days at a time under highly stressful conditions. Thorlund et al. (2011) found in a simulated surveillance mission of 8 days that highly trained Special Forces soldiers lost nearly 3 kg of fat-free mass. These soldiers decreased 11% in knee extension strength, 20% in maximal rate of force development, and 10% in jump height. Three hours of recovery with additional nourishment and light exercises had no or minimal effect on recovering performance, which the authors noted were comparable to performance declines after exhaustive training and malnourishment. These findings reveal that there is much to learn about training and a strong need for novel training strategies to enable maintenance of function even following high levels of inactivity.

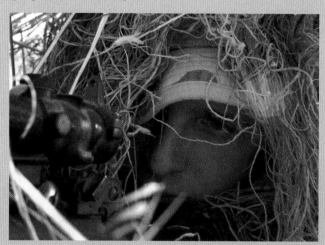

Photo courtesy of Department of Defense.

Research on functional training in nonathletic populations is mostly directed at persons with disabilities, the elderly, or those requiring extensive rehabilitation. Physical and occupational therapists have long used *added-purpose training*, *task-oriented training*, and other functional rehabilitation techniques to provide better results than generic rehabilitation (Chiung-Ju & Latham, 2011; Rensink et al., 2009; Shumway-Cook & Woollacott, 2005). This form of training is intended to provide purpose and meaning to enhance motivation and develop coordination mechanisms that are context specific and transfer better to real-world activities (Chiung-Ju & Latham, 2011). In addition to meaningful and motivating cognitive components, an effective functional training program may address other individual-specific psychological and psychosocial aspects of movement. For instance, the quality of life of frail elders may be more associated with confidence over fall prevention than actual physical performance, and thus, self-efficacy should be a target outcome of training programs in this population (Stretton et al., 2006). Other conditions, like heart failure, are accompanied by depression and anxiety and require use of psychological strategies that coincide with physical rehabilitation (Rutledge et al., 2006). Some authors have termed this the mind–body approach to rehabilitation (Casey et al., 2009).

For relatively healthy persons with nagging problems, subacute injuries and illnesses, or general decline due to aging, the available data regarding the success of functional training are abundant in some areas and scant in others. The widely diverse needs of relatively healthy persons prevent definitive and sweeping statements of what kinds of functional training work and for what purposes. Yet, it is well recognized that functional training for vocational and wellness purposes may reduce musculoskeletal pain and improve work performance (Elders et al., 2000; Gard et al., 2000), improve mobility function and activities of daily living of elders (Vluggen et al., 2009), and reduce falls in the elderly (Costello & Edelstein, 2008). Multimodal functional training interventions that include a cognitive component (i.e., psychophysical functional training) appear to be more effective than those without (Bethge et al., 2011; Gard et al., 2000) and may provide adherence benefits (Rejeski & Brawley, 2006). It has been further noted that measuring the effectiveness of any balance training program for elders should include dual-task challenges as they reveal real-world capabilities (Silsupadol et al., 2009).

There is an increasing amount of data showing that added-purpose training affects brain growth differences as well (see Thinking It Through box below). Some of the more successful functional training programs have risked going against conventional wisdom. For example, high-intensity, high-speed power, and eccentric training programs that were once thought to be off limits for elders have been shown to be more effective in some cases than less intense resistance training programs (Caserotti et al., 2008; Hazell et al., 2007; Pereira et al., 2012; Tschopp et al., 2011).

■ Thinking It Through 12.3 Training Body and Brain with Added-Purpose Training

Does it really matter how one trains or practices, as long as successful results are achieved? Consider a study by Filippi et al. (2010) who did brain imaging on their subjects during performance on the Purdue Pegboard Test: a test of hand/finger fine motor skills. Two groups of subjects trained daily over 2 weeks with hand manipulation exercises. One group trained with generic finger movement actions (flexion, extension, abduction, and finger sequencing) and the other group trained with functional, goal-oriented motor actions (guitar playing, drumstick rolling, juggling, manipulating weighted objects). At the end of the 2-week training period, as well as 3 months after training ceased, both groups improved the same on the pegboard test and neither group had significant a relapse after 3 months. Based on MRI scans, both groups improved similarly in overall brain gray matter volume and had specific brain areas with similar increases. However, there were fundamentally different areas in each group that increased in gray matter volume. In particular, the functional training group had larger gains in the hippocampus, and the generic training group had larger changes in parietal lobe regions. The hippocampus is an important area for memory consolidation and the parietal areas have vast connections among sensorimotor areas and helps interpret spatial attention information. The authors concluded that brain changes were made in neural network areas important to the training strategies. Given that the outcome performance was the same for both groups, it is reasonable to ask if it then matters how they trained or if it matters that different brain areas changed. Think through these questions and consider that it may matter on both accounts. Why? Think about transfer of skills and that the pegboard test was a closed skill. Also consider what may have happened in a group that trained both ways. There may be no definitive answers to these questions, but our lack of knowledge only underscores that we have much to learn.

The use and benefit of functional training for nonathlete populations can be understood by examining the **model of disablement** shown in Figure 12.5. The model of disablement tracks progression of health from pathology to disability. Pathology is the underlying disease or physiological abnormality, which contributes to impairment. Impairment is a dysfunction in how organs, tissues, or systems operate. Impairments may lead to a functional limitation, which are disruptions in one's day-to-day

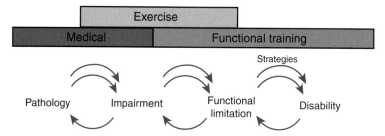

Pathologies are biological, but they may contribute to both physiological and psychological impairments. Pain, weakness, and attention deficit disorder are examples of impairments. Functional limitations may include slow walking speed, inability to sit for long periods of time, poor concentration, or inability to life boxes overhead. Individuals often adopt strategies to counter the functional limitations, such as driving rather than walking and adaptive postures.

Progression along the continuum is mostly left to right (hence the *double arrows*), but not always (*single arrow*). It is not always direct as indicated by the *curved arrows*. Numerous risk factors influence if and how one level of progresses to the next. Key risk factors are:
- Demographic (e.g., age, socioeconomic status, education)
- Physiological (e.g., body size, diet, gender)
- Psychosocial (e.g., anxiety, motivation, social networks)
- Environmental (e.g., housing, climate, occupation)
- Comorbidities (e.g., hypertension, diabetes, obesity, depression)

Notice the overlap among medical, exercise, and functional training interventions, but that functional training targets a broader scope than other methods. An important target for functional training is the development of effective strategies to prevent functional limitations from becoming disabilities.

Figure 12.5 • The model of disablement illustrates the progression of disease to disability. The goal of functional training, ultimately, is to stop impairments from becoming functional limitations and stop functional impairments from becoming disabilities. Improving functional health may increase one's activity level and psychological status, thereby having a positive effect on impairments and pathologies. (With permission from Ives & Keller, 2008).

functioning. Should this disruption impair how one can function in society, then it becomes a disability. Most people, particularly middle-aged and older, have some level of impairment and functional limitations. This could be joint and muscle pain including arthritis and low back pain, subclinical coronary artery disease, overweightness, disordered physiological and psychological stress response and coping skills, and more.

It is tempting to think that addressing the pathologies and impairments on the left side of the continuum would automatically have a positive effect on the "downstream" functional limitations and disability, but this is not necessarily the case. Improving some basic outcome measures and physiological measures may have no positive impact on disability scores (Latham et al., 2004). For this reason, it is necessary to also address the right side of the continuum by focusing on functional limitations. According to Ives and Keller (2008), functional training works best on the right side of the continuum, helping to overcome functional limitations, and conventional exercise works best on the left side of the continuum.

Functional training with a psychophysical component for relatively healthy persons and those with chronic disorders is within the scope of practice and tools of exercise science practitioners. Determining needs and prescribing a functional training program requires creativity and careful assessment of individual needs that are not always available in the existing literature, even for persons with common disorders (Haddad et al., 2012). The basic four-step guidelines presented earlier can be used, but with more latitude to reflect the diverse needs across nonathletic populations. One aspect of assessment should be a functional health evaluation or quality of life assessment, both of which are aimed at assessing individual-specific needs, physical function, and psychosocial characteristics. It should also evaluate the individual's task difficulties and environmental characteristics in which the individual often engages. Ives and Keller (2008) recommended using health-related quality of life questionnaires such as the SF-36 and population-specific physical performance test batteries as good starting points in a functional health evaluation.

Functional psychophysical training for nonathletes may look a bit different than for athletes. Successful *return-to-work programs* (*work hardening* programs) for individuals with musculoskeletal problems often incorporate multiple separate interventions that are then integrated. For example, Gard et al. (2000) used a combination of progressive and graded exercise training, occupational-specific motor training, and psychosocial interventions to vastly improve worker return to work and quality of life compared to standard treatments. These authors pointed out that the program covered fitness, specificity, and "spirit." These factors, along with individual-based programs, individual goals, and a purpose aimed at functionality, were instrumental in improved outcomes of increased motivation, improved functional coordination, and improved pain coping. This idea of spirit, which can be further described by terms such as vitality, enthusiasm, optimism, and encouragement, may be central to one's engagement in healthy behaviors and the quality of outcome results. These terms also describe the positive behaviors associated with better immune function, less illness, better recovery from cardiovascular disease, and an overall better quality of life (Richman et al., 2005; Rozanski et al., 2005) and impact one's response to exercise. In fact, in their extensive review of why aerobic exercise prescriptions have such a wide variation in effectiveness, Hautala et al. (2009) noted the importance of motivation and other neuropsychological factors and the effects of the autonomic nervous systems in regulating exercise responses. These authors concluded that the cognitive–emotional resources of an individual be assessed and used as part of an individually tailored exercise program and promoting lifestyle changes. In sum, effective exercise training for nonathletes aimed toward improving function, quality of life, and lowering disease risk should include a measure of psychophysical functional training.

Concepts in Action

An Integrated Psychophysical Approach

An extensive psychophysical functional training program is illustrated in the work of Bethge et al. (2011). These authors examined workers on disability for musculoskeletal disorders and engaged them in a multimodal work hardening program to prepare them to go back to work. The components included standard exercise, functional occupation-specific exercises, and several interventions to reduce stress and increase self-efficacy and empowerment and cope with pain during work. Though these components were administered side by side, the trainers and others involved regularly met to insure integration of the training components. The result were that the multimodal work hardening group was more than twice as likely than a "treatment as usual" group to have positive work outcomes after 6 months, better scores for mental and physical health-related quality of life, and better pain management. This multimodal program highlights the need for health care practitioners to not only understand what other health care workers are doing as part of a team effort but to integrate the other modalities into their own care. For instance, in the case presented here, exercise science clinicians can integrate pain management and postural control strategies during functional strength training exercises.

FUNCTIONAL PSYCHOPHYSICAL TRAINING VIA VIRTUAL REALITY

The potential complexities in manipulating environmental and task constraints within a functional psychophysical training program may prohibit complete program development. *Virtual reality* (VR) or *virtual environments* (VEs) may offer solutions to this complexity. VEs range from simple computer video games to full surround video immersive rooms that also monitor and react to body movements. Between these two extremes are VR headsets that project the VE on the inside of goggles worn by the user. Sensors in the headset detect head movement to which the VR display responds. More sophisticated systems include sensors affixed to gloves or body suits to monitor limb and body movement. Some of these sophisticated technologies have made their way into consumer products for fitness center and home use, such as the Wii Fit, X-box 360 Kinect, and the GameBike®. Nearly all of these consumer products fall under the heading of exercise gaming (*exergames*). Exergames require physical exercise, real-life–based motor/sport skills, or both, to interact and play within the computer environment. True VR exergaming requires the VE to be compatible with the exercise mode, such as a VR bicycle race on a cycle ergometer (Fig. 12.6). Some exergames, though, simply require physical exercise in place of joystick control to provide input responses to video games that are unrelated to the physical act. These exergames can be as simple as answering trivia questions based on pedaling cadence or following computer-generated movement instructions (e.g., Dance Dance Revolution [DDR]).

VEs are currently being used with some promise in training motor skills and tactics in sports (Portus & Farrow, 2011) and occupations such as surgery in which mistakes during actual practice have dire consequences (van Dongen et al., 2011). For similar reasons, the military has long used computer simulators to train pilots and more recently to train teams of soldiers in combat missions (Lampton et al., 2003) and to provide military stress inoculation (Popović et al., 2009). In their evaluation of

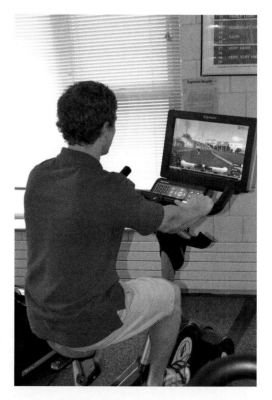

Figure 12.6 • This exergame setup has exercisers competing against the computer and against other online exergamers. (Photo courtesy of Jeffrey C. Ives.)

computer-simulated training for motor skill enhancement, Ward et al. (2006) maintained that the psychological and information processing reality of the simulated environments and tasks are likely of greatest importance, as evidenced by reports showing that realism and level of information available in the graphical displays may alter the user's movement biomechanics and strategies (Morice et al., 2010; Vignais et al., 2009). The use of VR in motor rehabilitation and movement skill retraining is now extensively used for a number of different conditions, most often for brain injuries, orthopedic rehabilitation, and training for functional activities of daily living (Fig. 12.7). Most patients can tolerate the VR and are able to take gains from the VE to real-world equivalent tasks (Holden, 2005).

The use of VR as an aid to physical training for relatively healthy persons has only been explored rigorously from the standpoint of adherence and mental health benefits. A majority of data suggest that VR exercise promotes exercise adherence (Annesi & Mazas, 1997) and positive mood states (Plante et al., 2006) and this may be particularly the case when the VR experience is in the form of exergaming (Barros et al., 2012; Plante et al., 2003b; Van Schaik et al., 2008). The particular benefits of the exergame environment may be due to competitive enjoyment as well as the requirement for an external focus

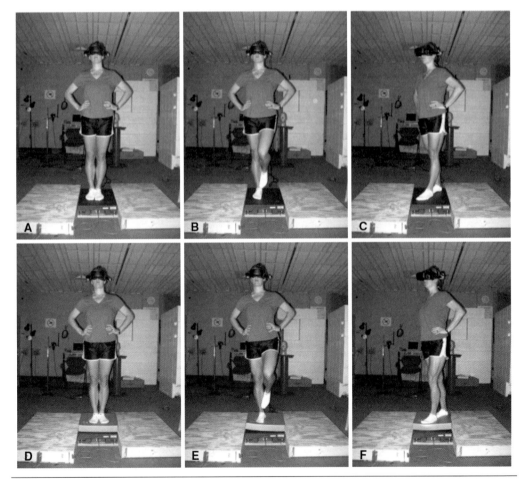

Figure 12.7 • A VR headset is being worn during balance assessment tests on firm (**A–C**) and foam (**D–F**) surfaces. The VR environment enables the use of context-specific challenges and may provide for more precise testing. (Image reprinted from Mihalik, J. P., Kohli, L., & Whitton, M. C. (2008). Do the physical characteristics of a virtual reality device contraindicate its use for balance assessment? *Journal of Sport Rehabilitation*, *17*(1), 38–49, with permission.)

SIDE**NOTE**	**EXERGAMING AND ELDER COGNITIVE FUNCTION**

Exergaming has been shown to improve cognitive function in older healthy adults over other forms of traditional exercise. In one of the largest studies to date on this topic, Anderson-Hanley et al. (2012) examined cognitive status in community-dwelling elders following 3 months of VR stationary bicycle touring that provided VR competition. VR cycling was significantly better than non-VR stationary cycling in promoting cognitive function and in reducing the risk of developing cognitive impairments, but was not better in terms of fitness development. The additional finding that the VR cyclists had significantly more neural growth factor proteins suggests that the VR enhanced neuroplasticity. How the VR results compare to actual touring and competitive cycling remains to be seen, but at least one other study has shown that VR training program for mobility and living skills is not superior to training in real environments (Richardson et al., 2000).

of attention and purposeful physical effort directed toward the constraints of the VR environment (Mestre et al., 2011). Note, however, that these findings of better mood states or adherence are in comparison to traditional indoor stationary exercise (e.g., treadmill, cycle ergometer) and likely do not hold true in comparison to outdoor nonstationary exercise (Plante et al., 2003a, 2006). What this means is that the VE still lacks in comparison to the real environment in terms of creating a positive exercise experience. Given the rapid advancement in computer simulation technology, it may not be long before the VR experience truly mimics the real-world experience.

The adherence benefit of VR exercise has been applied to training for weight control, where most authors suggest that VR training can promote exercise self-efficacy for sedentary and overweight children and adults (Ruiz et al., 2012). These effects are not necessarily universal, and factors such as gender, fitness level, physical intensity demands of the VR environment, VR viewing perspective (e.g., 1st person, 3rd person), amount of user-controlled interaction, and mode of exercise may influence the user's affinity for VR exercise and the potential VR benefits (Adamo et al., 2010; Bailenson et al., 2008; Foley & Maddison, 2010; Legrand et al., 2011; Ruiz et al., 2012; Skip Rizzo et al., 2011).

Though the informed use of VR can be used to advance fitness and motor skills, it remains to be seen if true functional training benefits are possible. There are only very limited data available, such as

Concepts in Action

Designing Your Own Game or Equipment

The growth of VR technology, exergames, and functional training equipment is exploding faster that catalogs can keep up. In our experience, few of these devices were created with a real understanding of functional training or motor behavior principles, but rather as games to meet specific needs. For instance, the icon of exergames, Dance Dance Revolution, was invented by an individual vacationing in Japan who felt constrained by too many people around him when trying to exercise. With a firm understanding of motor behavior principles, create a functional training program that involves both software/computers and specifically designed training equipment. Your program could be for sport training, general wellness, or occupation-specific training. You need not get into the engineering of the product, but simply describe what it does. Identify the precise purposes of your equipment and program and how it is designed to achieve these purposes. Consider the five essential features of practice and/or the four steps to psychophysical functional training.

VR rotational balance training to help ice dancers (Tornese et al., 2011). Physically rigorous games like DDR may help with laboratory measures of balance (Brumels et al., 2008), but it is unknown if actual dance performance is improved. Other devices (e.g., Parisi Speed School quickness trainer) have not been investigated. In sum, VR and VE functional training hold promise, but the newness of this kind of training prevents having sufficient data and making firm recommendations.

SUMMARY

Strength and power are seen as important components to athletic success and general wellness, yet the nature and extent of their association to performance has been difficult to quantify. In particular, the routine use of strength- and power-based training programs has not always been shown effective in improving athletic performance. Part of the difficulty in matching training with performance outcomes are the vast number of ways strength and power can be evaluated and trained. This has led to uncertainties in creating programs that transfer the abilities gained in the weight room to the playing field. Though functional training is purported to overcome these challenges and maximize transfer, without integration of psychological constraints effectiveness is limited. Functional training incorporating both physiological and psychological components, that is, functional psychophysical training, presents a framework to maximize transfer of abilities from the weight room to the playing field.

Functional psychophysical training brings the perceptual aspects of the task and the environment into the training program, such that physiological systems are stressed within both psychological and physiological constraints. A four-step process beginning with identification of perceptual factors alongside task and environmental constraints characterizes one approach to better functional training. The other steps involve incorporation of these constraints into the training environment and progressing through these obstacles in a discovery learning manner. Regardless of the specific approach used, incorporating physiological and psychological approaches simultaneously improves outcomes in rehabilitation, occupational settings, elderly slip and fall prevention and quality of life, and sport performance.

Using VR and other computerized training technologies holds promise in functional training. VR enables bringing "real-life" situational challenges to the training environment in a safe and entertaining manner. If nothing else, these technologies may enhance adherence to exercise. In sum, knowledgeable trainers and coaches are able to bring the appropriate task and environmental constraints into the training environment in order to maximize transfer and improve real-life performance. The use of VR to provide psychophysical training environments holds promise but is too new to offer firm conclusions.

STUDY QUESTIONS

1. What is the purpose of functional training compared to practice and conventional physical training?
2. How is functional training set up to maximize transfer of physiological abilities to real-world situations?
3. What are the physical and psychological contributors to the production of strength and power?
4. Identify and define the different modes of strength and power production.
5. What are the difficulties and controversies in strength and power testing and training?
6. Explain the relationship between laboratory measures of strength and power and athletic performance.
7. What is functional psychophysical training and how does it differ from conventional functional training?

8. What is the four-step approach to creating a psychophysical training program?
9. What is functional health, and how does it relate to functional training?
10. What is the model of disablement, and how does functional training fit within this model?
11. Explain the benefits and shortcomings of using virtual reality as a functional training mode.

References

Aagaard, P. (2010). The use of eccentric strength training to enhance maximal muscle strength, explosive force (RDF) and muscular power—consequences for athletic performance. *Open Sports Sciences Journal*, *3*, 52–55.

Aagaard, P. P., & Andersen, J. L. (2010). Effects of strength training on endurance capacity in top-level endurance athletes. *Scandinavian Journal of Medicine & Science in Sports*, *20*, 39–47.

Abernethy, P. P., Wilson, G. G., & Logan, P. P. (1995). Strength and power assessment: Issues, controversies and challenges. *Sports Medicine*, *19*(6), 401–417.

Adamo, K. B., Rutherford, J. A., & Goldfield, G. S. (2010). Effects of interactive video game cycling on overweight and obese adolescent health. *Applied Physiology, Nutrition and Metabolism*, *35*(6), 805–815.

American College of Sports Medicine. (1990). ACSM position stand: The recommended quality and quantity of exercise for developing and maintaining cardiorespiratory and muscular fitness in healthy adults. *Medicine and Science in Sports and Exercise*, *22*(9), 265–274.

American College of Sports Medicine. (1998). ACSM position stand: The recommended quantity and quality of exercise for developing and maintaining cardiorespiratory and muscular fitness, and flexibility in healthy adults. *Medicine and Science in Sports and Exercise*, *30*(6), 975–991.

Andersen, J. L., & Aagaard, P. P. (2010). Effects of strength training on muscle fiber types and size; consequences for athletes training for high-intensity sport. *Scandinavian Journal of Medicine & Science in Sports*, *20*, 32–38.

Anderson-Hanley, C., Arciero, P., Brickman, A., Nimon, J., Okuma, N., Westen, S., et al. (2012). Exergaming and older adult cognition: A cluster randomized clinical trial. *American Journal of Preventive Medicine*, *42*(2), 109–119.

Annesi, J. J., & Mazas, J. J. (1997). Effects of virtual reality-enhanced exercise equipment on adherence and exercise-induced feeling states. *Perceptual and Motor Skills*, *85*(3 Pt 1), 835–844.

Bailenson, J., Patel, K., Nielsen, A., Bajscy, R., Jung, S., & Kurillo, G. (2008). The effect of interactivity on learning physical actions in virtual reality. *Media Psychology*, *11*(3), 354–376.

Barros, M., Neves, A., Correia, W., & Soares, M. (2012). Exergames: The role of ergonomics and design in helping to control childhood obesity through physical and functional exercise program. *Work*, *41*, 1208–1211.

Behm, D. G., & Sale, D. G. (1993). Velocity specificity of resistance training. *Sports Medicine*, *15*(6), 374–388.

Bethge, M. M., Herbold, D. D., Trowitzsch, L. L., & Jacobi, C. C. (2011). Work status and health-related quality of life following multimodal work hardening: A cluster randomised trial. *Journal of Back and Musculoskeletal Rehabilitation*, *24*(3), 161–172.

Birrer, D. D., & Morgan, G. G. (2010). Psychological skills training as a way to enhance an athlete's performance in high-intensity sports. *Scandinavian Journal of Medicine & Science in Sports*, *20*, 78–87.

Bishop, D., Girard, O., & Mendez-Villanueva, A. (2011). Repeated-sprint ability—Part II: Recommendations for training. *Sports Medicine*, *41*(9), 741–756.

Bloomer, R. J., & Ives, J. C. (2000). Varying neural and hypertrophic influences in a strength program. *Strength and Conditioning Journal*, *22*(2), 30–35.

Bonacci, J., Chapman, A., Blanch, P., & Vicenzino, B. (2009). Neuromuscular adaptations to training, injury and passive interventions: Implications for running economy. *Sports Medicine*, *39*(11), 903–921.

Brumels, K. A., Blasius, T., Cortright, T., Oumedian, D., & Solberg, B. (2008). Comparison of efficacy between traditional and video game based balance programs. *Clinical Kinesiology*, *62*(4), 26–31.

Carpinelli, R. N. (2009). Challenging the American College of Sports Medicine 2009 position stand on resistance training. *Medicina Sportiva*, *13*(2), 131–137.

Carroll, T. J., Selvanayagam, V. S., Riek, S. S., & Semmler, J. G. (2011). Neural adaptations to strength training: Moving beyond transcranial magnetic stimulation and reflex studies. *Acta Physiologica*, *202*(2), 119–140.

Caserotti, P., Aagaard, P., & Puggaard, L. (2008). Changes in power and force generation during coupled eccentric–concentric versus concentric muscle contraction with training and aging. *European Journal of Applied Physiology, 103*(2), 151–161.

Casey, A., Chang, B., Huddleston, J., Virani, N., Benson, H., & Dusek, J. (2009). A model for integrating a mind/body approach to cardiac rehabilitation: Outcomes and correlators. *Journal of Cardiopulmonary Rehabilitation and Prevention, 29*(4), 230–240.

Chiung-Ju, L., & Latham, N. (2011). Can progressive resistance strength training reduce physical disability in older adults? A meta-analysis study. *Disability and Rehabilitation, 33*(2), 87–97.

Cormie, P., McGuigan, M., & Newton, R. (2010). Adaptations in athletic performance after ballistic power versus strength training. *Medicine and Science in Sports and Exercise, 42*(8), 1582–1598.

Cormie, P., McGuigan, M., & Newton, R. (2011a). Developing maximal neuromuscular power: Part 1—Biological basis of maximal power production. *Sports Medicine, 41*(1), 17–38.

Cormie, P., McGuigan, M., & Newton, R. (2011b). Developing maximal neuromuscular power: Part 2—Training considerations for improving maximal power production. *Sports Medicine, 41*(2), 125–146.

Costello, E., & Edelstein, J. E. (2008). Update on falls prevention for community-dwelling older adults: Review of single and multifactorial intervention programs. *Journal of Rehabilitation Research and Development, 45*(8), 1135–1152.

Cronin, J., & Sleivert, G. (2005). Challenges in understanding the influence of maximal power training on improving athletic performance. *Sports Medicine, 35*(3), 213–234.

Dudley, G. A., & Djamil, R. (1985). Incompatibility of endurance- and strength-training modes of exercise. *Journal of Applied Physiology, 59*, 1446–1451.

Elders, L., van der Beek, A., & Burdorf, A. (2000). Return to work after sickness absence due to back disorders—A systematic review on intervention strategies. *International Archives of Occupational and Environmental Health, 73*(5), 339–348.

Filippi, M., Ceccarelli, A., Pagani, E., Gatti, R., Rossi, A., Stefanelli, L., et al. (2010). Motor learning in healthy humans is associated to gray matter changes: A tensor-based morphometry study. *PLoS One, 5*(4), e10198.

Foley, L., & Maddison, R. (2010). Use of active video games to increase physical activity in children: A (virtual) reality? *Pediatric Exercise Science, 22*(1), 7–20.

Folland, J. P., & Williams, A. G. (2007). The adaptations to strength training. *Sports Medicine, 37*(2), 145–168.

Gabbett, T., & Benton, D. (2009). Reactive agility of rugby league players. *Journal of Science and Medicine in Sport, 12*(1), 212–214.

Garber, C., Blissmer, B., Deschenes, M., Franklin, B., Lamonte, M., Lee, I., et al. (2011). American College of Sports Medicine position stand. Quantity and quality of exercise for developing and maintaining cardiorespiratory, musculoskeletal, and neuromotor fitness in apparently healthy adults: Guidance for prescribing exercise. *Medicine and Science in Sports and Exercise, 43*(7), 1334–1359.

Gard, G., Gille, K., & Grahn, B. (2000). Functional activities and psychosocial factors in the rehabilitation of patients with low back pain. *Scandinavian Journal of Caring Sciences, 14*(2), 75–81.

Haddad, J., Rietdyk, S., & Claxton, L. (2012). Exercise training to improve independence and quality of life in impaired individuals. *Exercise and Sport Sciences Reviews, 40*(3), 117.

Handford, C., Davids, K., Bennett, S., & Button, C. (1997). Skill acquisition in sport: Some applications of an evolving practice ecology. *Journal of Sports Sciences, 15*(6), 621–640.

Harris, N., Cronin, J., & Keogh, J. (2007). Contraction force specificity and its relationship to functional performance. *Journal of Sports Sciences, 25*(2), 201–212.

Hautala, A., Kiviniemi, A., & Tulppo, M. (2009). Individual responses to aerobic exercise: The role of the autonomic nervous system. *Neuroscience and Biobehavioral Reviews, 33*(2), 107–115.

Hazell, T., Kenno, K., & Jakobi, J. (2007). Functional benefit of power training for older adults. *Journal of Aging and Physical Activity, 15*(3), 349–359.

Holden, M. (2005). Virtual environments for motor rehabilitation: Review. *Cyberpsychology & Behavior, 8*(3), 187–211.

Hortobagyi, T. T., Katch, F. I., & LaChance, P. F. (1989). Interrelationships among various measures of upper body strength assessed by different contraction modes. Evidence for a general strength component. *European Journal of Applied Physiology and Occupational Physiology, 58*(7), 749–755.

Ives, J. C., & Keller, B. A. (2008). Functional training for health. In J. K. Silver & C. Morin (Eds.), *Understanding fitness. How exercise fuels health and fights disease*. Westport, CT: Praeger Publishers.

Ives, J. C., & Shelley, G. A. (2003). Psychophysics in functional strength and power training: Review and implementation framework. *Journal of Strength and Conditioning Research, 17*, 177–186.

Jones, A. M. (2006). The physiology of the world record holder for the women's marathon. *International Journal of Sports Science & Coaching, 1*(2), 101–116.

Knapik, J., Harman, E., Steelman, R., & Graham, B. (2012). A systematic review of the effects of physical training on load carriage performance. *Journal of Strength and Conditioning Research, 26*(2), 585–597.

Lampton, D. R., Clark, B. R., & Knerr, B. W. (2003). Urban combat: The ultimate extreme environment. *Journal of Human Performance in Extreme Environments, 7*(2), 57–62.

Latham, N., Bennett, D., Stretton, C., & Anderson, C. (2004). Systematic review of progressive resistance strength training in older adults. *Journals of Gerontology. Series A, Biological Sciences and Medical Sciences, 59*(1), 48–61.

Lawton, T., Cronin, J., & McGuigan, M. (2011). Strength testing and training of rowers: A review. *Sports Medicine, 41*(5), 413–432.

Lee, G. L., Chan, C. H., & Hui-Chan, C. Y. (2001). Consistency of performance on the functional capacity assessment: Static strength and dynamic endurance. *American Journal of Physical Medicine & Rehabilitation, 80*(3), 189–195.

Legrand, F. D., Joly, P. M., Bertucci, W. M., Soudain-Pineau, M. A., & Marcel, J. (2011). Interactive-virtual reality (IVR) exercise: An examination of in-task and pre-to-post exercise affective changes. *Journal of Applied Sport Psychology, 23*(1), 65–75.

Marcovic, G. (2007). Poor relationship between strength and power qualities and agility performance. *The Journal of Sports Medicine and Physical Fitness, 47*(3), 276–283.

McGill, S., Karpowicz, A., Fenwick, C., & Brown, S. (2009). Exercises for the torso performed in a standing posture: Spine and hip motion and motor patterns and spine load. *Journal of Strength and Conditioning Research, 23*(2), 455–464.

Mestre, D., Ewald, M., & Maiano, C. (2011). Virtual reality and exercise: Behavioral and psychological effects of visual feedback. *Studies in Health Technology and Informatics, 167*, 122–127.

Moir, G., Sanders, R., Button, C., & Glaister, M. (2007). The effect of periodized resistance training on accelerative sprint performance. *Sports Biomechanics, 6*(3), 285–300.

Morice, A. P., François, M., Jacobs, D. M., & Montagne, G. (2010). Environmental constraints modify the way an interceptive action is controlled. *Experimental Brain Research, 202*(2), 397–411.

Newton, R. U., & Dugan, E. E. (2002). Application of strength diagnosis. *Strength and Conditioning Journal, 24*(5), 50–59.

Passos, P., Araújo, D., Davids, K., & Shuttleworth, R. (2008). Manipulating constraints to train decision making in rugby union. *International Journal of Sports Science & Coaching, 3*(1), 125–140.

Pereira, A., Izquierdo, M., Silva, A., Costa, A., González-Badillo, J., & Marques, M. (2012). Muscle performance and functional capacity retention in older women after high-speed power training cessation. *Experimental Gerontology, 47*(8), 620–624.

Plante, T. G., Aldridge, A., Su, D., Bogdan, R., Belo, M., & Kahn, K. (2003a). Does virtual reality enhance the management of stress when paired with exercise? An exploratory study. *International Journal of Stress Management, 10*(3), 203–216.

Plante, T. G., Cage, C., Clements, S., & Stover, A. (2006). Psychological benefits of exercise paired with virtual reality: Outdoor exercise energizes whereas indoor virtual exercise relaxes. *International Journal of Stress Management, 13*(1), 108–117.

Plante, T. G., Frazier, S. S., Tittle, A. A., Babula, M. M., Ferlic, E. E., & Riggs, E. E. (2003b). Does virtual reality enhance the psychological benefits of exercise? *Journal of Human Movement Studies, 45*(6), 485–507.

Popović, S., Horvat, M., Kukolja, D., Dropuljić, B., & ćosić, K. (2009). Stress inoculation training supported by physiology-driven adaptive virtual reality stimulation. *Annual Review of Cybertherapy and Telemedicine, 7*, 50–54.

Portus, M. R., & Farrow, D. (2011). Enhancing cricket batting skill: Implications for biomechanics and skill acquisition research and practice. *Sports Biomechanics, 10*(4), 294–305.

Protas, E. J., & Tissier, S. (2009). Strength and speed training for elders with mobility disability. *Journal of Aging and Physical Activity, 17*(3), 257–271.

Reilly, T., Morris, T., & Whyte, G. (2009). The specificity of training prescription and physiological assessment: A review. *Journal of Sports Sciences*, 27(6), 575–589.

Rejeski, W., & Brawley, L. (2006). Functional health: Innovations in research on physical activity with older adults. *Medicine and Science in Sports and Exercise*, 38(1), 93–99.

Rensink, M., Schuurmans, M., Lindeman, E., & Hafsteinsdóttir, T. (2009). Task-oriented training in rehabilitation after stroke: Systematic review. *Journal of Advanced Nursing*, 65(4), 737–754.

Richardson, J., Law, M., Wishart, L., & Guyatt, G. (2000). The use of a simulated environment (easy street) to retrain independent living skills in elderly persons: A randomized controlled trial. *The Journals of Gerontology. Biological Sciences and Medical Sciences*, 55(10), M578–M584.

Richman, L., Kubzansky, L., Maselko, J., Kawachi, I., Choo, P., & Bauer, M. (2005). Positive emotion and health: Going beyond the negative. *Health Psychology*, 24(4), 422–429.

Roig, M., O'Brien, K., Kirk, G., Murray, R., McKinnon, P., Shadgan, B., et al. (2009). The effects of eccentric versus concentric resistance training on muscle strength and mass in healthy adults: A systematic review with meta-analysis. *British Journal of Sports Medicine*, 43(8), 556–568.

Rozanski, A., Blumenthal, J., Davidson, K., Saab, P., & Kubzansky, L. (2005). The epidemiology, pathophysiology, and management of psychosocial risk factors in cardiac practice: The emerging field of behavioral cardiology. *Journal of the American College of Cardiology*, 45(5), 637–651.

Ruiz, J., Andrade, A., Anam, R., Aguiar, R., Sun, H., & Roos, B. (2012). Using anthropomorphic avatars resembling sedentary older individuals as models to enhance self-efficacy and adherence to physical activity: Psychophysiological correlates. *Studies in Health Technology and Informatics*, 173, 405–411.

Rutledge, T., Reis, V., Linke, S., Greenberg, B., & Mills, P. (2006). Depression in heart failure a meta-analytic review of prevalence, intervention effects, and associations with clinical outcomes. *Journal of the American College of Cardiology*, 48(8), 1527–1537.

Sell, T., Abt, J., Crawford, K., Lovalekar, M., Nagai, T., Deluzio, J., et al. (2010). Warrior model for human performance and injury prevention: Eagle Tactical Athlete Program (ETAP) part I. *Journal of Special Operations Medicine*, 10(4), 2–21.

Shumway-Cook, A., & Woollacott, M. H. (2005). *Motor control. Theory and practical applications* (2nd ed.). Philadelphia, PA: Lippincott Williams & Wilkins.

Silsupadol, P., Lugade, V., Shumway-Cook, A., van Donkelaar, P., Chou, L., Mayr, U., et al. (2009). Training-related changes in dual-task walking performance of elderly persons with balance impairment: A double-blind, randomized controlled trial. *Gait & Posture*, 29(4), 634–639.

Skip Rizzo, A., Lange, B., Suma, E., & Bolas, M. (2011). Virtual reality and interactive digital game technology: New tools to address obesity and diabetes. *Journal of Diabetes Science and Technology*, 5(2), 256–264.

Stratton, G. G., Jones, M., Fox, K. R., Tolfrey, K. K., Harris, J. J., Maffulli, N. N., et al. (2004). BASES position statement on guidelines for resistance exercise in young people. *Journal of Sports Sciences*, 22(4), 383–390.

Stretton, C., Latham, N., Carter, K., Lee, A., & Anderson, C. (2006). Determinants of physical health in frail older people: The importance of self-efficacy. *Clinical Rehabilitation*, 20(4), 357–366.

Thorlund, J., Jakobsen, O., Madsen, T., Christensen, P., Nedergaard, A., Andersen, J., et al. (2011). Changes in muscle strength and morphology after muscle unloading in Special Forces missions. *Scandinavian Journal of Medicine & Science in Sports*, 21(6), e56–e63.

Tomljanović, M., Spasić, M., Gabrilo, G., Uljević, O., & Foretić, N. (2011). Effects of five weeks of functional vs. traditional resistance training on anthropometric and motor performance variables. *Kinesiology*, 43(2), 145–154.

Tornese, D., Botta, M., Mattei, V., & Alpini, D. (2011). Self-experienced virtual reality to improve balance reflexes in ice dancers. A pilot study. *Sport Sciences for Health*, 6(2/3), 45–50.

Tschopp, M., Sattelmayer, M., & Hilfiker, R. (2011). Is power training or conventional resistance training better for function in elderly persons? A meta-analysis. *Age and Ageing*, 40(5), 549–556.

van Dongen, K., Ahlberg, G., Bonavina, L., Carter, F., Grantcharov, T., Hyltander, A., et al. (2011). European consensus on a competency-based virtual reality training program for basic endoscopic surgical psychomotor skills. *Surgical Endoscopy*, 25(1), 166–171.

Van Schaik, P., Blake, J., Pernet, F., Spears, I., & Fencott, C. (2008). Virtual augmented exercise gaming for older adults. *Cyberpsychology & Behavior*, 11(1), 103–106.

Vignais, N., Bideau, B., Craig, C., Brault, S., Multon, F., Delamarche, P., et al. (2009). Does the level of graphical detail of a virtual handball thrower influence a goalkeeper's motor response? *Journal of Sports Science and Medicine*, 8(4), 501–508.

Vluggen, T., Lexis, M., Schuurman, J., & Schols, J. (2009). The effect of functional training compared with resistance training on ADL performance and muscle strength in community dwelling elderly: A systematic review [Dutch]. *Nederlands Tijdschrift Voor Fysiotherapie*, 119(4), 122–128.

Ward, P., Williams, A., & Hancock, P. A. (2006). Simulation for performance and training. In K. Ericsson, N. Charness, P. J. Feltovich, R. R. Hoffman, K. Ericsson, N. Charness, et al. (Eds.) *The Cambridge handbook of expertise and expert performance* (pp. 243–262). New York: Cambridge University Press.

Yamamoto, L., Klau, J., Casa, D., Kraemer, W., Armstrong, L., & Maresh, C. (2010). The effects of resistance training on road cycling performance among highly trained cyclists: A systematic review. *Journal of Strength and Conditioning Research*, 24(2), 560–566.

Young, W. (2006). Transfer of strength and power training to sports performance. *International Journal of Sports Physiology and Performance*, 1(2), 74–83.

Young, W., & Farrow, D. (2006). A review of agility: Practical applications for strength and conditioning. *Strength and Conditioning Journal*, 28(5), 24–29.

Young, W., Farrow, D., Pyne, D., McGregor, W., & Handke, T. (2011). Validity and reliability of agility tests in junior Australian football players. *Journal of Strength and Conditioning Research*, 25(12), 3399–3403.

Ziv, G., & Lidor, R. (2010). Vertical jump in female and male volleyball players: a review of observational and experimental studies. *Scandinavian Journal of Medicine & Science in Sports, 20*(4), 556–567.

GLOSSARY

Ability: Refers to factors or characteristics that underlie the general capacity of an individual related to the performance of specific motor skills; these factors may be physiological, psychological, or psychomotor, as well as genetic or learned.

Absolute error (AE): The average over a given number of trials of the error absolute values; therefore, no plus or minus or direction of the scores is provided, just the error magnitude.

Action potential (AP): The bioelectrical signal by which neurons communicate information among each other and to muscles and other effector organs

Activation history: Term referring to the prior amount and type of muscle contractile activity, which may influence the mechanical and neural properties of the muscle and muscle spindle

Acuity: Refers to the ability to precisely localize or identify a stimulus; based on the size of area covered by a receptor and the density of receptors in the stimulus area. See sensitivity.

Affordances: Qualities or characteristics in the environment that give rise to specific movement or action responses; affordances limit the need for extensive sensory processing by reducing degrees of freedom.

Agonists: Muscles directly involved in producing desired movement; can be either prime movers or synergists

All-or-none principle: Refers to the activation of muscle fibers within each motor unit, in which all muscle fibers within a motor unit contract or none contract in response to the neuron's action potential

Ambient vision: Visual information implicitly gathered without conscious awareness or attention being specifically focused; involves both foveal and peripheral vision

Ankle strategy: A whole-body postural adjustment, under perturbed and normal stance conditions, using ankle movements to maintain standing balance

Antagonists: Muscles that oppose the action of the agonists

Anticipation timing: Whole-body or limb movements done in accord with the temporal patterns of an external reference, often for an interceptive action such as catching or hitting an oncoming ball

Anticipatory postural adjustments (APAs): Proactive postural control movements that accompany most planned movements, designed to stabilize joints, body segments, or the whole body prior to the execution of the motor skill

Arthrogenic muscle inhibition (AMI): An inhibitory effect on the musculature surrounding a joint from the combined actions of the joint's kinesthetic receptors, theorized to protect joints from overloading

Attention switch: To switch from one stimulus or information processing resource to another; may occur spatially or temporally

Attention: The mental process of concentrating on specific things, that is, an exclusive allocation of processing resources; can be focused on the external environment, the internal bodily environment, or on mental processes themselves

Attractor state: A preferred state of operation within a dynamic system that is stable and patterned and relatively resistant to change; a state of operation that the system will naturally organize itself to a given set of circumstances

Augmented feedback (AFB): Value-added information passed from instructor to learner regarding aspects of performance; feedback that enhances, modifies, or reveals information that the performer would not ordinarily receive

Autonomic nervous system: Division of the PNS that regulates visceral and bodily processes at the subconscious level (involuntary system) including heart rate, ventilation, digestion, and other systems involving smooth muscle and glands

Axon: A process extending from a neuron cell body that carries electrical impulses in the form of an action potential away from the cell body and out to synapses on its distal end

Bilateral transfer: Specific cases of transfer of learning from one limb to the other, such as cross-transfer of strength from one arm to the contralateral arm following unilateral strength training

Bimanual transfer: Specific case of bilateral transfer involving the wrist and hand

Biofeedback: Augmented sensory feedback, which is the use of electronic devices to amplify biological processes to make them noticeable to the learner

Brodmann areas: Groups of brain cells with similar structure and, because of that, similar function

Ceiling effect: Performance on a task that has stabilized at a maximal level because the criterion measure is so simple that the person maximizes the score easily and there is little room for improvement

Central nervous system (CNS): The brain and spinal cord parts of the nervous system; the integration and command center for the entire nervous system

Central pattern generators (CPGs): Innate nervous system pathways that when activated produce complex rhythmic movement patterns that can run independently of voluntary control

Cervicocollic reflex: A righting reflex initiated by neck movements and that act upon neck muscles to keep the head in an upright and stable position

Cervicospinal reflex: A righting reflex initiated by neck movements and that act upon arm and leg muscles with the purpose to prevent falling, keep the head upright, or prepare for falling

Closed skills: Skills performed in an environment that is stable and predictable, wherein the environment or objects in the environment wait to be acted upon by the individual

Cocontraction: Simultaneous contraction of antagonist muscles during agonist muscle activation, for example, to help stabilize the joint during very rapid or very forceful agonist contractions

Compartmentalization: Refers to smaller and independently controlled groups of muscle fibers contained within a single muscle or across a group of muscles

Concurrent movements: Movements, such as vertical jumping, in which an involved multijoint muscle is engaged in contractile shortening at one joint to move a load, while at the opposite joint is being stretched

Constant error (CE): The average of error scores over a given number of trials; provides information on the magnitude and direction of error

Constraint: An environmental or individual characteristic or feature that influences or dictates precisely how a movement must be done or what movement must be done; a barrier or restriction that must be used, avoided, or overcome for effective movement to take place

Contextual interference: A situation in which motor skill performance is hindered when it is practiced in the context of another task or within a different practice environment

Continuous skills: Repetitive skills such as swimming and running that have arbitrary beginning and endpoints

Contractility: Muscle tissue property enabling it to produce force by shortening.

Control parameter: Factors within a dynamic system that when disrupted or change cause a wholesale change throughout the entire system from one stable state to another

Coordination: Refers to the patterning of the body, limb segments, and muscles among themselves and to the external environment. See intramuscular coordination and intermuscular coordination

Coordinative structures: A form of neuromuscular synergy referring to the coupling between opposite limbs during bilateral movements

Core training: Exercise training for body segment stability involving muscles of the axial skeleton, including shoulder and pelvic girdles

Countercurrent: Movements in which an involved multijoint muscle is engaged in contractile shortening to move loads at the muscle's opposing joints or engaged in lengthening at both opposing joints; results in a rapid and large amount of shortening during contraction or a rapid and large amount of stretch during lengthening

Degrees of freedom: Refers to the large number of possible movement solutions for any given movement task; highlights the need for the nervous system to have mechanisms to determine which solution to use

Deliberate practice: A specific term describing practice activities with specific features, namely, high levels of motivation and effort, activities based on knowledge and characteristics of the performer, immediate and continual feedback, a large amount of repetition, and the intention to improve

Dendrite: A process extending from a neuron cell body that carries electrical impulses toward the cell body from synapses or sensory organelles on their distal ends

Depolarize: To change a cell's electrical potential to be more positive or less negative

Discharge patterning: Refers to specific manipulation of a motor neuron's firing rate to meet specific task demands, for instance, a sequence of two to three rapid action potentials sent to the muscle fibers may greatly increase the tension output of the muscle

Discovery learning: A learning process using a guided trial and error approach that requires learners to determine on their own their best movement solutions

Discrete skills: Motor skills having a definitive beginning and endpoint, such as a finger snap or throwing a punch

Domain selection: The identification of a particular field or area in which specific abilities may be more important; generally refers to choosing a particular sport or endeavor based on identifying an individual's strong and weak abilities that are related to performance in that sport or endeavor

Dynamic balance: The ability to maintain the body in equilibrium during body movement, such as walking on slippery surfaces or controlled landing from a jump

Dynamic systems: A term specifically describing interdependent assemblies of components (systems) that are in a constant state of flux and change in relationship to one another

Efference copy: Copying of a motor command to higher brain centers; enables the brain to have a record of the command to predict movement results and sensory inflow

Effort: Refers to the level of mental and physical engagement; strong effort is a product of intention and motivation and is necessary for effective learning and performance

Elasticity: The capability of the muscle and tendon to recoil from stretch

Electromyography (EMG): A technique to detect and record muscle electrical activity using electrodes within the muscle or on the skin over a muscle

EPSPs (excitatory postsynaptic potentials): Depolarizing stimuli on a postsynaptic neuron from a presynaptic neuron that can be summed to generate an action potential in the postsynaptic neuron

Excitable: A property of some biological tissues (e.g., muscle tissue) referring to the tissue's capability to respond to electrical impulses

Exploratory learning: See discovery learning.

Extensibility: The capability of muscle and tendon tissue to stretch

Externally paced: Refers to the timing and initiation of a motor skill being influenced by the environment; most often associated with open skills

Exteroreceptors: Sensory receptors located close to the outer surface of the body that provide information on the outside world, including tactile sensation (touch, pain, temperature) in the skin, and vision, hearing, taste, and smell

Facilitated: State of a neuron in which it has been excited by incoming action potentials to a subthreshold level that is insufficient to cause an action potential, but instead primes the neuron to fire

Feedback: Refers to sensory information arising from any sensory receptor and sent to the CNS for processing; including movement-related information arising during movement or available after the outcome of movement

Feedback control: Refers to motor commands using or allowing sensory information (feedback) to regulate and change the commands; the distinguishing feature of closed loop control

Feedforward: Refers to motor commands that are not influenced by sensory information (see feedforward control below); also refers to sensory information that does not arise as a consequence of movement or physiological processes, but rather provides advance knowledge on upcoming situations such as provided by visual and auditory information

Feedforward control/commands: Motor commands that originate in the major brain structures and proceed relatively unabated to their target muscles; sensory feedback is mostly used to plan subsequent motor commands and has little influence on the ongoing motor command.

Final common pathway: Motor units onto which is made a final converging of signals for all nervous system motor activity

Fine motor skills: Classification of motor skills that characteristically use small muscles and are precise, such as writing and sewing; are generally also categorized as psychomotor skills

Firing rate: The number of action potentials per second traveling down a neuron or along a muscle fiber; firing rate influences muscle force production and may range from a minimum of 5 to 8 Hz to a maximum of 120 Hz for ballistic contractions.

Fitts and Posner's 3-stage model: Learning stage theory describing the characteristics and changes in performance learners go through as they progress in learning from beginners to accomplished performers; the model begins with stage 1 that emphasizes cognitive learning and ends with stage 3 that emphasizes automatic performance of motor skills.

Fixator: Muscles that usually contract statically to stabilize a body part or other muscle against the pull of contracting muscles or movement of body parts; many categorized as postural muscles

Floor effect: Performance on a task that appears to have stabilized at a poor level; often a result of a criterion measure being inappropriate or so difficult to achieve that even strong or improving performance is measured as poor

Focal vision: Vision based on the most visually sharp information gathered from the center of the visual field; considered a consciously aware process controlled by voluntary processing and is primarily used to identify objects and detail

Focus of attention: Refers to the quality of concentration on stimuli or ongoing situations

Force–velocity curve: The relationship between muscle contraction velocity and force output; illustrates that high forces can only be generated at slow speeds

Free dendritic endings: A type of mechanoreceptor having multiple dendrites that freely intertwine with the surrounding tissue and respond to mechanical disturbances within the tissue

Functional training: Physiological training designed to bring real-life situational needs and constraints to the training environment, with the goal of maximizing transfer of abilities to improved performance on the field, at work, or in activities of daily living.

Functional psychophysical training: Functional training with an emphasis on using psychological challenges, such as decision making, to maximize the transfer of training gains to the real-world environment

Gamma motor neurons: Small motor neurons that innervate intrafusal fibers in the muscle spindle

Generalized motor program (GMP): A theory of how movement plans are stored in the brain; it postulates that movement actions are stored as an abstract or general representation of a class of actions that have with similar characteristics.

Gentile's 2-stage model: A learning stage theory describing the changes learners go through as they progress along the learning continuum; the model focuses on the learning process and instruction occurring during the stages, ranging from getting an idea of movement to a fixation and diversification stage.

Goal-directed movements: Intentional and voluntary acts with an outcome in mind; used synonymously with the term motor skills

Golgi tendon reflex (aka the inverse stretch reflex): Stimulation of the Golgi tendon organ via contraction of the muscle or external forces resulting in inhibition of the homonymous muscle and its synergists and facilitating contraction of the antagonist muscle and its synergists

Gross motor skills: Motor skills that use large muscle groups, often use whole-body movements, and characteristically have little precision; includes many fundamental motor skills like running and jumping that are learned early in development and are foundational to other motor skills

Heterarchical: Refers to a motor command structure in which the many components, namely, the CNS and PNS, provide codependent and distributed commands

Hierarchical: Refers to a strict top-down motor command structure in which the highest levels of the brain control lower levels, which in turn control even lower levels and the spinal cord

Hip strategy: A whole-body postural adjustment made by hip flexion and extension; enables a large amount of correction and affords a different biomechanical profile than an ankle strategy

Homunculus: The topographical map of a specific brain area, namely the motor cortex or somatosensory cortex, that corresponds to a body region.

Hysteresis: A property of connective tissue and muscle tissue describing the difference between the stretch force and stretch length and the amount of any subsequent recoil force and shortening

Identical elements: Similarity among different motor skills in terms of the skill components or context under which the skills are performed; more similarity facilitates transfer of learning.

Information processing: The essential job of the brain; to take in information and interpret it, store it, manipulate it, and eventually use it

Inhibited (or Inhibition): State of a neuron in which generating an AP is more difficult; generally occurs as a result of IPSPs acting on the neuron

Innervation ratio: The ratio of one neuron to the number of muscle fibers it innervates; smaller innervation ratios enable finer movement control.

Intention: A psychological process that provides a goal, a purpose, or a reason for action; for motor skill production that includes the what, why, and how of a movement

Intermuscular coordination: The patterning of muscle groups, limbs, and body segments to produce efficient and purposeful movements in the context of environmental and task demands

Interneurons: Neurons that interconnect among other neurons; interneurons lie between motor and sensory neurons to link the sensory and motor divisions of the PNS.

Interoreceptors: Sensory receptors located within the viscera and blood vessels that feed information back to the CNS regarding internal bodily processes, such as core temperature, acid balance, and smooth muscle movement. Also called visceroreceptors

Intrafusal fibers: The small muscle fibers within the muscle spindle; innervated by gamma motor neurons

Intramuscular coordination: The patterning and use of motor units within a muscle or motor unit task groups across muscles to produce effective and efficient forces and movements

Invariant characteristics: Those features of a generalized motor program for a class of actions that do not change and includes relative force, relative timing (rhythm) of the skill components, and sequencing of the components

Inverted-U principle: The relationship between arousal and performance depicted by an upside-down U; illustrates that performance is optimized when arousal is neither too high nor too low

IPSPs (inhibitory postsynaptic potentials): Stimuli from a presynaptic neuron that causes an inhibitory action on the postsynaptic neuron that decreases the chance for the postsynaptic neuron to generate an action potential

Kinesthesia: The perception of movement-based sensory information (vestibular, somatosensory) leading to awareness of body and limb positioning and movement in space

Labyrinthine receptor: Sensory receptor detecting the movement of fluid contained in the labyrinth of the inner ear; provides information on body and head movements relative to gravity. Also called vestibular receptor

Learning style: Defined as a learner's preferred way of responding to a learning task, in terms of how one learns and the quality of one's learning

Learning variable: Characteristics of the learner or learning environment that affect learning but not necessarily performance; includes factors such as motivation, fatigue, and amount of time spent in practice

Learning: Defined as a relatively permanent improvement in one's potential, or capability, to perform a skill as a result of practice or experience; is often associated with but not necessarily reflected in improvement in the actual performance

Length–tension curve: A model of the relationship between the force a muscle can generate or store to the length of the muscle's contractile and elastic elements

Limbic system: A widespread and interconnected network of regions of the brain largely devoted to regulation of emotional behaviors, including those behaviors related to movement

Long-term memory: The brain's permanent repository of stored information that includes procedural (how to do something), declarative (what to do), semantic (general knowledge from experience), and episodic (personally experienced events and the times they occurred) information

Mastery goal: An achievement goal adopted by a learner wherein the intention is to improve and learn, and comparisons are made to oneself regarding achievement.

Mechanomyography (MMG): A technique used to assess muscle activity by detecting minute vibrations during contractions using special vibration sensors placed on the skin surface

Mind–body connection: A concept describing the interconnected and bidirectional relationship between one's thinking and psychological behaviors and how the body functions; in motor behavior the mind–body connection is highlighted by the relationship between motor learning and motor control.

Mirror neurons: A particular group of brain neurons that fire when an individual makes an action and when the individual visually observes someone else making the action; they work in a system called the motor resonance system.

Model of disablement: A conceptual model that tracks progression of health from pathology to impairment to functional limitation to disability

Modeling: A common method of instruction in which the instructor or model demonstrates the skill in person or on video, and the learner then mimics the skill; otherwise known as demonstration or observational learning

Momentary intention: A quick and transient switch in attention

Motor (efferent) division: Division of the PNS that sends signals from the CNS to effector organs, namely, the muscles; includes both somatic and autonomic divisions

Motor (efferent) neurons: Neurons in the PNS that have their cell bodies and dendrites in the spinal cord and connect to muscle fibers at the distal end of the axon

Motor behavior: Term describing the reasons, mechanisms, and outcomes of one's movement actions; includes the behavioral and physiological and biomechanical factors responsible for voluntary and nonvoluntary movements

Motor control: Term describing the neural, physiological, and biomechanical components of motor behavior

Motor learning: Term describing the behavioral component of motor behavior, emphasizing the mental processes of acquiring (i.e., learning), planning, initiating, and modifying movement

Motor memory: The capacity to remember motor skills acquired through learning or experience; indicated by the ability to recall and repeat large numbers of motor skills over and over again even after long periods of time

Motor redundancy: The existence of multiple movement solutions capable of solving a movement problem; redundancy enables a wide range of choices to meet specific task demands but also poses a problem in selecting just one solution from many.

Motor resonance system: A brain neural system that is activated when movements are executed and when they are observed (live or video); appears to function to enable the brain to (1) understand the action, (2) understand the intention, (3) enable imitation, and (4) understand behavioral state

Motor set: Attentional strategy in which focus of attention is placed on the movement response rather than on the stimuli the prompts the movement response

Motor skills: See **goal-directed movements**.

Motor time (aka electromechanical delay or EMD): Component of reaction time that includes time from the onset of muscle electrical activity to the initiation of the motor response, reflecting peripheral neuromuscular delays

Motor unit (MU): A single lower motor neuron and all the muscle fibers it innervates; the PNS component responsible for the final execution of the movement plan initiated by the brain

Motor unit pool (or motoneuron pool): A grouping of motor units in the spinal cord that activate a particular muscle or muscle group

Movement time (MvT): The duration of a movement; defined as the time from the onset of movement to the movement completion

Multimodal or multimodal sensory input: The convergence of incoming sensory signals into the CNS arriving from multiple sensory sources

Multiple resource theory: Posits that a variety of resources or capabilities exist in the brain to process specific types of information, but that these resources are limited and when exceeded cause poor information-processing performance

Muscle spindle: Important sensory receptors located throughout a muscle that function to detect muscle stretch and contraction characteristics; provide muscle function feedback to the CNS and initiate the myotatic stretch reflex

Muscle tone: Refers to the force with which a muscle resists lengthening, that is, its stiffness; serves to provide an underlying level of muscle control to help maintain postural control

Muscle wisdom: A form of discharge patterning that refers to the change (slowing) in discharge rates during fatigue.

Negative transfer: A form of motor skill transfer wherein previous learning impedes or interferes with learning of the secondary skill

Nerve: A cluster of neuron fibers enclosed within a connective tissue sheath; may contain only afferent or efferent fibers, but typical spinal nerves contain both.

Neuromuscular control: Term describing the neural, physiological, and biomechanical components of motor behavior; used synonymously with motor control

Neuromuscular mechanics (aka neuromechanics): A component of motor control that refers to the relationship between the neural control of movement and the mechanical output of muscle

Neuron: The basic building blocks of the nervous system; specialized nerve cells that process and transmits information by electrical or chemical signaling

Neutralizers: Muscles acting to prevent an undesired action of other active muscles

Open skills: Motor skills performed in a changing and unpredictable environment, wherein the performer acts according to what is happening in the environment

Optical flow: A feature of the ambient visual system in which sensory information is provided by the changing patterns of light striking the retina due to eye and head movements and the movement of objects in the environment.

Order parameters: Components of a system that define or characterize the system; in a motor skill context order parameters are those characteristics that may give rise to a movement classification or movement type.

Overlearning: Continual practice even past a point where performance seems to have peaked, the benefits of which include modifying brain structures to be more resistant to forgetting and to enhance movement adaptability and flexibility

Pacinian corpuscle: Type of sensory ending found beneath the skin and in ligaments and tendon sheaths; stimulated by rapid joint angle changes that put pressure on the corpuscle

Parameters: Parameters are features of a generalized motor program that are modifiable and include overall force, overall duration, and specific muscles used

Parasympathetic: Division of the autonomic system of the peripheral nervous system; stimulates activities of the body at rest; generally opposes effects of the sympathetic system

Part practice: A method of simplification of motor skills to facilitate learning; requires breaking down the motor skill into its constituent components and practicing the components separately

Perception: A type of central nervous system information processing in which sensory feedback is interpreted and understood

Perception–action coupling: The linking between interpretation of sensory information and a subsequent motor action; both an innate and learned behavior that links a motor action with environmental and task-related sensory inflow

Perceptual motor skill: A type of psychomotor skill with specific characteristics; typically requires a large amount of interpreting environmental cues and decision making

Performance goals: An achievement goal adopted by a learner wherein the intention is to win or be better than others or a set of standards

Performance measure (or criterion measure): A variable or factor that when measured can be used to evaluate motor skill performance or abilities

Performance variables: Characteristics of the learner or learning environment that affect performance on a motor task, but not necessarily learning of the task

Performance: The observable and measurable outcome of executing a motor skill

Peripheral nervous system (PNS): The component of the nervous system that is outside the central nervous system; may be further divided into sensory and motor divisions

Plateau: Describes a point on the performance-time curve when performance levels off with little or no improvement; may be caused by numerous learner-based factors, instructor-based factors, or task-based factors

Plyometrics: A form of high effort power training emphasizing a forceful eccentric phase of the stretch-shorten cycle followed by an explosive rapid reversal of the concentric phase of movement

Positive transfer: Form of transfer of learning wherein previous learning facilitates the learning of the secondary motor skill

Postural control: A motor behavior function that maintains body alignment and spatial orientation to subserve effective motor skill performance

Practice: Dedicated effort toward improving upon a skill or task, aimed at improving mental performance, tactics, strategies, team play, and motor skills

Premotor time: A time period reflecting pure information processing during a reaction time task; measured as the time from a stimulus to the onset of muscle electrical activity

Proprioceptors: Sensory mechanoreceptors located in muscles, joints, ligaments, and tendons that detect stimuli related to body movement and provide the CNS with movement-related information

Psychological refractory period (PRP): The information-processing delay of one task while another task is being carried out; it occurs when two tasks arrive simultaneously or closely spaced in time.

Psychomotor skill: A term describing motor skills with specific features that require large amounts of cognitive effort or sensory feedback to execute; typically include high degrees of precision, dexterity, fast reactions, and control of timing

Psychophysics: A term referring to the sensitivity and relationship between the detection of sensory stimuli and subsequent interpretation and use of the stimuli information

Rate-coding: Regulation of the firing rate of action potentials to modify muscle force output

Reaction time (RT): Measure of the time from a stimulus to the onset of a response; is generally used to measure the information-processing time involved in a task

Receptive field: The area surrounding a sensory ending that when stimulated produces a response in the sensory ending

Reciprocal inhibition: A process through which sensory information arising from a muscle services to inhibit the action of antagonist muscles

Recruitment (aka motor unit recruitment): A mechanism to change muscle force output by increasing or decreasing the number of active motor units.

Reflexes: Stereotyped and repeatable muscle actions that are initiated by stimulation of sensory receptors and without conscious involvement.

Relative age: A concept referring to the observation that older or more mature children within an age group will be more likely to succeed within their age cohort and may be more likely to advance to higher levels of performance

Response (or performance) outcome measure: A criterion measure that evaluates the result of a particular motor skill, revealing what happened, not how it happened

Response (or performance) production measure: A criterion measure that reveals how, or even why, a motor skill was produced

Ruffini ending: Sensory receptor located in the deep skin and in the collagenous fibers of the joint capsule; responds to continual states of mechanical deformation and provides information on joint position and joint position changes

Schemata: A component of the generalized motor program that involves decision making and learning; involves memory components in which movements are recognized and recalled

Selective attention: An aspect of attention referring to identification of something purposeful and specific in which to place attention; it is one of the keys to avoid overburdening information-processing resources.

Self-organizing properties: A feature of dynamic systems in which the systems' components naturally interact with other components to find a stable and preferred method of functioning.

Self-paced: An aspect of closed skills, meaning that the individual chooses the pace or timing of their actions

Sensitivity: The ability of a sensory receptor to detect or discriminate a stimulus; low sensitivity means that a large stimulus is required to elicit a response from the receptor, and small changes in stimulus strength may not be detected.

Sensorimotor integration: A process involving the convergence and processing of sensory information and motor commands; may involve the use of motor commands and movements to enhance sensory information and the coupling and relationship between incoming sensory information and outgoing motor actions

Sensory (afferent) division: Division of the PNS that detects stimuli in the periphery with sensory endings and sends signals from these endings through neurons to the CNS

Sensory (afferent) neurons: Neurons in the sensory division of the PNS; have sensory endings at their distal end and send sensory information to the CNS

Sensory integration: The process of filtering and encoding multiple sources of sensory information in order to better interpret and understand events; necessary for such information to be used effectively in the process of planning coordinated movement actions

Sensory set: Attentional strategy in which focus of attention is placed on the stimuli and reacting as fast as possible to the stimuli, rather than on the movement response

Serial (or sequential) skills: A large or compound motor skill made up of a series of discrete movements or smaller component motor skills

Similarity of information processing: A factor contributing to the effectiveness of transfer of motor learning; refers to better transfer occurring among motor skills that have similar requirements involving decision making, perception, and other information-processing functions

Size principle of recruitment: A property of motor unit activation in which motor units are recruited in order from small units to large units, largely due to the neuron size and the stimulation energy needed to reach threshold

Skill: A term referring to the quality of motor performance

Somatic system: Division of the PNS that controls voluntary motor behavior; carries motor commands from the CNS to activate effector organs (e.g., muscles) in the PNS

Somatoreceptors: Term used to describe sensory receptors in the musculoskeletal system (proprioceptors) and skin

Spatial summation: A physiological process to generate an action potential by the adding of EPSPs from multiple presynaptic neurons

Stability (postural): Defined as a postural position that is resistant to disturbance or returns to its normal state after disruption; the primary outcome of postural alignment and orientation

Stabilizer: See fixator.

Static balance: Defined as the ability to maintain the center of mass within the base of support during static or relatively steady body positions; may include challenging body positions such as single leg stance and environmental challenges such as unstable support surfaces

Stepping strategy: A technique to maintain balance during a perturbation by taking a step; one of the change-in-support strategies that may be adopted in more extreme balance challenges

Stretch reflex (aka myotatic stretch reflex): A reflex muscle contraction initiated by a stretch to the muscle spindle in the homonymous muscle

Supraspinal: Referring to processes and commands occurring above the level of the spinal cord

Suspensory strategy: A technique to maintain balance that involves going into a crouching and flexed behavior to lower the center of mass; most often done by those afraid to fall or when in unfamiliar environments

Sympathetic system: A division of autonomic system in the PNS; serves to mobilize autonomic functions and tends to oppose effects of the parasympathetic system

Synapse: Electrical or chemical connections between neurons or between neurons and effector organs; allows transmission of the AP from one to the other

Synchronization: A motor unit discharge pattern whereby activation of different motor units, especially the firing rates of already active units, become timed to fire all at the same time

Synergies: Ensembles or groupings of muscles and limbs that work together as a functional unit and by their actions also constrain one another

Synergists: Muscles that work with agonist muscles to perform specific joint or limb movements

Tactical training: A form of functional training designed for persons in physically and psychologically demanding activities, particularly the military, police, fire, and rescue work; often aimed at high-stress environments, interpersonal engagement, and equipment use

Talent: Refers to the specific genetic abilities contributing to performance of a particular motor skill or task; in some usage includes all abilities and component motor skills that contribute to success at a particular sport or activity (see talent identification)

Talent identification: The practice of predicting future performance or possibility of success based on the assessment of one's specific abilities and component skills that are considered important to success at a particular sport or activity

Tau: An optical flow characteristic referring to the rate of change of the size of object's image projected onto the retina due to the object's movement toward the eye.

Temporal summation: A physiological process to generate an action potential by increasing the firing rate of individual presynaptic neurons so as to enable adding together of EPSPs

Threshold: A specific level of current needed to create an action potential in a postsynaptic neuron

Total response time (RpT): A measure of the total time to execute a motor skill involving both reaction time and movement time; measured from a stimulus to the completion of the motor response

Training: Often used interchangeably with practice, but refers specifically to dedicated effort aimed at improving physiological functioning and physical proficiency abilities

Transfer of learning: An information-processing phenomenon whereby previous learning and experiences influence the learning—positive, negative, or both – of subsequent motor skills

Transition phase: The change from one stable state to a new stable state in a dynamic system; generally describes change from one movement type to another when the original state is sufficiently destabilized by a perturbation to the control parameter

Variable error (VE): A measurement of the consistency of motor skill responses; is measured by the standard deviation of a number of error scores

Vestibulocollic: Refers to righting reflexes initiated by the vestibular receptors and acting on neck muscles to maintain head position in response to head movements

Vestibulospinal: Refers to righting reflexes initiated by the vestibular receptors and acting on limb (arm and leg) muscles to maintain head and body position to prevent falls or ready for falls

Visceroreceptors: See interoreceptors.

Visual search: Voluntary and automatic behaviors to visually scan the environment for important information that will enable an individual to anticipate actions and thereby effectively and rapidly plan their own motor actions

Working memory: The temporary use and storage system for information (or short-term memory); the active system for information processing, especially for immediate situational needs such as decision making and problem solving

INDEX

Note: Page numbers in *italics* indicate figures; page numbers followed by a "t" indicate tables.